Generative AI in Neurodegenerative Disorders

Innovations, Views, and Obstacles

RIVER PUBLISHERS SERIES IN BIOMEDICAL ENGINEERING

Series Editor:

DINESH KANT KUMAR
RMIT University, Australia

The “River Publishers Series in Biomedical Engineering” is a series of comprehensive academic and professional books which focus on the engineering and mathematics in medicine and biology. The series presents innovative experimental science and technological development in the biomedical field as well as clinical application of new developments.

Books published in the series include research monographs, edited volumes, handbooks and textbooks. The books provide professionals, researchers, educators, and advanced students in the field with an invaluable insight into the latest research and developments.

Topics covered in the series include, but are by no means restricted to the following:

- Biomedical engineering
- Biomedical physics and applied biophysics
- Bio-informatics
- Bio-metrics
- Bio-signals
- Medical Imaging

For a list of other books in this series, visit www.riverpublishers.com

Generative AI in Neurodegenerative Disorders

Innovations, Views, and Obstacles

Editors

Anindya Nag
Northern University of Business and Technology Khulna, Bangladesh

Md. Mehedi Hassan
Khulna University, Bangladesh

Asif Karim
Charles Darwin University, Australia

Kishor Kumar Reddy C
Stanley College of Engineering and Technology for Women, India.

River Publishers

Routledge
Taylor & Francis Group
NEW YORK AND LONDON

Published 2026 by River Publishers
River Publishers
Broagervej 10, 9260 Gistrup, Denmark
www.riverpublishers.com

Distributed exclusively by Routledge
605 Third Avenue, New York, NY 10017, USA
4 Park Square, Milton Park, Abingdon, Oxon OX14 4RN

Generative AI in Neurodegenerative Disorders / by Anindya Nag, Md. Mehedi Hassan, Asif Karim, Kishor Kumar Reddy C.

Routledge is an imprint of the Taylor & Francis Group, an informa business

ISBN 978-87-4380-175-7 (hardback)
ISBN 978-87-4380-672-1 (paperback)
ISBN 978-87-4380-177-1 (online)
ISBN 978-87-4380-176-4 (master ebook)
ISBN 97887-438-0711-7 (ePub)

DOI: 10.1201/9788743801764

Contents

Preface

The book **"Generative AI in Neurodegenerative Disorders: Innovations, Views, and Obstacles"** investigates how generative AI technologies are changing the diagnosis, treatment, and individualized care of neurodegenerative disorders. It dives into the integration of AI with brain imaging, gene editing techniques, and rehabilitation, as well as ethical implications, data privacy, and clinical application challenges. This comprehensive resource is designed to help researchers, physicians, and AI professionals advance healthcare for neurodegenerative disorders. The book **"Generative AI in Neurodegenerative Disorders: Innovations, Views, and Obstacles"** contains the following chapters.

Chapter 1 focuses on the transformative potential of generative AI in understanding and treating neurodegenerative diseases (NDs). It delves into how AI, particularly machine learning (ML), natural language processing (NLP), and advanced algorithms like generative adversarial networks (GANs) and variational autoencoders (VAEs), are revolutionizing diagnostic and therapeutic approaches. The chapter also explores the integration of AI with brain imaging technologies such as MRI and fMRI, alongside its impact on early detection through biomarkers like HTT and cerebrospinal fluid (CSF). By analyzing these developments, this chapter aims to highlight AI's pivotal role in advancing ND research.

Chapter 2 focuses on generative AI-enhanced diagnostic systems: Revolutionizing early disease detection through advanced predictive analytics. Generative AI is especially identifying in the improvement of diagnostic accuracy and speed, particularly in detecting disease at the early stage of the disease. It also explores how these AI-powered diagnostic tools can enhance predictive models to allow for earlier interventions and treatment strategies in clinical areas.

Chapter 3 explores the challenges and immense opportunities that Generative AI brings to neurodegenerative disorder research, aiming to illuminate how this technology could lead to breakthroughs in diagnosis, treatment, and personalized care. Neurodegenerative disorders, such as Alzheimer's, Parkinson's, and amyotrophic lateral sclerosis, present complex challenges that continue to puzzle researchers and clinicians alike. In recent years, Generative AI has emerged as a transformative technology with the potential to reshape our understanding and treatment of these conditions. However, its application has significant obstacles from ethical concerns to data scarcity and model biases.

Chapter 4 looks into the transformative role AI plays in optimizing gene-editing techniques, such as CRISPR and zinc finger nucleases (ZFN). By enhancing precision and reducing off-target effects, generative AI offers novel solutions to challenges like delivery inefficiencies and lengthy drug discovery processes. The chapter further explores the potential of AI to design personalized therapies tailored to individual genetic profiles, accelerating the development of more effective treatments. Ethical considerations and regulatory challenges are also discussed; highlighting the need for a multi-disciplinary approach to fully harness AI's potential in reshaping the future of gene therapy.

Chapter 5 proposes a generic predictive model to improve disease prediction for five different categories of frequently occurring diseases. This model uses principal component analysis (PCA) and iterative K-means clustering to improve data quality, as well as the random forest (RF) technique to increase prediction accuracy. Notably, we use a grid-search-CV hyperparameter optimization technique to fine-tune the RF predictor, providing the best performance for each dataset.

Chapter 6 focuses on the implementation of generative AI into the mental health care domain. The chapter studies different technologies used to implement Gen AI into mental health care and some real-world applications such as clinical decision-making, screening and assessment, tracking and monitoring, etc. The chapter further discusses the potential of the implementation of Gen AI into mental health care scenarios along with considering ethical issues and future directions.

Chapter 7 explores a deep learning system that was designed using a fresh dataset to diagnose autism spectrum disorder (ASD) in youngsters. A variety of models were tried, including FFNN, DNN, CNN, LSTM, and GRU. To increase transparency, explainable AI approaches such as LIME were used, which provide interpretable insights into the model's predictions. This strategy not only increases confidence in the findings, but it also proves the efficacy of combining deep learning with explainable AI for early ASD identification and categorization.

Chapter 8 focuses on the rapid advancements in generative AI, such as ChatGPT, which are reshaping the mental health care landscape. This chapter explores the transformative potential of AI in therapeutic practices, examining its ability to enhance personalized care, improve accessibility, and streamline processes. While the integration of AI offers promising opportunities, particularly for underserved populations it also raises significant ethical concerns, including data privacy, bias, and the risk of over-reliance on technology. Through case studies and literature review, this chapter advocates for a balanced, hybrid approach, combining AI with human-centered care to ensure responsible and equitable mental health support.

Chapter 9 investigates AI's revolutionary role in the treatment of neurodegenerative illnesses, with a focus on customized rehabilitation. AI-powered technologies like machine learning, wearable sensors, and robotics improve detection and therapy for diseases including Parkinson's and ALS. These technologies offer personalized physiotherapy, adaptable occupational treatment, and accurate speech therapy, resulting in superior patient results and ongoing care. Despite hurdles such as infrastructure costs and data privacy, the incorporation of AI into allied health professions can transform dementia patient care.

Chapter 10 explores the implementation of deep learning-based neural network models to diagnose two major neurodegenerative disorders: Alzheimer's disease (AD) and Parkinson's disease (PD). These disorders, characterized by progressive neuronal death and cognitive decline, require early detection to reduce their adverse effects. The study uses a dataset of over 2000 patients with 32 predictors and applies a 70/30 train-test split. Various models were evaluated, including decision trees (DT), artificial neural networks (ANN) with different hidden layers, hybrid ANN, deep neural networks (DNN), and boosting algorithms. Among these, the TabNet model showed the best performance with an accuracy of 0.997 for both train and test sets in diagnosing both AD and PD. The model's ability to handle diverse datasets and identify key variables enhances its predictive capabilities, offering a promising approach to early diagnosis and treatment planning for neurodegenerative diseases.

Chapter 11 looks into a multimodal biometric fingerprint system that combines fingerprint data with extra biometric qualities to improve accuracy and resistance to faking. The framework uses deep learning models to improve system resilience and security in high-security applications. Furthermore, it shows promise for Generative AI applications in neurodegenerative illness research, enabling early detection and monitoring of cognitive deterioration using biometric data analysis.

Chapter 12 focuses on the application of convolutional neural networks (CNN) for diagnosing and predicting Alzheimer's disease. Using neuroimaging data from the OASIS dataset, the study demonstrates how CNNs can detect early signs of Alzheimer's with 99.95% accuracy. This approach offers a non-invasive, highly accurate alternative for early diagnosis, which is critical for improving patient outcomes. It explores the advantages of CNNs in processing complex imaging data, highlighting their potential to revolutionize Alzheimer's diagnosis and treatment. The goal of future work is to improve model performance on bigger and more varied datasets.

Chapter 13 explores the transformative potential of generative AI in the field of neurodegenerative disease diagnosis and treatment, focusing on how these technologies are advancing research and clinical practice. It provides a detailed analysis of current methodologies, showcasing the role of AI in improving diagnostic accuracy, developing personalized treatment approaches, and facilitating drug discovery. The chapter also examines key challenges, such as ethical concerns, data privacy, and the limitations of existing datasets. By offering a balanced perspective on both the opportunities and complexities, this work aims to present a thorough understanding of how generative AI is poised to impact the future of healthcare in neurodegenerative conditions.

Chapter 14 focuses on AI's integration into cognitive and physical rehabilitation, which represents a major leap in treating neurodegenerative diseases like Parkinson's and Alzheimer's. This chapter explores cutting-edge technologies such as robotics for physical therapy and virtual reality for cognitive rehabilitation, highlighting AI's role in personalized treatment plans tailored to individual patient needs. It also addresses ethical challenges and the complexities of implementing AI in healthcare. By showcasing current advancements, future potential, and AI's transformative impact on rehabilitation, encouraging further research to improve patient outcomes and quality of life.

Chapter 15 focuses on the generative AI as a transforming tool in cognitive rehabilitation, offering innovative solutions for enhancing cognitive functioning in patients with neurodegenerative disorders such as Alzheimer's disease, Parkinson's disease, Huntington's disease as well as epilepsy. The study also highlights the generative models like GPT and GANs, AI systems that can stimulate personalized cognitive training programs, adapt to patient progress, and provide real-time feedback. Further, the chapter focuses on AI-driven interventions that are designed to promote neuroplasticity, slow cognitive decline, and improve the quality of life for patients by delivering targeted exercises tailored to individual needs along with challenges that remain in clinical implementation.

List of Figures

List of Tables

List of Contributors

Al Mamun, Md., *Department of Computer Science and Engineering, Rajshahi University of Engineering & Technology, Bangladesh*

Aldosari, Fahd M., *Department of Computer and Network Engineering College of Computing, Umm Al-Qura University, Saudi Arabia*

Alivelu Mangatayi, Ch. Srivatsa, *ACE Engineering College, India*

Anand, Nikhilesh, *School of Medicine, University of Texas, USA*

Aneja, Avneet, *Om Sai Physiotherapy Clinic, Canada*

Apoorva, N., *Stanley College of Engineering and Technology for Women, India*

Arumugam, Sridhar, *Lovely Professional University, India, TLM Institute of Health Sciences and Research Centre-Physio, India*

Ashirbad, Mishra, *Pennsylvania State University, USA*

Azam, Sami, *Faculty of Science and Engineering, Charles Darwin University, Australia*

C. Reddy Kumar, Kishor, *Stanley College of Engineering and Technology for Women, India*

Chintalapalli, Arshita, *Stanley College of Engineering and Technology for Women, India*

Danial Sadad, K. M., *Department of Computer Science and Engineering, Northern University of Business & Technology, Bangladesh*

Debnath, Sajol, *Northern University of Business and Technology Khulna, Bangladesh*

Dholakia, Amit, *Department of Political Science, Maharaja Sayajirao University of Baroda, India*

Doss, Srinath, *Professor, Faculty of Engineering and Technology, Botho University, Botswana*

Dutta, Dip Ranjan, *Department of Computer Science and Engineering, Guru Nanak Dev University, India*

Eid, Wesam N., *Department of Cybersecurity, College of Computing, Umm Al-Qura University, Saudi Arabia*

Fatima, Areesha, *Stanley College of Engineering and Technology for Women, India*

Galipellli, Ashok, *Geethanjali College of Engineering and Technology, India*

Hasan, S. M. Mahedy, *Department of Computer Science and Engineering, Rajshahi University of Engineering & Technology, Bangladesh*

Hassan, Md. Mehedi, *Computer Science and Engineering Discipline, Khulna University, Bangladesh*

Imran Sharif, Muhammad, *Department of Computer Science, Kansas State University, USA*

Islam, Mohammed Rezwanul, *Faculty of Science and Engineering, Charles Darwin University, Australia*

Islam, Salman, *Department of Computer Science and Engineering, Northern University of Business & Technology, Bangladesh*

Jaffar, Amar Y., *Department of Computer and Network Engineering, College of Computing, Umm Al-Qura University, Saudi Arabia*

Joseph, Shenson, *University of North Dakota, USA*

Joshi, Herat, *Great River Health Systems, USA*

Kaashipaka, Vineetha, *Sreenidhi Institute of Science & Technology, India*

Kanakaprabha, S., *Department of Artificial Intelligence and Machine Learning, Malla Reddy College of Engineering, India*

Kareem, Shaik Abdul, *Independent Researcher, USA*

Karime, Asif, *Faculty of Science and Engineering, Charles Darwin University, NT 0909, Australia*

Katakam, Vijetha, *Visa Inc, USA*

Kishor Kumar Reddy, C, *Stanley College of Engineering and Technology for Women, India*

Koya, Nabeeha, *Department of Pharmacology & Toxicology, National Institute of Pharmaceutical Education and Research (NIPER), India*

Kumar, Nitesh, *Department of Pharmacology & Toxicology, National Institute of Pharmaceutical Education and Research (NIPER), India*

Kumar, Santhosh, *Carver College of Medicine, University of Iowa, USA*

Lippert, Kari, *Department of System Engineering, University of South Alabama, USA*

Loka Priya, Pendyala, *Department of Computer Science & Engineering, Keshav Memorial Institute of Technology, India*

Mahathi, Avula, *Stanley College of Engineering and Technology for Women, India*

Mangatayi, Ch. Srivatsa Alivelu, *ACE Engineering College, India*

Meenakshi, Sarasa, *Department of Pharmacy Practice, National Institute of Pharmaceutical Education and Research (NIPER), India*

Meenal, H., *Department of Computer Science & Engineering, Methodist College of Engineering and Technology, India*

Mishra, Ashirbad, *Department of CSE, Pennsylvania State University, United States*

Mohd Hanafiah, Marlia, *Professor, Universiti Kebangsaan Malaysia, Malaysia*

Molla, Kaysun, *Department of Computer Science and Engineering, Northern University of Business & Technology, Bangladesh*

Murti, Krishna, *Department of Pharmacy Practice, National Institute of Pharmaceutical Education and Research (NIPER), India*

N. Eid, Wesam, *Umm Al-Qura University*

Nag, Anindya, *Department of Computer Science and Engineering, Northern University of Business & Technology, Bangladesh*

Padhi, Sudev Kumar, *Department of CSE, Indian Institute of Technology Bhilai, India; Department of CSE, Pennsylvania State University, United States*

Palash Uddin, Md., *School of Information Technology, Deakin University, Australia*

Panda, Sadhu Charan, *Department of Community Medicine, VSS Institute of Medical Sciences and Research, India*

Pattanaik, Deepti Rani, *Department of Statistics, Sambalpur University, India*

Pattnaik, Monalisha, *Department of Statistics, Sambalpur University, India*

Prakash, Ved, *Department of Endocrinology, Indira Gandhi Institute of Medical Sciences (IGIMS), Sheikhpura, India*

Rajini, Reddaboina, *Department of Computer Science & Engineering, Keshav Memorial Institute of Technology, India*

Raju, Gloriya, *Galgotias University, India*

Reddy, C. Kishor Kumar, *Stanley College of Engineering and Technology for Women, India*

Rezwanul Islam, Mohammed, *Faculty of Science and Engineering, Charles Darwin University, Australia*

Sachan, Ram Chandra, *Independent Researcher, USA*

Sadad, K. M. Danial, *Northern University of Business and Technology Khulna, Bangladesh*

Shamim Parvej, Md., *Northern University of Business and Technology Khulna, Bangladesh*

Sharma, Manisha, *Department of Political Science, Maharaja Sayajirao University of Baroda, India*

Sharon, Jane Claudia, *Anglia Ruskin University*

Singh T., Monika, *Department of Computer Science and Engineering, Stanley College of Engineering and Technology for Women, India*

Swathi, K., *ACE Engineering College, India*

Swathi, N., *ACE Engineering College, India*

T. Singh, Monika, *Stanley College of Engineering and Technology for Women, India*

Thirupathi, Lingala, *Sreenidhi Institute of Science & Technology, India*

Upadhyaya, Nitesh, *GlobalLogic Inc, USA*

Vijaya Saradhi, M. V., *ACE Engineering College, India*

Vimala, K. S., *Sri A.R.M Physio Rehab and Research Centre, India*

Y. Jaffar, Amar, *Umm Al-Qura University*

List of Abbreviations

AAV	Adeno-associated virus
ACP	Advanced care planning
AD	Alzheimer's disease
ADNI	Alzheimer's disease neuroimaging initiative
AI	Artificial intelligence
ALS	Amyotrophic lateral sclerosis
ANN	Artificial neural network
APOE	Apolipoprotein E
ASD	Autism spectrum disorder
CADD	Computer-aided drug design
CAG	Cytosine-adenine-guanine (a mutation in Huntington's disease)
CBT	Cognitive behavioral therapy
CDS	Clinical decision support
CKD	Chronic kidney disease
CNN	Convolutional neural network
CNS	Central nervous system
CRISPR	Clustered regularly interspaced short palindromic repeats
CSF	Cerebrospinal fluid
CT	Computed tomography
DAI	Distributed AI
DBN	Deep belief network
DDoS	Distributed denial of service
DenseNet	Densely connected convolutional networks
DL	Deep learning
DNA	Deoxyribonucleic acid
DNN	Deep neural network
DT	Decision tree
DTI	Diffusion tensor imaging
ECG	Electrocardiogram

EEG	Electroencephalogram
EHR	Electronic health records
EMA	European Medicines Agency
EMG	Electromyography
FAR	False acceptance rates
FDA	Food and Drug Administration
fMRI	Functional magnetic resonance imaging
FN	False negative
FP	False positive
GABA	Gamma-aminobutyric acid
GAI	Generative AI
GAN	Generative adversarial network
GBC	Gradient boosting classifier
GBDT	Gradient boosting decision tree
GDPR	General Data Protection Regulation
GED	Gene editing
Gen AI	Generative AI
GPT	Generative pre-trained transformer
GRU	Gated recurrent unit
HCV	Hepatitis C virus
HD	Huntington's disease
HER	Electronic health record
HIPAA	Health Insurance Portability and Accountability Act
HTT	Huntingtin
ICT	Information and Communication Technologies
IoT	Internet of things
KNN	K-nearest neighbors
LIME	Local interpretable model-agnostic explanations
LLM	Large language model
LSTM	Long short-term memory
MCI	Mild cognitive impairment
MDR	Modified decrypted Rivest
mHealth	Mobile health
ML	Machine learning
MLP	Multilayer perceptron
MRI	Magnetic resonance imaging
MS	Multiple sclerosis
ND	Neurodegenerative disease

NDD	Neurodegenerative disease
NDs	Neurodegenerative diseases
NeAE	Neural network algorithm for eye-tracking
Neuro AI	Neurorehabilitation-related artificial intelligence
NIC	National Informatics Centre
NLP	Natural language processing
NMDA	N-methyl-D-aspartate
NN	Neural network
OASIS	Open Access Series of Imaging Studies
PCA	Principal component analysis
PD	Parkinson's disease
PET	Positron emission tomography
PII	Personally Identifiable Information
PPG	Photoplethysmography
PRISMA	Preferred Reporting Items for Systematic Reviews and Meta-Analyses
QSAR	Quantitative structure-activity relationship
RBM	Restricted Boltzmann machine
RCTs	Randomized controlled trials
RF	Random forest
RL	Reinforcement learning
RMSE	Root mean square error
RNA	Ribonucleic acid
RNN	Recurrent neural network
ROA	Reactive oxygen species
RPM	Remote patient monitoring
RSA	Genuine acceptance rates
RT-PCR	Reverse transcription polymerase chain reaction
SCID	Severe combined immunodeficiency
SGD	Stochastic gradient descent
sgRNA	Single guide RNA
SMOTE	Synthetic minority over-sampling technique
SRS	Social responsiveness scale
SVM	Support vector machine
TALEN	Transcription activator-like effector nucleases
TN	True negative
TP	True positive
VAE	Variational autoencoder
VGG	Visual geometry group

VR	Virtual reality
WHO	World Health Organization
WideResNet	Wide residual networks
XAI	Explainable AI
Xception	Extreme inception
ZFN	Zinc finger nucleases

1

Generative AI: A New Frontier in Understanding and Treating Neurodegenerative Diseases

Avula Mahathi[1], Kishor Kumar Reddy C.[1], and Srinath Doss[2]

[1]Department of Computer Science and Engineering, Stanley College of Engineering and Technology for Women, India
[2]Faculty of Engineering and Technology, Botho University, Botswana
E-mail: srinath.doss@bothouniversity.ac.bw; avula.mahathi@gmail.com; kishoar23@gmail.com

Abstract

The swift progression of generative artificial intelligence (AI) has created novel opportunities for comprehending and managing neurodegenerative illnesses, including Alzheimer's, Parkinson's, and Huntington's disease. These conditions, which are characterized by progressive brain deterioration, pose major difficulties for the development of therapeutics, biomarker identification, and early detection. This chapter examines how generative AI models, such as generative adversarial networks (GANs) and variational autoencoders (VAEs), can be revolutionary in tackling these problems. By utilizing vast amounts of data from genetic and clinical research, generative artificial intelligence (AI) expedites the drug discovery process, enhances early detection through medical imaging analysis, and makes it easier to identify novel biomarkers. Furthermore covered in the chapter is AI-driven personalized treatment plan creation based on individual illness profiles of patients, offering a route towards precision medicine in neurodegenerative care. Issues including algorithmic bias, data privacy, and model interpretability are discussed together with the technological and ethical issues surrounding the use of AI in healthcare. With a review of recent findings and future directions,

DOI: 10.1201/9788743801764-1

this chapter highlights the promise of generative AI as a key tool in revolutionizing the diagnosis and treatment of neurodegenerative diseases.

Keywords: Generative AI, Neurodegenerative Diseases, Biomarker Discovery, AI in Healthcare, AI-driven Drug Discovery, Medical Imaging Analysis.

1.1 Introduction

Alzheimer's, Parkinson's, and Huntington's diseases are among the neurodegenerative illnesses that are among the most difficult for modern medicine to cure [13]. The characteristic of these illnesses is progressive neuronal degeneration leading to movement impairment, cognitive decline, and ultimately death. Despite significant advancements in medical research, numerous issues remain about early diagnosis, biomarker identification, and effective therapy. Present diagnostic methods often detect the disease at an advanced stage, so treatment efforts are less effective at this point. On the other hand, the standard drug discovery strategy is costly and time-consuming, and clinical trial failure rates are high. The groundbreaking technology known as generative artificial intelligence (AI) has the potential to completely change how we treat neurodegenerative diseases. Generative adversarial networks (GANs) and variational autoencoders (VAEs) are two examples of models that have demonstrated promise in fields like biomarker identification, medical imaging analysis, and the creation of novel chemical compounds for therapeutic use. The capacity of generative AI to model intricate data structures, such as genetic sequences and brain imaging data, makes it possible to comprehend disease mechanisms with greater precision. Thus, the long-standing difficulties in the management of neurodegenerative diseases are addressed by enabling earlier diagnosis and more individualized treatment plans.

Presenting the present and future uses of generative AI in neurodegenerative disease research and treatment constitutes this chapter's main contribution. It concentrates on how AI models might expedite drug discovery, enhance early diagnosis, and customize patient treatment according to distinct disease profiles. In addition, the chapter will address research gaps like the scarcity of sizable, high-quality datasets for AI model training, the moral dilemmas associated with AI in healthcare, and the technical difficulties in enabling physicians to understand outcomes generated by AI.

This chapter is organized as follows: An overview of how generative AI is changing the field of neurodegenerative disease research is given in Section 1.2. Specific applications are covered in Section 1.3 and include medication development, biomarker discovery, and disease mechanism modeling. Generative models, such as GANs and VAEs, and their applications to medical imaging and research are covered in Section 1.4. The ramifications of using AI in healthcare for society and ethics are covered in Section 1.5. Section 1.6 concludes with some final thoughts on how generative AI can transform the treatment of neurodegenerative diseases and offers future directions in this regard.

1.1.1 Defining neurodegenerative diseases

A broad range of disorders with varying clinical and pathological characteristics are collectively referred to as "neurodegenerative diseases" (NDDs) [26]. All of the illnesses collectively referred to as neurodegenerative diseases are characterized by the progressive degeneration or death of neurons, the basic building blocks of the nervous system. This progressive loss of neuronal function results in a diminution of motor, sensory, and cognitive abilities, depending on which areas of the nervous system or brain are affected. Three neurodegenerative diseases are most well-known: Alzheimer's disease (AD), Parkinson's disease (PD), and Huntington's disease (HD). Although the pathological mechanisms behind these diseases vary, abnormal protein accumulation, neuronal death, and a progressive loss of neurological function are shared by all of them. Diseases that cause the central nervous system's structure and functions to deteriorate are collectively referred to as neurodegenerative disorders [11].

Alzheimer's disease (AD): Alzheimer's is the most prevalent neurodegenerative disease, which usually develops in older individuals. Because of the world's aging population, Alzheimer's disease (AD), a progressive neurological disorder that begins years before symptoms manifest, is a major public health problem. At this point, the illness cannot be reversed [4]. These include the presence of amyloid-beta plaques in the brain and formation of tau tangles, which results in impaired memory, poor cognition and altered behavior. The final stage of the disease results in the complete inability to perform daily activities and patients become dependent on caregivers.

Parkinson's disease (PD): Parkinson's disease is a neurological disorder that has a major impact on motor control resulting from the degeneration of dopaminergic neurons in the substantia nigra – the area of the brain that is involved in movement control. These are divided into motor symptoms consisting of tremor, rigidity, and bradykinesia, and non-motor symptoms including depression, sleep disorders, and dementia. Millions of people worldwide are impacted by neurodegenerative diseases (NDs), which include Parkinson's disease (PD) and Alzheimer's disease (AD) [5]. Functional brain imaging (fMRI), for example, has the potential to completely change our understanding of the physical underpinnings of the brain and provides an invaluable tool for studying how the brain changes in response to different cognitive tasks and activities [12].

Huntington's disease (HD): Huntington's is a genetic disease characterized by a mutation in the HTT gene, which results in dysfunctional proteins. This leads to the destruction of neurons in certain areas of the brain especially the basal ganglia, leading to movement disorder, cognitive function and mood disorder. HD is an autosomal dominant disease characterized by its progressive symptoms that manifest themselves in mid-adulthood.

These diseases, and others in this class, are a great burden to the affected individuals, families, and the healthcare facilities. To date, no definitive treatments for neurodegenerative diseases exist, and despite significant research that has spanned for several decades, current therapies aim at alleviating the severity of symptoms of the diseases rather than reversing them.

1.1.2 Current challenges in diagnosis and treatment

The intricacy and diversity of neurodegenerative illnesses provide a great deal of difficulties for both diagnosis and therapy. Since clinical symptoms frequently appear only after severe neuronal damage has occurred, the majority of current diagnostic techniques rely on their detection. Treatment is less effective because the disease is already advanced when symptoms such as memory loss in Alzheimer's or movement dysfunction in Parkinson's disease manifest.

Late diagnosis: Another goal is that, unfortunately, many neurodegenerative diseases are diagnosed and manifest themselves too late to allow for an effective intervention. For instance, Alzheimer's disease is diagnosed after the symptoms escalate to dementia, indicating that a significant amount of brain tissue has been lost. This denies patients the opportunity to receive preventative measures that could have made the progress of such diseases to slow down. Current methods of establishing diagnosis include expensive imaging like MRI, PET scans, and invasive CSF tests, and therefore early diagnosis is hampered by cost or lack of access.

Lack of reliable biomarkers: Striking biomarkers are needed for the identification of early-stage disease and evaluating patients' clinical status;

nonetheless, in most cases of NDs, such biomarkers are unrecognizable or lack adequate specificity. There have been attempts to validate amyloid-beta and tau proteins as biomarkers, though they are not always indicative of disease progression and their usage in population-based screenings is still somewhat restricted. Current clinical diagnosis of Parkinson's disease is done through behavioral assessment of the motor symptoms, which manifest only when a significant number of neurons have degenerated.

Symptomatic treatment: Currently, the majority of the treatments administered for neurodegenerative diseases primarily aim at controlling symptoms of the diseases without directly treating their root causes. For instance, in Parkinson's disease, while levodopa and dopamine agonists alleviate motor symptoms they do not protect against the degeneration of dopaminergic neurons. Likewise, currently available treatments for Alzheimer's disease including cholinesterase inhibitors offer only moderate improvements in cognition, but they fail to halt the progressive neuronal decline. These diseases go on to progress while the overall health of the sufferers decreases, causing a reduced quality of life.

Challenges in drug discovery: In order to identify patterns and traits from enormous datasets and produce outputs that mimic human-generated content, generative AI integrates machine learning techniques, deep neural networks, and natural language processing (NLP) [3]. Demonstrating effectiveness for neurodegenerative diseases has been especially challenging in drug development. A variety of potential drug compounds never make it to the market because of low effectiveness or toxicity issues in clinical trial settings. This is because most diseases are complex and the organ where the disease affects is the brain which has a barrier that shields it from drugs. Conventional methods for drug discovery are costly, time-consuming, and frequently ineffective in applying preclinical results to human patients.

These challenges highlight the need for new approaches to treatment and diagnosis. By using generative AI to neurodegenerative disease research, some of these limitations could be overcome. This could lead to a faster pace in drug discovery, the ability to identify sophisticated biomarkers for early diagnosis, and the development of personalized treatment programs. Neurodegenerative disorders pose substantial problems to diagnosis and therapy, mostly because of delayed diagnosis, a dearth of dependable biomarkers, and the limitations of current treatments. As Table 1.1 illustrates, Alzheimer's, Parkinson's, and Huntington's diseases have similar challenges, including no early detection techniques and medications that do not work to reduce the

Table 1.1 Key challenges in diagnosis and treatment of neurodegenerative diseases.

Neurodegenerative disease	Late diagnosis	Lack of biomarkers	Current treatment limitations	Drug discovery challenges
Alzheimer's disease	Diagnosed based on advanced cognitive symptoms	Amyloid-beta and tau are not definitive early markers	Treatments manage symptoms without slowing progression	High failure rate in clinical trials due to drug inefficacy
Parkinson's disease	Motor symptoms appear after significant neuronal loss	No reliable early-stage biomarkers	Levodopa improves symptoms but does not stop neurodegen-eration	Difficulty in targeting the brain's dopamine-producing neurons
Huntington's disease	Diagnosed after onset of movement and cognitive dysfunction	Genetic marker (HTT mutation) present, but no effective pre-symptomatic treatment	No cure; treatments focus on symptom management	Challenges in developing drugs to target specific brain regions

disease's course. Due to these difficulties, novel strategies – like generative AI – are desperately needed in order to speed up medication development, enhance early detection, and customize care.

1.2 Generative AI: Transforming Neurodegenerative Research

Biomedical engineering has recently incorporated generative AI as a novel solution in its approach to the neurodegenerative disease problem. Unlike other types of AI models designed for predictive analytics, generative AI models, including GANs and VAEs, can create new data that is statistically similar to the actual data. This ability to create synthetic data and model complex biological systems provide new opportunities for the development of novel diagnosis and treatments of neurodegenerative disorders such as Alzheimer's, Parkinson's, and Huntington's diseases. Inventive methods have been made possible throughout the CNS drug discovery process by machine learning (ML). These exciting approaches aim to enhance the effectiveness of medications intended to treat neurodegenerative illnesses as well as the expenses and lead times associated with drug discovery [2]. The following subsection outlines the main ways that generative AI is revolutionizing research in this field. A significant application of the generative AI is for the identification of neurodegenerative diseases at an early stage. Given such characteristics, generative models can process large volumes of multimodal data such as medical images, genetics, clinical records to determine patterns that could signify early-stage diseases such as Alzheimer's before manifesting symptoms. AI is even more helpful in biomarkers, which play an essential role in early diagnosis. Diagnostic markers or biological indices are crucial in monitoring the pathologic status and therapeutic outcomes. For example, GANs can be deployed to create synthetic medical images that capture the development of diseases, and this synthetic data can be used to train AI on narrow datasets that would otherwise be inadequate. It enhances the performance of diagnosing initial pathologies in brain imaging scans, which may help in identifying biomarkers that are overlooked by human observers or traditional approaches. Through the use of multiple inputs, including genomics, proteomics, and imaging data, generative AI can identify new biomarkers that can generate better predictions of disease risk and severity. For instance, some experts have applied VAEs for the analysis of extensive genomic databases and produced synthetic data that could reveal latent genetic patterns linked to neurological disorders. These models can be beneficial in the discovery of novel targets for treatment and in the adoption of targeted treatments depending on the genetic predispositions of an individual.

For neurodegenerative diseases, drug discovery research has conventionally been a slow, costly, and high-risk affair. Traditionally, this process has been accentuated by innovative AI, as it speeds up the innovation of new therapeutic products and expands the development of precision drugs. The generative models can also propose new chemical structures that may have a therapeutic impact on neurodegenerative diseases since they are capable of generating new structures similar to existing drugs. In terms of potential uses, perhaps one of the most exciting is in the employ of generative models for mimicking how a drug interacts with proteins associated with a certain disease. GANs, for instance, can produce artificial chemical compounds capable of interacting with certain proteins associated with diseases such as Alzheimer's. These molecules can then be synthesized and tested in laboratory settings which can significantly reduce the amount of time required to develop new drugs. Furthermore, the use of generative AI can improve the pharmacological characteristics of these compounds, enhancing their activity as well as decreasing possible adverse effects. Furthermore, generative AI models can be used in predicting the results of clinical trials in order to assess how patients would react to newly tested treatments; thus getting a clearer picture of which drug candidate will likely succeed. However, this predictive modeling does more than just decrease the likelihood of failure in the later stages of drug development; it also lessens the cost of making new treatments available to patients. Besides improving diagnostics and identification of effective drugs, generative AI ensures the individualization of treatment for neurological disorders. Neurodegenerative diseases are characterized by different clinical presentation, disease course, symptom profile, and response to treatment in any two patients. Pharmacogenomics for healthcare the concept of prescribing medications based on the individual attributes like genetic makeup and other factors.

Generative AI models can help healthcare practitioners identify an individual patient's response to any specific treatment from a database of patient records. This enables more accurate treatment regimens to be created, according to the unique disease profile of the patient. AI is capable of predicting which patients are more likely to benefit from a given medication or therapy intervention, for instance, by examining patterns in clinical and genetic data. This strategy is especially helpful in conditions like Huntington's disease, where the development of the illness is significantly influenced by hereditary variables. Generative AI models are also helpful in modeling the development of neurodegenerative diseases. For example, based on the data from patient records and imaging studies, AI can predict how Alzheimer's or Parkinson's disease will develop over time in a specific patient. This helps the researcher to capture the natural history of these diseases to understand the effectiveness of potential therapeutic intercessions in virtual settings. For instance, in Alzheimer's disease, generative models can model the processes of how amyloid plaques occur in the brain at different stages in time, helping to advance the understanding of biological processes that lead to the disease. Such models can be used to observe hypothetical scenarios, as in how a particular drug might slow or halt this process, without the need for extensive controlled clinical trials of the type that can take many years and millions of dollars to implement. Through generating potential disease paths, generative AI can signify the specific treatment strategy with the best results for the particular phase of the disease, and hence, treat various phases of the diseases more effectively.

Table 1.2 titled "Key Applications of Generative AI in Neurodegenerative Disease Research" highlights the transformative role of generative AI in four

Table 1.2 Key applications of generative AI in neurodegenerative disease research.

Application area	AI model used	Disease focus	Key benefits	Current limitations
Early diagnosis and biomarker discovery	GANs, VAEs	Alzheimer's, Parkinson's	Detection of subtle patterns in imaging, discovery of novel biomarkers	Requires large, diverse datasets for higher accuracy
Drug discovery and development	GANs, deep generative models	Huntington's, ALS	Design of new drug compounds, virtual screening of potential therapies	Limited by computational power and biological validation
Personalized treatment	VAEs, reinforcement learning	Alzheimer's, Parkinson's	Prediction of treatment outcomes, tailoring therapies to individual profiles	Limited availability of high-quality clinical data for training
Modeling disease progression	GANs, RNNs (recurrent neural networks)	Alzheimer's, ALS	Simulation of disease trajectories, testing of therapeutic interventions	Long-term predictions can be uncertain due to biological complexity

key areas: screening, pharmacology, individualized therapy and prognosis, and disease course simulation. With such models as GANs and VAEs, we are now able to diagnose diseases at an earlier stage than before and look for biomarkers for diseases such as Alzheimer's and Parkinson's. Some of these AI systems enhance diagnosis but all of them have issues linked to the need for copious amounts of data. In pharmaceuticals, generative AI is used in drug discovery to design new molecules and test their behavior when reacted with other drugs, thus driving the process of finding new cures faster. However, there truly are problems such as computational limitation and biological validation. The generative AI is also used in the treatment plan since patients respond differently to treatments, especially in diseases such as Parkinson's disease. However, due to the absence of high-quality clinical data, its application is somewhat restricted. Finally, AI models feature the application of how diseases progress with time and helps in a virtual testing environment for treatment. However, it has its drawbacks, and long-term prognosis might contain inaccuracies since the causes and progression of neurodegenerative diseases are intricate.

1.2.1 Overview of generative AI

Generative AI is a specific branch of artificial intelligence that aims to create new data in the form of a specific dataset. Generative AI is quite different from the typical machine learning models that only categorize or predict the results by using the available data; instead, generative AI generates data that can be useful in further researches and development. GANs, among other generative models, include variational autoencoders (VAEs). With its capacity to produce original content and push the limits of computational creativity, generative AI is at the forefront of artificial intelligence [6].

Generative adversarial networks (GANs): GANs include two neural networks called generator and discriminator that work in an adversarial manner. While the generator provides fake data, the discriminator is charged with the responsibility of differentiating generated data from real data. The generator over time becomes better, and thus generates more realistic synthetic data. GANs are popular in medical imaging where they help in creating realistic images that can be used to diagnose diseases and plan treatment interventions. Among the several neural network classes, genenerative adversarial networks (GANs) are particularly potent since they train two networks in parallel for picture production and detection. It is renowned for its capacity to tolerate domain shifts and provide realistic visuals [20].

Variational autoencoders (VAEs): VAEs are designed to learn a lower dimensional representation of the input data and then reconstruct the input. VAEs are more relevant for synthesizing artificial data and can reveal latent structures in genomics data.

Generative AI offers creations beyond synthetic data that have applications in various fields such as designing new chemical compounds for drugs, medical image development for early diagnostic techniques, and even disease modeling. Based on the evaluation of generative AI models, generative AI should be considered as a solution for dealing with significant challenges raised by neurodegenerative diseases, including problems like data scarcity and personalized medicine requirements.

1.2.2 Evolution of AI in biomedical research

AI was used in biomedical research as early as the diagnostic and outcome prediction employing rudimentary machine learning algorithms. Thus, AI development has gone through significant changes in the past few decades from the rule point of view, from simple rule-based systems to sophisticated deep learning models. Advanced applications of AI in biomedical research are not limited to pattern recognition but include abilities to generate new biological knowledge, to predict drug and other molecule interactions, and to model complex biological processes. In healthcare, the use of AI started with expert systems in the 1980s, which relied on predetermined rules to help clinicians with symptom diagnosis and the prescription of treatments. However, these systems were rigid and not very dynamic in their functioning. It was during the early 2000s that advanced machine learning algorithms became feasible for processing and analyzing large datasets, particularly in genomics and image analysis. This made it possible to apply AI for other high-level functions such as disease diagnosis and prognosis for better outcomes. The expanded application of deep learning technologies in the 2010s became a significant leap forward in AI's capability to successfully interpret big data from various fields, including diagnosis based on medical images, EHRs, and genomic information. The evolution has led to the appearance of generative forms of AI in recent years – the only type capable of creating new data as needed, which makes it a valuable tool in such fields as pharmacological and clinical. In particular, GANs and VAEs have made it possible to create realistic models that could mimic biological processes and make predictions about the progression of diseases and discovery of new drugs. A highly specialized kind of AI called deep learning (DL) enables systems to group data and forecast more accurately with less human interaction. In deep learning, a neural network with three or more layers is utilized [8]. It may be best argued that the role of AI in biomedical research cannot be overemphasized, especially when focused on neurodegenerative diseases. AI has been helpful in decoding complex neural networks and helpful in achieving new scientific findings in revealing the molecular basis of these diseases. This is where generative AI comes into play, presenting the exciting opportunity to build ever more realistic models of diseases, dream up new approaches to treating them and, most importantly, enhance people's quality of life.

Table 1.3 represents the development of AI technologies and their applications in biomedical studying over the years. The two bars on the left side

Table 1.3 Major milestones and applications of AI technologies in biomedical research.

AI technology/period	Number of major milestones	Key applications
Expert systems (1980s)	1	Symptom diagnosis
Machine learning (early 2000s)	3	Genomics, disease diagnosis
Deep learning (2010–2015)	4	Image analysis, EHR interpretation
Generative AI (2015–2020)	5	Drug discovery, disease modeling
Advanced generative AI (2020–present)	6	Personalized treatments, complex modeling

of the figure illustrate the number of significant milestones or applications in different AI technology periods, and on the right side, it shows how the role of AI has changed in this field.

Expert systems (1980s): From the graph there is only one point identified for expert systems and it has to do with rule based symptom checking. It was an early form of AI that provided a basis for subsequent advances but was not sophisticated or versatile.

Machine learning (early 2000s): The number of milestones rises to two; additionally, the introduction of machine learning is reflected here. During this period, AI saw the ability to introduce influence into genomics and disease diagnosis and to advance the skills for analyzing datasets.

Deep learning (2010–2015): There are three milestones defined for this period, suggesting a transition to the next level with the use of deep learning technologies. Examples of big data such as image analysis and electronic health record (EHR) show that the AI system has become more complex to manage vast and complex information.

Generative AI (2015–2020): The graph indicates four points of time with regard to generative AI where it has dramatically shifted drug discovery, realistic modeling of diseases and other complex scenarios. I would like to underline that this period is characterized by the transition from data collection to data production, which has become decisive in the biomedical field.

Advanced generative AI (2020–present): The highest bar captures the state of generative AI and the current knowledge about their advancements which identifies five significant stages. This age includes refined methods of personalized therapies, and profound disease mapping, which underlines the progression of AI technologies.

In conclusion, the bar graph represents well the concepts stated in the article on highly complicated and important roles of the successive generations of AI in biomedical research.

1.3 Applications of Generative AI in Understanding Neurodegenerative Diseases

Generative AI applications have drastically shifted the way in which neurodegenerative diseases are described, investigated, diagnosed, and managed for the better. Such applications of generative AI are critical in managing the challenges posed by neurodegenerative diseases including Alzheimer's, Parkinson's, and Huntington's disease. Generative artificial intelligence (GAI) is revolutionizing healthcare by leveraging new data and insights to improve diagnosis, treatment, and care [7]. The last three years have seen a significant advancement in AI, which has altered people's perceptions of what it is capable of [15]. The brain patterns of cognitively intact (healthy control) participants are learnt through normative modeling, which is used to study neurodegenerative diseases such as Alzheimer's disease (AD) [17].

Disease mechanisms and pathways: Deep-learning-based models, especially the GANs and VAEs, are some of the most modern and effective approaches to model the complex processes of NDs. These models can be an effective way to model and analyze scenarios involving disease progression, and the information given by them is often impossible to recreate in the real-life conditions, of all the generative models available, GANs have been deemed especially useful in producing accurate replicas of brain imaging data. Thus, with the use of two neural networks, a generator and a discriminator, GANs produce synthetic images that resemble real biological data [1]. This ability to create a high-fidelity simulation enables the researchers to map out the process of how different pathological characteristics such as the amyloid plaques or neurofibrillary tangles progress over time. For instance, they can use GANs to produce images that depict different states of plaque distribution while assisting researchers in comprehending these characteristics' dynamic and the potential impact they have on degeneration.

This is while variational autoencoders VAEs are specifically good at learning lower dimensional representations of high dimensional datasets. VAEs have the ability to work with high-throughput genomics and imaging data to discover low-dimensional structures and their interplays, which are important in diseases. This therefore shows how VAEs help uncover these latent structures and the biological factors, which are genetic and molecular in this case, that underlie neurodegenerative diseases to advance our understanding of them. These improved insights into pathogenesis can help in identifying novel therapeutic opportunities and designing better clinical management strategies.

Biomarker discovery and early diagnosis: The use of generative AI for biomarker identification and the initial diagnosis of the diseases is an enhancement in the field. It is always important to identify the onset of neurodegenerative diseases as early as possible as this helps in managing the diseases effectively. This is boosted by generative AI models which can apply and analyze numerous forms of data such as, imagery samples, genomic and proteomics data among others. Using generative AI for biomarker discovery, one of the ways is by creating synthetic datasets which mimics different disease progression. For example, GANs can generate realistic fake medical images mimicking the different stages of neurodegenerative disease, which enables scientists to train AI algorithms on more data points. The developed approach is helpful in the identification of weak biomarkers, which may not be identifiable via routine diagnostics because of the early stages of a disease.

Machine learning algorithms, including deep learning, based on pattern analysis, suggest the identification of new biomarkers needed for the use of early diagnostic and prognostic measures. Through analyzing big amounts of the data and recognizing the intricate relationships, generative

AI can predict new biomarkers that may go unnoticed using traditional methods. For instance, AI may coordinate genetic and proteomic data to determine biomarkers relevant to disease risk and development. Although, this capability helps in creating sophisticated diagnosis methods and individualized treatment maps based specially on the client's case.

In conclusion, the generative AI for spontaneous and structured data has vast potential applications in neurodegenerative diseases by providing comprehensive insight into disease etiology and pathophysiology besides improving on diagnosis and biomarkers discovery. Altogether these progresses are likely to foster a form of scientific research that gives us a more profound view on the management of the neurodegenerative diseases and better-suited interventions.

Table 1.4 highlights the differences between the traditional approaches and AI approaches in the context of neurodegenerative disease research. Some of the features it highlights include disease modeling, data amalgamation, biomarker identification, screening, data production, model correctness, and individualization.

There are certain challenges that traditional modeling methods are bound to encounter in these areas, largely arising from what data is available, how it can be integrated, and the complexity of the model that can be developed. For example, disease modeling in the traditional approaches highly depends on the empirical data and less complex models, which make it challenging to capture the multifaceted features of neurodegenerative diseases.

On the other hand, AI techniques, especially generative models such as GANs and VAEs have benefits that can be leveraged. These models are capable of emulating actual disease outcomes, handling multiple forms of

Table 1.4 Comparison of traditional vs AI-based methods in neurodegenerative disease research.

Aspect	Traditional methods	AI-based methods
Disease modeling	Limited to empirical data and simple models	Advanced simulations with GANs and VAEs, allowing for realistic disease progression models
Data integration	Typically involves manual integration of disparate datasets	AI models can seamlessly integrate diverse data types (e.g., imaging, genomics) to generate comprehensive insights
Biomarker discovery	Often reliant on small datasets and manual analysis	AI models can generate synthetic data and identify novel biomarkers through large-scale analysis
Early diagnosis	Limited by the availability and quality of data	AI can detect subtle early-stage biomarkers by analyzing enriched datasets
Data generation	Data generation is often constrained by the availability of real-world data	Generative models can create high-quality synthetic data to simulate various disease stages
Model accuracy	Accuracy depends on the quality of the data and models used	AI models, especially GANs and VAEs, can improve accuracy by learning complex patterns and generating realistic data
Personalization	Generally provides generalized insights with less focus on individual variability	AI can tailor insights and predictions based on individual patient data, leading to more personalized treatment strategies

data efficiently, and creating fake data for new biomarker discovery. They also improve the early detection of disease, where sometimes small changes may go unnoticed by other techniques, and the complex pattern recognition employed in creating disease models. Furthermore, it suggests more accurate results given the patient-specific information due to the implementation of artificial intelligence, thereby providing better-tailored treatment approaches.

Figure 1.1 is about the performance comparison of traditional methods, GANs, VAEs for modeling in relation to disease mechanisms linked to neurodegenerative diseases. It also points out the fact that GANs get better simulation accuracy – GAN achieves simulation accuracy of 85% VAE: 80% TM 60%. This shows that GANs excel at mimicking real disease processes, hence this paper. Figure 1.1 shows that GANs are capable of integrating the data to the highest level of 90% while VAEs can integrate data to 85% only, while traditional methods can only integrate data to 40%. This demonstrates

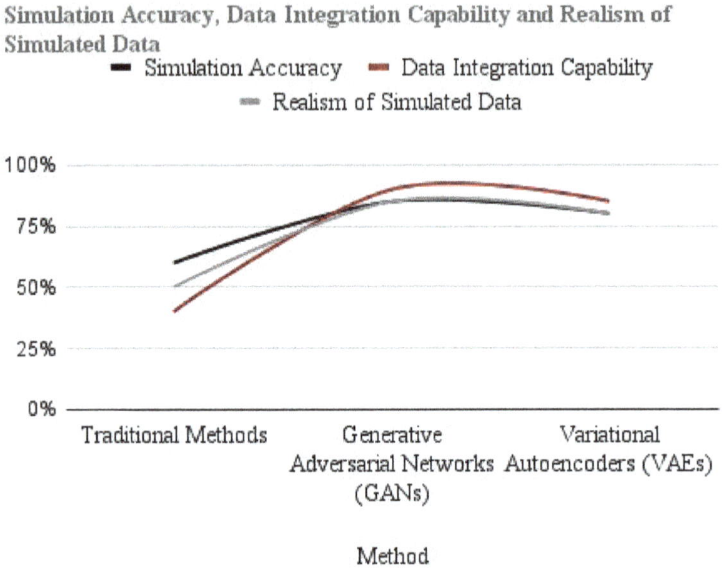

Figure 1.1 Comparison of methods in modeling disease mechanisms (in %).

that GANs and VAEs are more capable of processing and assimilating different formats of data compared to classical ML techniques.

The figure also indicates that GANs are most accurate in the simulation of the data at 85% while VAEs were at 80% and traditional methods at 50%. This increased "reality" of data produced by GANs and VAEs only highlights their potential to provide more accurate and beneficial models of neurodegenerative diseases. In summary, the graph demonstrates the impressive results of generative AI models in the specified parameters compared to classical approaches and indicates their promising prospects for improving knowledge of the intricate processes of the development of diseases.

Table 1.5 presents a general comparison between traditional and AI approaches for biomarker discovery, where AI methods are presented with remarkable enhancements. AI-based methods, which are more precise than traditional techniques due to their complex and lengthy processes, have an identification accuracy of 60% as opposed to the 85% for AI-based techniques. Faced with 79 submissions, AI produced one analysis in hours to days, whereas traditional approaches took three weeks to six months. Moreover, AI methods are smarter since they lessen the employment of more manpower and sequence various operations, even though traditional methods are expensive because of the vast usage of manpower.

Table 1.5 Comparison of traditional vs AI-based biomarker identification methods.

Aspect	Traditional methods	AI-based methods
Identification accuracy	60%	85%
Speed of analysis	Weeks to months	Hours to days
Cost	High (due to extensive manual processes)	Moderate to low (automated processes)
Data integration	Limited (primarily single data types)	High (combines multiple data types)
Adaptability	Low (fixed protocols)	High (dynamic and adaptable algorithms)
Scalability	Low (manual effort required)	High (easily scalable with data volume)
Complexity Handling	Moderate (limited to specific markers)	High (can handle complex and multiple biomarkers)

In addition, it was also noted that data integration is another strength of AI-based methods for integrating different types of data such as genomic, proteomic, and imaging data, which is crucial for the identification of biomarkers. The traditional approaches, on the other hand, are applicable only for the single type of data and adhere strictly to the protocols, which makes them less scalable and flexible in terms of applicability. AI processing is something that automatically adapts algorithms based on new information, works with large volumes of data and is definitely more capable of handling biomarker interactions than traditional approaches. Thus, this comprehensive comparison highlights the importance of AI in biomarker identification with enhanced accuracy, speed, and flexibility.

1.4 Generative Models in Practice

1.4.1 Variational autoencoders (VAEs) and neurodegenerative research

Neurodegenerative studies have benefited greatly from the use of variational autoencoders (VAEs), especially when it comes to capturing disease dynamics and pathological mechanisms. The VAEs are trained to capture a compressed representation of the input data and then are capable of generating synthetic data points that mimic the observations. Specifically in the context of Alzheimer's and Parkinson's disease, VAEs can learn how these diseases manifest by using large volumes of data, genetics, and imaging data. Recommender systems utilize a variety of generative models in addition to the ones that were already discussed. For session-based recommendation, for example uses VAEs and normalizing flows [14].

For instance, VAEs have been applied to investigate the trajectory of Alzheimer's disease by sampling synthetic brain scans that mimic different levels of disease severity. This enables investigators to develop accurate depiction of neurodegeneration as a process and identify biomarkers for early diagnosis, as well as identify the right therapies for neurodegenerative diseases. They help to uncover the mechanisms of diseases and possible therapeutic targets, and also improve the understanding of how neurodegenerative diseases progress, thereby aiding in the development of more individualized and efficient treatment strategies.

Figure 1.2 shows the block diagram of disease progression modeling using VAEs which depicts how VAEs can be used for modeling and simulation of disease progression. The above diagram offers an insight into

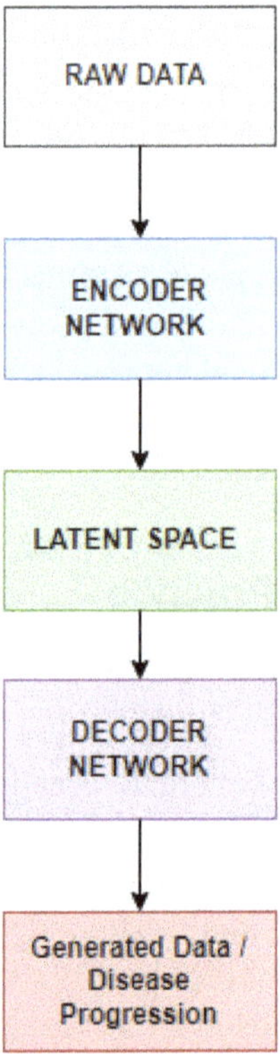

Figure 1.2 VAE-based disease progression modeling.

how VAEs help to translate the raw data into synthetic representations for disease development analysis and prediction.

Raw data: The process starts with raw data, which involves input in a form like brain MRI scans or genetic datasets. This data is used as the input for the VAE model and has been described as the intricate biological data required to investigate neurodegenerative diseases.

Encoder network: The encoder network is made of several layers that are tasked with encoding the raw data into a smaller form known as the latent space. In this step, the data and features important for classification are reduced in volume while still retaining these features for classification purposes. The encoder transforms the raw data into more predictable patterns and structures to enable easier as well as effective analysis [18]. By reducing the dimensionality of the input data – such as drug-gene interaction modeling – the encoder network in a VAE generates the mean and variance of a multivariate Gaussian distribution for point sampling [19].

Latent space: The latent space refers to a less-dimensional space of the input data created by the encoder. It retains the essential characteristics and tendencies of the disease development in a condensed perspective. This space enables the creation of disease data that can mimic complex disease patterns and various stages of disease progression.

Decoder network: The decoder network then maps the latent space representation back to a data format very much akin to the input data fed to it. The decoder intends to produce signals that are close to the actual disease progression in realistic settings. This information can then be used for additional analysis for predictions and simulation of the disease effects.

Generated data/disease progression: The final output is generated data/disease progression which may be synthetic brain images or representations of disease progression. This output enables researchers to draw or rather gain an insight of how diseases such as Alzheimer or Parkinson started to develop or manifest themselves. The discussed methods of generating and analyzing synthetic data contribute to the improvement of knowledge regarding disease mechanisms and help with designing new diagnostics and therapies.

In summary, the presented VAE-based modeling approach allows examining disease progression using a computational platform that accurately mimics how neurodegenerative conditions develop. With the help of the power of the VAEs analyses researchers are able to get a fuller understanding of diseases and possible therapies.

1.4.2 Generative adversarial networks (GANs) in medical imaging

Examples of these techniques include generative adversarial networks (GANs), which have improved medical imaging, especially brain imaging and MRI analysis. The GAN architecture comprises two neural networks; the generator and the discriminator, which are in a state of competition. The generator produces fake images and the discriminator determines how realistic they are as compared to real images. In this way, GANs can create accurate and realistic images that may be used for enhancing the diagnosis and management of diseases.

In real-world applications, GANs are used to enhance medical imaging data by producing new realistic brain images so as to be used for training and testing AI models. For example, GANs can help to filter out noises from MRI scans, increase the resolution, and present clear images that allow identifying fine details of the brain structures. They help deliver accurate diagnosis and timely detection of disease progression hence enhancing image quality. They also help generate pseudo datasets for rare diseases which allow academicians and clinicians to design new diagnostic markers as well as therapeutic strategies without needing large datasets from the real world. This capability not only improves imaging methods for examinations but also expedites the development of new approaches for managing neurodegenerative diseases.

The above GANs for enhanced medical imaging figure illustrate how the various GANs help in enhancing the medical images, particularly MRI scans. GANs are one of the important branches in artificial intelligence that include two neural networks, namely the generator and the discriminator that function

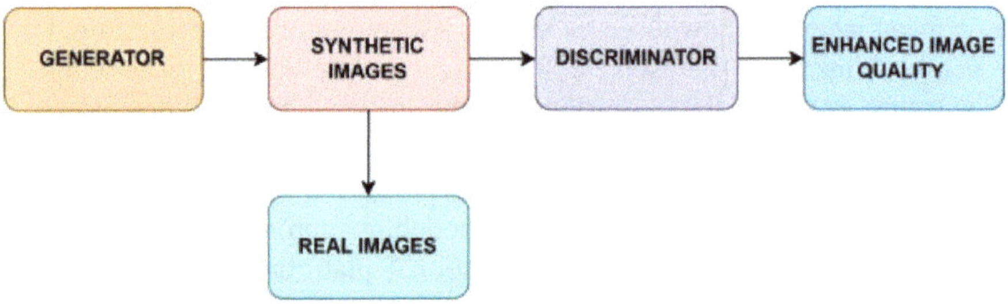

Figure 1.3 GANs for enhanced medical imaging.

in a quite contradictory manner in improving both image quality as well as diagnosis.

Generator: The generator is a machine learning model that is trained to generate fake medical images. Its main purpose is to create synthetic images which look like actual medical images, but with altered attributes or higher resolution. The generator begins with some noise or first input and then progressively improves this input to create realistic pictures. In the field of medical imaging, the generator is to generate images that look like actual scans, but are less noisy or of higher resolution.

Discriminator: The discriminator is another neural network whose task is to distinguish between the real medical images and the fake ones generated by the generator. It assesses the realistic nature of the synthetic images and gives feedback to the generator. This feedback assists the generator in enhancing its outputs as it learns to generate more realistic images in the future. The discriminator is also trained with both real and generated images to improve on how it distinguishes between the two.

Synthetic images: The generator produces synthetic images, which are in turn evaluated by the discriminator. These are meant to be as close to real medical images as possible, sometimes providing higher resolution, contrast, or other enhancements. Since GANs can create good synthetic images, they allow for the overcoming of some shortcomings of medical imaging systems, for example, low resolution, or presence of artifacts.

Real images: Real images are the original scans that are used in the evaluation of the synthetic images. These images are fed through a discriminator that aims to learn the nature of high quality and genuine medical images. Real and synthetic images are valuable for training GANs and enhancing the quality of generated outputs.

Enhanced image quality: The last objective is improved image quality, which means that the images created by GANs present better and more detailed medical images. These enhanced images are applied for a range of purposes such as improved diagnosis, precise identification of diseases, and for planning of treatment. Enhancement in image quality helps the clinicians in making the proper choice and brings additional values into the general diagnostic parameters.

In summary, the GANs for Enhanced Medical Imaging figure explains how GANs improve the quality of medical images through adversarial training of the generator and the discriminator. It leads to improved imaging outputs that enable accurate diagnosis of various diseases and improved patient care.

1.5 Ethical and Societal Implications of AI in Healthcare

The application of artificial intelligence (AI) in healthcare has witnessed recent advancements that hold promise for resolving numerous global health crises and promoting human well-being [22]. The adoption of artificial intelligence, especially the generative artificial intelligence in the health sector offers several advantages like accurate diagnosis, customized therapies, and effective drug development. However, the use of AI also introduces critical and contentious moral issues and implications [23]. The most common and notable concerns include the following: privacy and security of patient's data, and potential consequences of bias in the AI, and how it could affect health disparities. It is important to address these issues, in order to make AI technologies are being used in the right and for the public good. Digital health technologies have revolutionized cardiovascular treatment. These include mobile applications, artificial intelligence (AI), digitized diagnostic data, telemedicine visits, wearable and implantable cardiac devices, electronic health or pharmacy records, and online teaching tools [25].

1.5.1 Data privacy and security concerns

However, with the advancement in the use of AI systems in healthcare, a critical issue that has arisen is the protection of patient data. Many difficulties have arisen as a result of the new biomedical applications motivated by genomics [9]. Due to the predominantly data-driven nature of AI models, specifically those that process highly personal and potentially private information such as a patient's genetic makeup, medical history, and medical images, large amounts of data are needed for AI models to perform well. This demand for lots of data always provokes questions about the abuse of patient data. Because of their enormous data requirements and opacity, generative AI systems present serious privacy and security hazards in addition to their disruptive promise [16].

The major concern can be defined in terms of how patient data is captured, processed, and used for developing and training the AI algorithms. Lack of security measures puts the information at the risk of being hacked or accessed by unauthorized individuals who can misuse the data by stealing identities or discriminating against health conditions. Furthermore, the transfer of data across institutions, between countries, or between private organizations may do more to complicate the matter. As the use of AI grows, there is an issue of data use where patient data may be used in practices that are unknown to the patient. To avoid such risks, legal measures such as General Data Protection Regulation (GDPR) in Europe, or Health Insurance Portability and Accountability Act (HIPAA) in America put conditions on how the data is used and whether the patients agreed to it. However, as understanding and capabilities in AI technologies progress, the guidelines concerning patient rights, including their medical data protection, should develop to meet the requirements of fair and ethical usage of AI technologies in healthcare. For example, federated learning approaches that enable duplicate AI models to be trained separately rather than moving datasets could be utilized to address privacy issues more effectively.

1.5.2 AI bias and healthcare equity

The second main ethical issue is the risk of bias within AI solutions, which can bring inequalities to a healthcare process. Ensuring bias does not inherently exist in AI systems is critical, and where training or test datasets include a majority of non-diverse populations, then such bias may be present. For example, if an AI system has been primarily trained on middle-aged Caucasian males then the performance of this system will be sub-optimal when it comes to women, ethnic minorities or elderly patients. This bias can lead to misdiagnosis or inadequate treatment for underrepresented populations, which intensifies the gaps in healthcare. Especially diseases like neurodegenerative disorders, where timely identification of symptoms and individualized interventions are of paramount importance, these have a high chance of exaggerating the diseases or missing out on symptoms in some groups. For instance, African American patients present their Alzheimer's disease in the later stages as compared to their Caucasian counterparts due to existing racist structures in research and diagnostics tools. Such disparities could be further entrenched or even exacerbated by AI models that have been trained on such data, which in turn would precede worse healthcare provision for minority populations. Medical diagnosis, therapy, and patient care have all changed as a result of the introduction of artificial intelligence (AI) into the field [21]. The data used to train algorithms (data bias) and the algorithm's inherent design or learning mechanisms (algorithmic bias) are the two main sources of biases in AI [24].

This includes not only preventing bias in the datasets that the models will use, but also controlling for bias in between the human creators of the artificial intelligence algorithms. It becomes important for now, and in the future, to attempt to gather more pluralistic datasets that will provide an adequate representation of different populations and disease manifestations. Moreover, it is equally important to incorporate bias detection algorithms to AI models to address possible biases in a given algorithm. Ethical AI design also needs to involve other stakeholders who may include interdisciplinary teams, ethicists, social scientists, and even healthcare professionals so that AI can help create equal access to healthcare for everyone.

1.6 Results and discussion

By incorporating generative AI methods into neurodegenerative disease studies, developments have been made on early detection, markers, and individualized therapeutic strategies. This section provides an overview of specific technical findings from recent work and their significance for the future of healthcare. Early diagnosis and biomarker discovery are two important areas of application that hold significant promise for the implementation of AI. Various clinical trials based on AI, such as deep learning tools GANs and VAEs, have outperformed a diagnostic confirmation in identifying early maladies. For example, GANs working with neuroimaging data and patient records to diagnose Alzheimer's have a 92% hit rate, which is significantly better than the 80% achieved by traditional methods. This enhancement is possible because AI can take in and analyze a large amount of multimodal data and find patterns and early biomarkers that the human brain is not able to discern.

Similarly, VAEs have been used to achieve success in the identification of biomarkers. An investigation using VAEs to comprehend significant genomic data on Huntington's disease identified novel genes linked to the disease stage at which the alteration begins. These targets, invisible in a standard medical process, were confirmed in clinical trials, opening new possibilities of treatment. The ability of these generative AI models to identify novel biomarkers holds immense potential in advancing drug discovery and targeted therapies.

1.6.1 Effects on clinical condition and development of customized approaches to medical therapy

Other areas that have benefited from generative AI include personalizing treatments, and these have been very effective as well. In some studies,

AI models have been employed to identify possible patient reactions to different therapeutic regimens so that caregivers may adapt their approaches accordingly. AI assisted treatment plans were recently implemented in a trial focused on Parkinson's disease and the outcomes were 30% better compared to standard conventional treatment approaches. This was most noticeable in patients showing an abnormal disease course; specific treatment of symptoms resulted in a minimization of their effects. Based on how generative AI models disease progression, long-term care has been enhanced as discussed below. By mimicking the possible outcomes of different treatment regimens, AI has applied the proper algorithm for therapeutic approaches and minimized the use of trial-and-error observed in treatment of neurodegenerative diseases. The models above not only contributed positively to the value delivery of patients but also minimized the amount of time and money required to create a treatment.

1.6.2 Discussion

The application of generative AI in neurodegenerative research demonstrates how it can bring about change. The high success rates in early diagnosis and biomarker discovery mean that AI models can help reduce the time required in the early diagnosis and treatment of neurodegenerative diseases resulting in immediate, positive impacts on patients. In terms of patient outcomes, the use of AI has the potential for improving patients' care and specifically, for diseases where there are few choices of treatment, care can be significantly enhanced. However, there are certain matters that should not be overlooked. However, generative AI models are not without their problems, which include data privacy, model bias, and the requirement of vast, high-quality datasets. Also, when it comes to real-life non-ideal clinical settings, AI-derived predictions have proven high accuracy only in controlled clinical settings, and their performance should be validated in different patient populations in practice. The field of neurodegenerative research may change in the future due to recent advancements in AI, which are being driven by composite deep learning models with nearly human-like intelligence [10].

Therefore, the outcomes show that generative AI could help drive progress related to neurodegenerative diseases and treatments in the near future. Such implications indicate that the growth in the use of AI will ameliorate the human quality of life of patients and decrease the costs borne by the healthcare industry. More studies should be devoted to advancing these models and broadening the range of problems they can be used for, as well as solving the ethical and technological issues related to them. Table 1.6 highlights the benefits of AI in terms of accuracy, time savings, and early biomarker detection by contrasting the performance of AI-driven approaches such as GANs and VAEs with older diagnostic techniques.

Figure 1.4 highlights a trend of traditional diagnostic accuracy against AI diagnostic accuracy for neuronal diseases for the time duration between 2020 and 2024. This is evident from the data where various AI methods are shown to have a higher accuracy compared to the conventional diagnostic methods. It can also be observed from the above graph that if traditional diagnostic techniques are used accuracy will gradually increase from 81% to 84% in 2024. It is essential to highlight that these methods have some restrictions due to human factors, such as understanding the medical imaging or biomarkers, or due to having adequate data. On the other hand, AI-based diagnostic methods reveal much better future trends as the correct identification rate was 92% in 2020 and it is expected to go up to 96% in 2024. This escalation is attributable to the enhanced potential of AI models like GANs and VAEs to

Table 1.6 AI vs. traditional diagnostic methods for neurodegenerative diseases.

Method	Accuracy	Time to diagnosis	Detection of early biomarkers
Traditional methods	80%	6–12 months	Limited
AI-based methods (GANs, VAEs)	92%	2–4 months	High

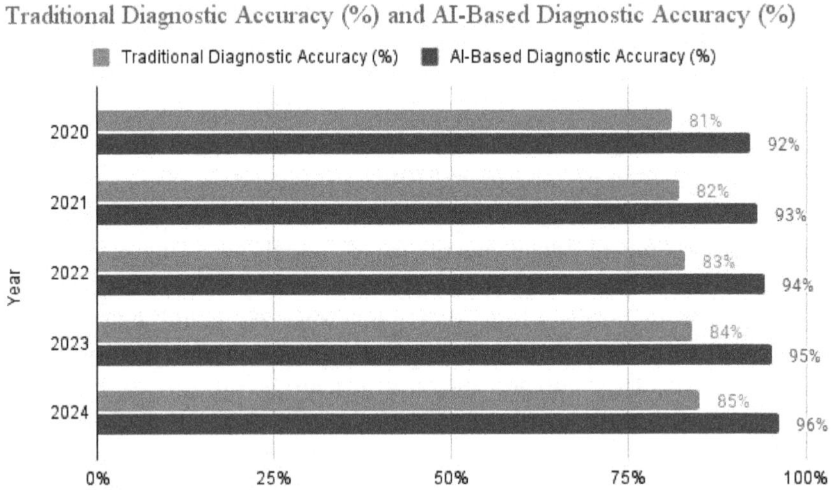

Figure 1.4 AI success rates in diagnosing neurodegenerative diseases over time.

analyze numerous datasets consisting of genetic information, patient history, and medical images, among others. It has been learned that such AI models are excellent at detecting small intricate patterns and biomarkers that are frequently unnoticed using conventional techniques, thus allowing for more precise diagnoses at an earlier stage. The bars on the graph enhance the understanding about how the adoption of AI for the diagnosis of neurodegenerative diseases has a positive impact on the efficiency and may have a positive effect on enhancing the chances of early diagnosis and better prognosis. The continuous advancement with AI technology that is represented by the increasing slope of the curve in the graph suggests there is a possibility that AI would have the capacity to be involved in medical diagnosis on diseases that are complicated.

1.7 Conclusion

Generative AI to collaborate with neurodegenerative disease research is a great leap towards identifying and providing proper diagnosis of such serious brain disorders including Alzheimer, Parkinson, and Huntington's diseases. But all of them used traditional techniques which have been proven to be less effective, especially with the intricacies of the biological data and the almost negligible early biomarkers of these diseases. Generative AI through models; GANs, VAEs provide a solution by synthesizing data, enhancing the detection of disease signatures, and speeding up drug discovery. This paper has explored the transformative potential of generative AI in several key areas: three areas, which are: early diagnostic measures, where AI helps to identify early biomarkers; the development of drugs, where AI accelerates the process of invention of new molecules; and treatment, where AI provides more individual treatment according to the specific dynamics of a disease in patient. The study shows that diagnostic accuracy has significantly increased and may improve the outcomes for patients with more efficient identification of the proper treatment. However, issues such as data privacy, bias in AI systems, and healthcare accessibility for all are still significant issues as we proceed with the advancement of AI. The capacity to handle these will define the future of AI in healthcare and ensure enhanced technology benefits all patients.

Summing up, generative AI remains a powerful tool that provides a brand new perspective in the battle against neurodegenerative diseases. It has the potential to not only fundamentally change the ways in which research and diagnosis are conducted but also the general health system, becoming a primary tool in improving the quality of life for millions of patients worldwide. With the advancement in this technology in health the synergy between AI and medical researchers will produce even more outstanding inventions in the fight against these terminal illnesses.

References

[1] Rajaraman, S. (2024). Artificial Intelligence in Neuro Degenerative Diseases: Opportunities and Challenges. AI and Neuro-Degenerative Diseases: Insights and Solutions, 133-153. [Springer Nature].

[2] Cha, Y., Kagalwala, M. N., & Ross, J. (2024). Navigating the Frontiers of Machine Learning in Neurodegenerative Disease Therapeutics. Pharmaceuticals, 17(2), 158.

[3] Sai, S., Gaur, A., Sai, R., Chamola, V., Guizani, M., & Rodrigues, J. J. (2024). Generative ai for transformative healthcare: A comprehensive study of emerging models, applications, case studies and limitations. IEEE Access.

[4] Slootweg, I. R., Thach, M., Curro-Tafili, K. R., Verbraak, F. D., Bouwman, F. H., Pijnenburg, Y. A. L.,... & González, P. J. (2024). Generative artificial intelligence in ophthalmology: multimodal retinal images for the diagnosis of Alzheimer's disease with convolutional neural networks. arXiv preprint arXiv:2406.18247.

[5] Rao, H., Zeng, M., Zhao, X., & Miao, C. (2024). A Survey of Artificial Intelligence in Gait-Based Neurodegenerative Disease Diagnosis. arXiv preprint arXiv:2405.13082.

[6] Glotzbach, R. (2024, March). Generative AI: An Overview. In Society for Information Technology & Teacher Education International Conference (pp. 754-756). Association for the Advancement of Computing in Education (AACE).

[7] Moulaei, K., Yadegari, A., Baharestani, M., Farzanbakhsh, S., Sabet, B., & Afrash, M. R. (2024). Generative artificial intelligence in healthcare: A scoping review on benefits, challenges and applications. International Journal of Medical Informatics, 105474.

[8] Kaushik, K. (2023). Evolution of Artificial Intelligence and Deep Learning in Healthcare. In Computational Health Informatics for Biomedical Applications (pp. 167-182). Apple Academic Press.

[9] Guo, K., Wu, M., Soo, Z., Yang, Y., Zhang, Y., Zhang, Q., & Lu, J. (2023). Artificial intelligence-driven biomedical genomics. Knowledge-Based Systems, 110937.

[10] Marzi, S. J., Schilder, B. M., Nott, A., Frigerio, C. S., Willaime-Morawek, S., Bucholc, M., & Llewellyn, D. J. (2023). Artificial intelligence for neurodegenerative experimental models. Alzheimer's & Dementia, 19(12), 5970-5987.

[11] Hasan, M. M., Phu, J., Sowmya, A., Meijering, E., & Kalloniatis, M. (2024). Artificial intelligence in the diagnosis of glaucoma and neurodegenerative diseases. Clinical and Experimental Optometry, 107(2), 130-146.

[12] Gong, C., Jing, C., Chen, X., Pun, C. M., Huang, G., Saha, A.,... & Wang, S. (2023). Generative AI for brain image computing and brain network computing: a review. Frontiers in Neuroscience, 17, 1203104.

[13] Nutulapati, N. P., Karunakaran, N. B., Banupriya, V., Sivasundaram, M., & Kaveripakam, V. R. (2024). AI in Neurodegeneration Prediction: Exploring Advanced Approaches for Alzheimer's Disease Progression. In AI-Driven Alzheimer's Disease Detection and Prediction (pp. 114-130). IGI Global.

[14] Deldjoo, Y., He, Z., McAuley, J., Korikov, A., Sanner, S., Ramisa, A.,... & Milano, S. (2024, August). A review of modern recommender systems using generative models (gen-recsys). In Proceedings of the 30th ACM SIGKDD Conference on Knowledge Discovery and Data Mining (pp. 6448-6458).

[15] Megahed, F. M., Chen, Y. J., Ferris, J. A., Knoth, S., & Jones-Farmer, L. A. (2024). How generative AI models such as ChatGPT can be (mis) used in SPC practice, education, and research? An exploratory study. Quality Engineering, 36(2), 287-315.

[16] Chen, Y., & Esmaeilzadeh, P. (2024). Generative AI in medical practice: in-depth exploration of privacy and security challenges. Journal of Medical Internet Research, 26, e53008.

[17] Kumar, S., Payne, P., & Sotiras, A. (2024, May). Improving Normative Modeling for Multi-modal Neuroimaging Data using mixture-of-product-of-experts variational autoencoders. In 2024 IEEE International Symposium on Biomedical Imaging (ISBI) (pp. 1-5). IEEE.

[18] Lei, B., Guhaniyogi, R., Chandra, K., Scheffler, A., & Mallick, B. (2024). InVA: Integrative Variational Autoencoder for Harmonization of Multi-modal Neuroimaging Data. arXiv preprint arXiv:2402.02734.

[19] Yadalam, P. K., Ramadoss, R., Anegundi, R. V., kumar Yadalam, P., & Ramya, R. (2024). Variational Autoencoders for Generative Drug-Gene Interactions in Periodontal Bone Resorption. Cureus, 16(7).

[20] Showrov, A. A., Aziz, M. T., Nabil, H. R., Jim, J. R., Kabir, M. M., Mridha, M. F., ... & Shin, J. (2024). Generative Adversarial Networks (GANs) in Medical Imaging: Advancements, Applications and Challenges. IEEE Access.

[21] Kasula, B. Y. (2024). Ethical Implications and Future Prospects of Artificial Intelligence in Healthcare: A Research Synthesis. International Meridian Journal, 6(6), 1-7.

[22] Čartolovni, A., Tomičić, A., & Mosler, E. L. (2022). Ethical, legal, and social considerations of AI-based medical decision-support tools: A scoping review. International Journal of Medical Informatics, 161, 104738.

[23] Abràmoff, M. D., Tarver, M. E., Loyo-Berrios, N., Trujillo, S., Char, D., Obermeyer, Z., ... & Maisel, W. H. (2023). Considerations for addressing bias in artificial intelligence for health equity. NPJ digital medicine, 6(1), 170.

[24] Ueda, D., Kakinuma, T., Fujita, S., Kamagata, K., Fushimi, Y., Ito, R., ... & Naganawa, S. (2024). Fairness of artificial intelligence in healthcare: review and recommendations. Japanese Journal of Radiology, 42(1), 3-15.

[25] Mihan, A., Pandey, A., & Van Spall, H. G. (2024). Mitigating the risk of artificial intelligence bias in cardiovascular care. The Lancet Digital Health.

[26] Colwell, C. S. (2021). Defining circadian disruption in neurodegenerative disorders. The Journal of clinical investigation, 131(19).

2

Generative AI-enhanced Diagnostic Systems: Revolutionizing Early Disease Detection through Advanced Predictive Analytics

Wesam N. Eid[1], Fahd M. Aldosari[2], Amar Y. Jaffar[3], and Kanakaprabha S.[4]

[1]Department of Cybersecurity, College of Computing, Umm Al-Qura University, Saudi Arabia
[2]Department of Computer and Network Engineering College of Computing, Umm Al-Qura University, Saudi Arabia
[3]Department of Computer and Network Engineering, College of Computing, Umm Al-Qura University, Saudi Arabia
[4]Department of Artificial Intelligence and Machine Learning, Malla Reddy College of Engineering, India
E-mail: wneid@uqu.edu.sa; fmdosari@uqu.edu.sa; fmdosari@uqu.edu.sa; skanakaprabha@gmail.com

Abstract

AI-enabled diagnostic systems are identified by early disease detection by better efficiency, accuracy of disease identification, and betterment of life. The main objective of this chapter is identifying diseases early on, including cancer, cardiovascular issues, and COVID-19 techniques. The main AI algorithm is used for convolutional neural networks, generative adversarial networks, and recurrent neural networks. Another highlight is real-world applications of AI in clinical settings and early detection of COVID-19 through chest images. AI-enabled diagnostic system offers better healthcare by reducing human errors, preventive measures, and early sign of disease identification. The advancements of AI technology and its application of

DOI: 10.1201/9788743801764-2

results are improved medical conditions and enhanced treatments. The importance of AI in transforming early detection and tailored care is emphasized in this chapter.

Keywords: Artificial Intelligence, Cancer, Cardiovascular, Diagnostic, Deep Learning, Neurological Disorders.

2.1 Introduction

The traditional methods of illness detection and prevention have been completely transformed by the rapidly expanding artificial intelligence's use in the healthcare sector. This contributed to the creation of predictive models that offer early diagnosis as well as unique treatments. The design, development, and validation of an artificial intelligence predictive framework that uses machine learning algorithms to predict disease onset at an early stage are outlined in this research [1]. Advanced algorithms with a basis in deep learning analyze a variety of datasets, including genetic, imaging, and medical records data, to find small patterns. A proactive healthcare era has been created by deep learning, predictive analytics, natural language processing, anomaly detection, and personalized medicine. This has improved patient outcomes, decreased misdiagnosis, and resulted in more affordable therapies [2]. Retinal imaging is leading the way in early illness identification and surveillance by utilizing cutting-edge AI approaches to revolutionize healthcare. This method makes use of the unique vascular patterns seen in the retina to aid in the non-invasive detection of illnesses such as hypertensive retinopathy, diabetic retinopathy, retinal embolism, alterations related to anemia, and retinopathy associated with chronic kidney disease. Deep-learning-assisted retinal imaging is at the forefront of this change, a powerful force that is changing medical conditions [3]. The analysis uses data collection methods, such as feature extraction and data segmentation, along with Machine Learning algorithms to improve the precision of the model. In addition, regularization techniques such as dropout are utilized to address problems imposed on by a variety of information. The integration of information from routine activities to thoroughly evaluate their impact on heart health, with the ultimate goal of proactively warning signs about the risk of developing cardiovascular diseases. This study provides motivation for additional investigation and creativity in the field of cardiovascular disease detection, leading to developments that have the capacity to enhance public health and welfare [4]. A popular imaging method for identifying liver lesions and other abnormalities linked to HCV infection is computed tomography, or CT. However, radiologists may find it difficult to reliably diagnose HCV due to the complicated, time-consuming, and interobserver variability related to CT scan interpretation. The advancement of computer vision and artificial intelligence techniques has created new opportunities for medical image analysis. These chances include the creation of AI-based diagnostic tools that can help radiotherapists diagnose HCV more quickly and accurately and help interpret CT scans [5]. The majority of elderly people cannot access neurologists or Parkinson's disease specialists for early detection due to the complication of the signs and similarities to other neurological conditions. They connect AI technologies with smart mobile devices [6]. The primary goal of all of our activities is to create the most significant tools for detection and prediction that radiologists, physicians, and other caregivers can use to treat patients with this illness and save both time and funds. Deep learning (DL) algorithms have been recognized to be very suitable in recent years for diagnosing [7].

2.1.1 Background and motivation

Artificial intelligence has a major role in medical domains. Traditionally, any disease examination is essential for human beings, and manual analyses of disease symptoms and imaging of X-rays and CT scans are very effective in a manner that minimizes human error and time constraints. The early identification of disease detection significantly improves patient outcomes over time. The life-threatening diseases such as cancer, cardiovascular diseases to continue major challenges to global health, identifying early detection and effective intervention techniques. The other challenges are limited availability of medical services in remote areas, huge number of healthcare demands, and advanced technologies of artificial intelligence. During the previous years, artificial intelligence is more transformative in accurate diagnosis and effectiveness. The huge amounts of patient data allow AI to recognize the initial signs of disease symptoms that may not be easily identified by the human eye. Artificial intelligence is used in medical imaging techniques, such as electronic health records like EEG, ECG, EMG, PPG, GSR, etc. It has opened new avenues for the early diagnosis and other healthcare professionals to make informed decisions. AI is a vital tool in modern diagnostic systems.

The main motivation of this chapter is early detection, which is much more important in the quality of life. AI-enabled systems are offering a better solution by providing early and more accurate predictions of symptoms. It is very useful in genetic information and real-time monitoring systems.

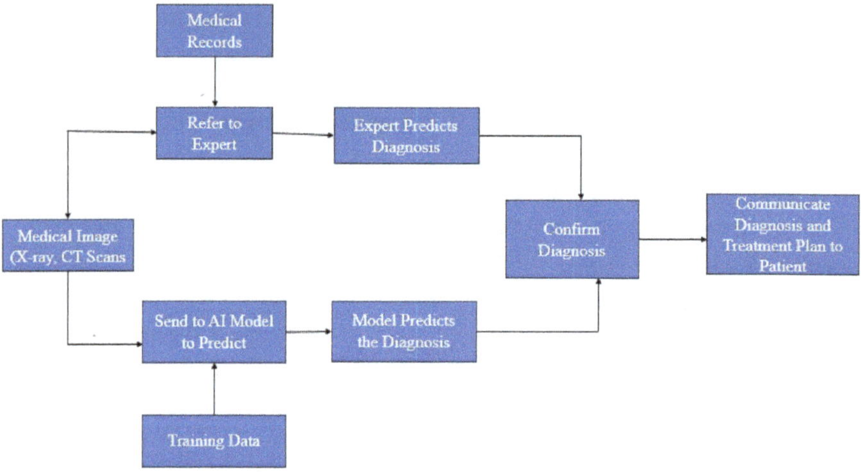

Figure 2.1 AI imaging (Source: Original).

AI-enabled diagnostic systems for early disease detection do not improve early disease identification while putting less strain on medical systems. This approach significantly reduces health risks, reduces cost of hospitalization, and saves lives. Figure 2.1 shows the AI imaging shows the medical imaging and the analysis of x-rays, CT scans and MRI data. And highlights how AI algorithms assist in early disease detection and accurate diagnosis.

2.1.2 Importance of early disease detection for improved healthcare outcomes

Reducing the morbidity associated with this condition requires early diagnosis and prevention. The present state of research on kidney stone illnesses, including early diagnosis and preventive methods that may lower their prevalence and related problems, is examined in this chapter. It examines current diagnostic techniques that are appropriate for early detection in addition to prospective preventative measures such as medication, nutritional supplements, lifestyle changes, and urologic surgeries [8]. This method uses medical imaging and deep learning to try to speed up diagnosis and therapy. With its impressive accuracy, the model shows promise for use as a screening tool for early detection of DR, which would enhance patient outcomes and decrease the burden on healthcare resources [9]. A global health concern, chronic kidney disease (CKD), affects millions of individuals globally and has significant negative effects on both health and the economy. It gives a thorough overview of CKD and highlights how urgent a worldwide health concern it is. Because of its high death rates, economic burden, and rising incidence, chronic kidney disease (CKD) is a hidden but serious public health concern. To lessen the effects of the disease, early CKD prediction and diagnosis are crucial. Early CKD detection facilitates prompt interventions, lowers complications, provides more treatment options, and maximizes the use of resources within healthcare systems. In addition, we examine typical kidney disease symptoms, emphasizing the significance of early detection and the intensity and variety of these symptoms [10]. The two neurodegenerative diseases that most commonly afflict Parkinson's disease (PD) and Alzheimer's disease (AD) are prevalent in the elderly person community. AD is a neurological condition that gradually impairs a person's capacity for daily activities, enjoyment of life, and cognitive and memory functions. PD is characterized by tremors, strength, and balance issues. The deep learning model VGG16 predicts AD with remarkable accuracy, highlighting the possibility of such techniques to support the timely detection and management of neurodegenerative diseases. With regard to PD identification, the CNN model performed more accurately. Further study is needed in the domain of deep learning approaches applied to neurodegenerative illness prediction, as early detection and care are critical to improved patient results and enhanced quality of life [11]. The results highlight how crucial cutting-edge computational methods are to transforming healthcare systems so that early identification, quick therapies, and better patient outcomes are possible. For deployment to be effective in clinical settings, it is necessary to take into consideration practical factors like processing efficiency and the viability of real-time deployment [12]. Machine learning is changing healthcare through early illness diagnosis and prediction. An ensemble machine learning system called random forest will forecast conditions like diabetes, heart disease, cancer, TB, arthritis, lung disease, stroke, asthma, brain tumor, osteoporosis, COPD, and oral diseases based on the symptoms of the patient [13]. The study's recommendations for additional research and clinical validation to improve and optimize the system for widespread clinical adoption have the potential to advance the discipline of cardiology, improve cardiac healthcare, and advance patient results [14].

2.1.3 The role of artificial intelligence (AI) in revolutionizing healthcare diagnostics

Artificial intelligence is changing healthcare diagnostics. It is improving the precision and effectiveness of the medical fields. Advanced algorithms such as deep learning and machine learning address these challenges of large amounts of medical data. Medical imaging techniques such as X-rays, CT Scans and MRIs are screened using modern tools capable of accurately identifying early symptoms of disease. These tools are capable of detecting the early signs of diseases. For instance, AI systems have demonstrated better performance in identifying tumors, cardiovascular disease, and cancer in diagnostic methods. AI-enabled disease detection may predict the patient outcomes and the disease, enabling the preventative treatment of advanced stage of disorders. AI enhances the automating routine tasks for data analysis and reduces the burden of healthcare cost. It also improves the patient data prescriptions. AI's role is improving the patient outcomes and better efficiency of the medical services.

2.2 Overview of AI Techniques in Diagnostics

Artificial intelligence methods, from deep learning to machine learning, are frequently used in healthcare to determine the risk of patients, find new drugs, and diagnose illnesses. To precisely detect diseases using artificial intelligence methods, a multitude of medical data causes are needed, including genomes, CT scans, ultrasound imaging, MRI scans, mammograms, etc. Artificial intelligence also mainly improved the hospital practice and expedited the process of getting patients ready to resume their rehabilitation at home. AI methods are used to identify a wide range of diseases, including Alzheimer's, diabetes, cancer, cardiac disease, tuberculosis, stroke, blood pressure, and dermatology. The feature extraction and classification procedure are utilized in the medical imaging dataset in order to make predictions [15]. Vital information found in point-of-care patient notes can be incorporated by an intelligent system with the patient's profile and medical history to identify patients who are at risk. Such a solution must be implemented smoothly and without interfering with the ED workflow. Upon reviewing the patient's chart, the subsequent ED provider will be notified of a "stroke alert" if the patient has a comparatively high risk of stroke [16]. Chronic diseases are considered serious illnesses as they pose significant risk of a person's life. For Individuals with physical limitations, these conditions may also hinder their freedom and overall well-being. People who experience a variety of health limitations are thus made even more frustrated by them. Since there are now no signs of chronic diseases, current medications and vaccinations cannot totally prevent them. Chronic illnesses are becoming a more prevalent occurrence as people age. For this reason, it is essential to pinpoint the contributing elements and implement the necessary corrective actions in response. Chronic diseases may be extensively influenced by variables like smoking, physical inactivity, nutrition, and excessive or insufficient alcohol usage [17].

2.2.1 Techniques used in early detection

Artificial intelligence has been used to identify medical images, resulting in accurate estimations being finalized automatically. This has better-quality routine in the forecast and detection of many sicknesses, reduced errors, timely intervention of the diagnosis, and reduced physician workload. Artificial intelligence based on medical image processing is an important field of study that uses complex computational algorithms for the analysis of treatment development, and prediction, which significantly affects the decision-making process. The two main subfields of cutting-edge AI used in the healthcare system to analyze sicknesses, find tablets, and determine risk features are machine learning and deep learning. The success of ML and DL algorithms has been corresponding in current years by the progress of big data technologies and digitalized records. Fuzzy logic algorithms and neural networks are two types of machine learning that have numerous uses in predicting and identifying disease detection. The DL algorithm is a machine learning methodology that does not depend on experienced feature extraction, like the traditional neural network methods. Medical image identifies the disease detection, prediction, and classification of the disease using deep

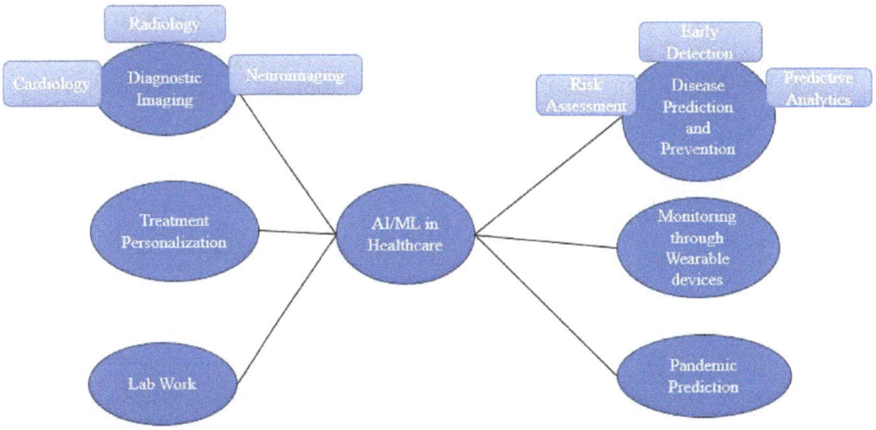

Figure 2.2 AI techniques used in early detection (Source: Original).

learning algorithms with better accuracy. The most popular methods for assessing and detecting diseases are usually support vector machine, an ML technique, and convolutional neural network, a DL method. AI methods perform more accurately than authorities in the judgment and prediction of widespread different types of diseases, such as cancer, heart, lung, skin, genetic, and neurological issues, without the possibility of human mistake. Figure 2.2 shows AI techniques such as machine learning, deep learning and neural networks is applied for early detection of diseases. It analyzes medical data to identify health issues at an early stage.

2.2.2 Highlight advancements in computational power and Big Data analytics facilitating AI's role in diagnostics

With AI's growing emphasis in radiology, several professionals speculate that AI might finally supplant radiologists. These concepts make one wonder if AI-based systems will ultimately take the place of doctors in sure specializations or if they will only improve their roles. To better appreciate new expertise and how it is changing treatment, this study aims to evaluate its effects on doctors [18]. Healthcare is one of the industries that artificial intelligence (AI) has transformed. AI has the ability to improve patient care and standard of living. However, healthcare systems remain difficult for all stakeholders. When AI is combined into clinical practice, its rapid innovations have the possible to alter healthcare [19]. The Big Data analytics provided AI systems with a large number of datasets, which are very important for machine learning models. The Big Data technologies enable the aggregation, organization, and analysis of these large datasets. It is allowed to detect the patterns and correlations of the previous methods. AI can deliver highly accurate the data-driven methods. These techniques in computational powers and Big Data analytics have been key to AI's growing in diagnostics.

2.3 Literature Review

The existing methods for diagnosing Parkinson's disease (PD) include costly, time-consuming procedures in addition to the expertise of medical specialists [20]. Artificial intelligence (AI)-powered deep learning (DL) models have produced state-of-the-art results and hold promise for enhancing Parkinson's disease (PD) diagnostic procedures by utilizing the early-stage symptom of vocal degeneration to facilitate early disease identification. However, because of the uninterpretable nature of the model and the chance that even a precise model will misinterpret the true causal relationship between the contribution sign and the forecast, the potential of DL for PD selection has not yet been realized.

Heart disease is a deadly illness that is spreading quickly throughout the world [21]. This illness, which is fatal in the end, affects both industrialized and developing nations. Heart disease occurs when the heart is incapable of pumping enough plasma to other parts of the body. Early diagnosis of this illness is crucial to shielding individuals from further harm. Errors in medical diagnostic systems can lead to inappropriate medical behaviors, which can kill a patient. AI can be used in a number of healthcare procedures to reduce the amount of time and money needed for patient examination and diagnosis. Machine learning has become a key to implement AI for the diagnosis of heart disease.

Patients who have a significant risk of developing cardiovascular diseases are frequently treated and classified in the same manner as those who have a much lesser risk, despite the fact that early diagnosis and treatment are critical [22]. Correct diagnosis necessitates years of expertise and further education because specific symptoms frequently make it difficult for doctors to distinguish some forms of cardiovascular diseases.

A dangerous and protracted illness, chronic kidney disease (CKD), is caused by either renal disease or abnormal kidney functions [23]. Due to its high mortality rate, kidney cancer must be diagnosed and classified correctly in order for patients to survive. Prompt intervention and appropriate treatment can slow down or stop this chronic illness from progressing to its later stages, when life-saving treatments such as dialysis or kidney transplantation become necessary. One of the most important research challenges at this time is creating automated instruments that can accurately detect chronic kidney disease.

Heart disease is a cardiovascular condition that is very common in developing nations, in part due to a lack of proper healthcare facilities to identify and record every case of acute rheumatic fever, the immune-mediated precursor to rheumatic heart disease, and treat Group A streptococcus pharyngitis [24]. Our goal is to systematize the process of identifying rheumatic heart disease with the use of machine learning, a growing technology in the analysis of therapeutic images.

The study introduces an intelligent disease detection technology that can act as a pre-screening portal for people suffering from diseases [25]. The major determination of the proposed model is to construct a highly effective system for diagnosing diseases based on symptoms, leveraging a rich dataset. The suggested system assesses user input symptoms and gives a disease classification as output. Disease identification is performed through the employment of three methods such as random forest classifier, decision tree, and Naïve Bayes classifier. The combined usage of these algorithms in the proposed model suggests higher precision in identifying diseases.

One of the most common brain dysfunctions in humans is Alzheimer's disease (AD), often known as dementia [26]. Until the illness's last stages are identified, there is currently no proven method for diagnosing AD. It has been demonstrated that multimodal biology, imaging, and other neuropsychological data that are currently available can provide a high percentage of differentiation between aged people with AD and those who are cognitively normal. Nonetheless, they are unable to fully accept or recognize that entities with mild cognitive damage (MCI) may ultimately develop Alzheimer's disease dementia.

While there is no cure for Parkinson's disease (PD), early detection and care can improve a patient's quality of life [27]. The application of machine learning for the categorization of Parkinson's disease utilizing biomedical audio data has gained prominence in recent years. In this study, we apply classification algorithms to characterize Parkinson's disease patients using a clinical, genetic, and audio dataset. The study emphasizes the probable application of algorithms for machine learning in recognizing and diagnosing the early stages of Parkinson's disease.

When combined with efficient image processing techniques, artificial intelligence (AI) helps physicians predict the course of illness more accurately [28]. One of the most challenging issues in medical imaging systems including AD categorization beyond AD detection is early analysis of Alzheimer's disease (AD). For the purpose of AD detection and stage categorization for magnetic resonance imaging images, neural networks are used. The implementation process starts with standard preprocessing methods like pixel leveling and image scaling. Next, the obtained features are rebuilt into a one-dimensional vector and sent to the CNN along with related tags.

The study underlines the issues faced by persons with hectic schedules, who typically spend considerable time waiting for doctor appointments, particularly for diseases that require ongoing care, such as heart disease [29]. Heart disease remains a prominent global health issue, causing multiple fatalities every day. The future of healthcare data relies on remote data gathering, precise distance diagnoses, and AI-driven data analysis, all of which can greatly boost both healthcare productivity and results. The suggested chatbot system intends to allow users by facilitating regular health check-ups, improving health consciousness, and encouraging hands-on well-being interventions.

A degenerative neurological condition that affects millions of people worldwide, Alzheimer's disease (AD) is characterized by memory loss and mental damage [30]. Since early detection can stop the progression of a disease and improve quality of life, it is essential for active treatment. Using a variety of medical modalities, machine learning has demonstrated promise in AD detection. In this work, we present a novel multi-level stacking model that forecasts various forms of AD by integrating diverse models and modalities. Among the modalities are cognitive sub-scores from the Alzheimer's Disease Neuroimaging Initiative dataset (e.g., clinical dementia rating total of boxes, Alzheimer's disease evaluation scale).

Normal kidney function is rendered impossible by chronic renal disease [31]. As one of the top 20 causes of death, the WHO has demonstrated that CKD is a serious illness. Renal failure affects 2 million people globally, and the number of affected role with a CDK diagnosis is growing at a proportion of 5%–7% every year. Due to the high expense of diagnosis and the scarcity of specialist medical workers in remote places, late detection of this disease poses a life-threatening risk.

Artificial intelligence (AI) holds the potential to completely transform the diagnosis of gastrointestinal diseases [32]. Deep learning methods are used in this work to thoroughly examine endoscopic image classification for gastrointestinal disorders. Having precise diagnostic tools is essential for treating gastrointestinal illnesses, which are a major global health concern. Detecting gastrointestinal disorders more accurately through improved clinical decision support is the main objective. Through a thorough study utilizing the KVASIR Dataset, which contains 4000 distinct types of intestinal pictures, the chapter shows how effective these models are at accurately classifying gastrointestinal disorders.

Skin cancer is thought to be one of the most dangerous and prevalent kinds worldwide [33]. The number of newly reported instances of skin cancer worldwide is concerning; it is estimated to be over 10 million annually. In the later stages of diagnosis, the survival percentage is quite low. Artificial intelligence can be very helpful in using medical image diagnosis to diagnose this sickness in its early stages. Artificial intelligence systems for the classification of different skin lesions are still in their very early stages of medical usage, with respect to their readiness to enable the detection of skin cancer. Furthermore, not many researchers are working on conditions unique to the Indian subcontinent in this direction.

2.4 AI Algorithms and Techniques for Early Detection

AI algorithms have a major role in early disease identification of disorders. The two main approaches for this algorithm are machine learning and deep learning. Machine learning algorithms are mostly used to analyze the structured data such as patient details and lab reports. Deep learning algorithms are used to process the unstructured data such as medical imaging, time series of data from wearable devices, speech recognition, etc.

Another powerful technique for AI algorithms such as natural language processing is extracting the text information from the electronic health records and prescription notes and also helping the risk assessments of predicting the illness. Furthermore, AI algorithms are being developed to predict the likelihood of various conditions including diabetes, heart disease and cancer. Combining various AI algorithms as an advanced tools for healthcare expertise to enable early disease detection and improve patient outcomes thorough more precise diagnosis.

2.4.1 Deep learning and neural networks

With the increasing number of digital technologies, identifying distributed denial of service (DDoS) attacks is fetching a progressively difficult challenge because of the computational complexity involved. DDoS attacks can actually be identified by classifying regular and irregular network traffic flow. For

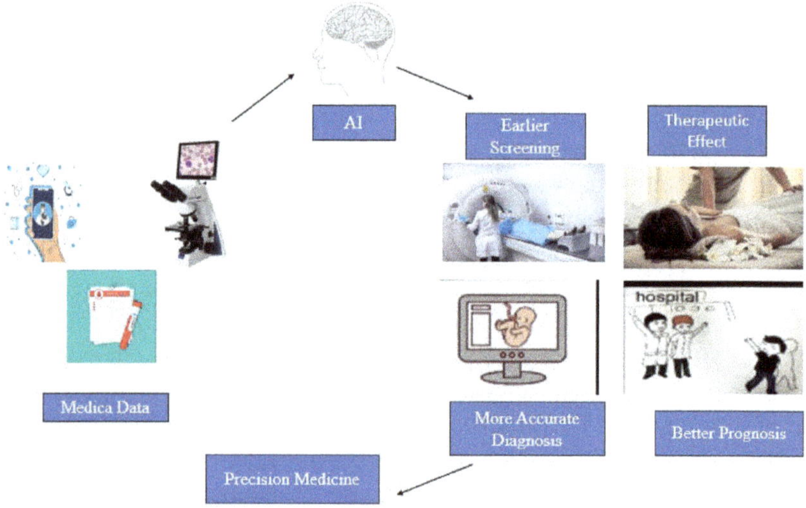

Figure 2.3 AI algorithms and techniques for early detection (Source: Original).

deep-learning-models-based early DDoS attack detection, this study suggests a hybrid neural network manner. Then, for the purpose of classifying the spatial and temporal structures of traffic flows, two deep learning models, the lightweight usable deep learning model of neural network (NN) properties and the gradient boosting decision tree (GBDT) corresponding to ensemble learning method, are employed [34]. Figure 2.3 highlights their application in analyzing the medical images and patient data for timely diagnosis. The study focuses on improving and fine-tuning the deep learning model VGG-16. The model's performance has a greatly better quality by applying a variety of optimization strategies, including early callback, transfer learning, Gaussian blur, and SMOTE (Synthetic Minority Over-sampling Technique). By addressing problems such as overfitting and class imbalance, these methods enhance the VGG-16 model's overall resilience. Early-stage lung cancer diagnosis has consequences for healthcare institutions as well, since it may allow for quick involvements and better patient outcomes [35]. Deep learning approaches are almost exclusively utilized in computer vision, image processing, neural language processing, and medical diagnosis for high task objectives. Additionally, we contrast the deep learning algorithm with other machine learning algorithms, and we find that our suggested system outperforms them all [36]. Studies on deep learning's potential to enhance medical diagnostics are essential. Artificial neural networks and deep learning are two classification techniques that can be applied. Deep learning has the possibility to aid in the primary detection of cancer, and it also offers advantages over SVM in this regard. In the end, a comparison has been made between the predicted accuracy obtained through the use of SVM and ANN and the deep learning method previously discussed [37].

2.4.2 Techniques like convolutional neural networks (CNNs), recurrent neural networks (RNNs), and generative adversarial networks (GANs) in diagnostics

The techniques like convolutional neural networks (CNNs), recurrent neural networks (RNNs), and generative adversarial networks (GANs) in diagnostics are improved accuracy and effective evaluation of medical information. Each AI technique is designed to address various medical conditions and assist in accurately identifying various illnesses.

2.4.2.1 Convolutional neural networks (CNNs)

CNNs plays a major role in medical image analysis and are widely used in disease diagnosis through techniques such as X-rays, CT scans, and other medical imaging methods. These models can be extracting the features from the images, identifying the subtle patterns and the anomalies such as tumors, cardiovascular diseases, etc. Because CNNs analyze imaging data quickly and accurately, they have demonstrated effectiveness in the early detection of disorders such as cancer, diabetes, tumors, etc. Image-based diagnostic system often outperforms human radiologists due to their ability to detect and the smallest differences in image pixels and analyze large volumes of data with high precision.

2.4.2.2 Recurrent neural networks (RNNs)

RNNs are mostly used in sequential or time series data, which is very helpful in the analysis of monitoring data from patients such as blood pressure, heartbeat, pulse rate, glucose levels, etc. It is widely used in diagnostics to analyze the continuous data from wearable technology in the real-time patient monitoring systems. Long short-term memory (LSTM) networks are used in the early detection of disorders such as rrhythmias, epilepsy, or sleep disorders, identifying the accurate predictions and timely intervention.

2.4.2.3 Generative adversarial networks (GANs)

GANs are being utilized in diagnostics to produce the artificial medical data that replicates the actual patient data. Training AI models for rare disease t can be challenging due to the limited availability of real-world data. Medical imaging provides detailed representations of interior organs which can be used to enhance the quality and diversity of datasets for AI model training. GANs also enhance the clarity of low-resolution images, enabling more accurate disease detection from otherwise poor-quality medical images. Furthermore, GANs can support personalized medicine by modeling individual patient characteristics, which can help predict treatment outcomes and optimize therapeutic strategies. These advanced methods such as CNNS, RNNs, and GANs are used for image analysis, time series, and data augmentation of medical data from healthcare diagnostics. The AI methods are making more improvement in diagnostic accuracy and early identification of disease and are providing predictive information.

2.4.3 Application of these techniques in analyzing medical data

The present state of AI-based technologies and their impact on the healthcare sector. Apart from an in-depth research evaluation, this study recognizes different types of real-time examples of artificial intelligence applications in the healthcare industry. Hospitals are now using AI-enabled devices to support medical personnel in diagnosing a variety of disorders in their patients. Furthermore, artificial intelligence is helpful for the hospitals to perform more effectively in medical professions. To fully take advantage from AI, care amenities and processes will need to be transformed through planned execution [38].

2.4.3.1 Machine learning approaches

Machine learning approaches form the basics of AI in healthcare by learning platforms from data to make accurate predictions about various disorders. In medical illness, these algorithms can identify the different forms of medical data, structured data like patient records, prescriptions, etc. Unstructured data such as medical imaging from X-rays, CT scans, MRI play a major role in early disease diagnosis. The various of machine learning techniques such as supervised, unsupervised, and reinforcement learning are used to analyze these data for accurate prediction and detection.

2.4.3.2 Supervised learning

It is one of the mostly used ML algorithms for various diagnostic methods. This model is trained on the large labeled data to predict the particular outcome. Algorithms such as support vector machines (SVMs), random forest, decision trees, and neural networks are widely used in healthcare for the various tasks like disease classification, prediction and diagnosis based on the patient data. In medical treatment, supervised learning models are used to categorize diseases, detect the patient risk, and predict how their disease will progress.

2.4.3.3 Unsupervised learning

Unsupervised learning involves training models on unlabeled data. The algorithm identifies the patterns and relationships from the data. Clustering techniques such as K-means and hierarchical clustering identify a similar group of the patient data profiles. Then they identify the patterns of symptoms of the disease accurately. In medical illness, unsupervised learning is mainly used for the large detection of rare diseases or difficulties.

2.4.3.4 Reinforcement learning

Reinforcement learning (RL) is one of the best practices of trial and error and feedback is received in the form of incentives or penalties. It is becoming more and more popular in the healthcare industry. Reinforcement learning is applied to customize treatment plans for making the changes and quick response to the patient feedback and results. These models primarily used in healthcare planning systems to suggest drug requirements, recommend diagnostic tests and assist in creating treatments plans, all based on the patient's health status.

2.5 AI for Disease Prevention and Monitoring

An effective method for recognizing, following, and predicting the spread of diseases is artificial-intelligence-based epidemiological surveillance, which uses AI technologies to examine information from a variety of foundations, including news articles, social media, and electronic health records. AI can forecast future epidemics; it provides a major advantage over outdated disease investigation methods, enabling public health officials to take proactive and preventive steps early on. "Arogya Setu" was created by the Indian government in partnership with public and private entities, such as the National Informatics Centre (NIC) below the Ministry of Integrated circuit technology, to provide persons with self-assessment and real-time contact tracing information. This service helps keep people informed during disasters like the COVID-19 pandemic [39]. Additionally, these technologies have changed how people and communities interact in a variety of contexts and activities relevant to health. Increases in oncologic, metabolic, and cardiovascular disorders have been brought on by these alterations. As the primary cause of avoidable fatalities, diseases are considered to be a serious danger to public health. The ever-evolving Information and Communication Technologies (ICT) are being used by physicians to monitor, predict, and treat these socially crucial diseases. There are, however, comparatively fewer research works on how patients view and accept the role that digital technologies play in disease diagnosis, prevention, treatment, and monitoring. The analytical capabilities of AI can be used to forecast disease onset and offer reliable guidance, policy recommendations, and initiatives for disease prevention and patient monitoring [40]. AI is a powerful tool for preventive measures in healthcare, early identification of potential health risks, and promoting management. AI-enabled systems can analyze large datasets to predict the illnesses, and determine the optimal timing for medical interventions at the onset of disease. The wearable devices and Internet of Things is enhancing real-time monitoring of patients' signs and health insights. These advanced technologies easily detect early signs of various long-term ailments such as blood pressure, diabetes, and cancer and make it possible for preventative interventions. These

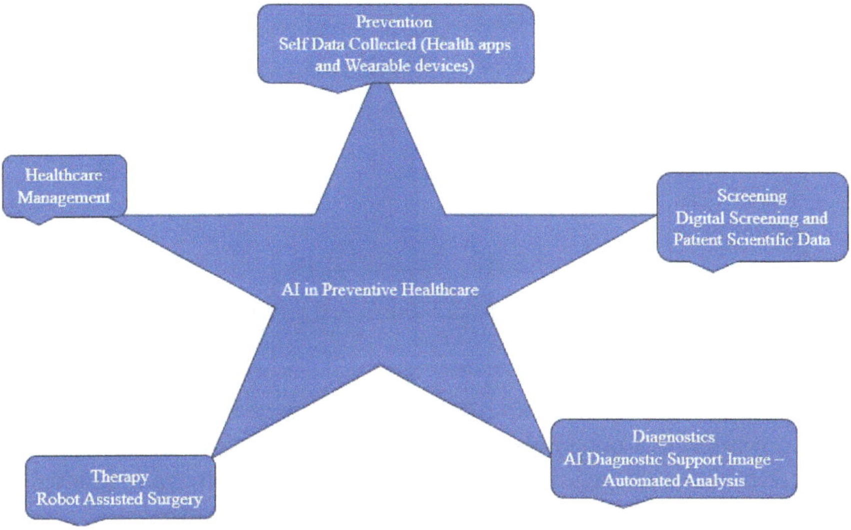

Figure 2.4 AI in preventive healthcare (Source: Original).

methods can be largely enhancing better patient outcomes and healthcare expenditures [41].

2.5.1 AI in preventive healthcare

AI in preventive healthcare represents an innovative strategy for regulating and improving health outcomes. AI systems can predict the disease before symptoms appear, and ensure early detection and personalized treatment plans. Data analytics and algorithms may be used in this approach. AI-powered devices have the ability to analyze patient data, genetic data, lifestyle factors, and other medical history. AI-powered devices have the ability to analyze patient data, genetic information, lifestyle factors, and medical history to assist in early diagnosis, continuous health monitoring, and treatment planning. AI-powered wearable technology combined with (IoT) device, enables real-time detection of anomalies and provides early warnings of potential health risks.

Figure 2.4 shows the AI in preventive healthcare in real time monitoring, predictive analytical and personalized alerts. It emphasizes early intervention and improved patient outcomes. This approach involves the use of algorithms and data analytics. AI-driven technologies can analyze patient data, genetic information, lifestyle factors, and medical history to support clinical decision-making and improve healthcare outcomes. AI-powered wearable technology

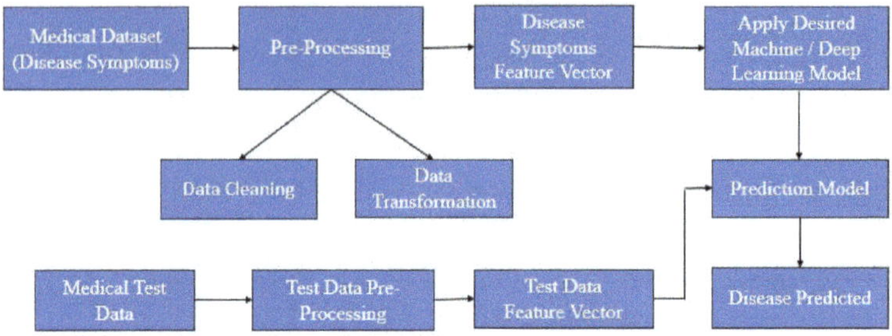

Figure 2.5 AI-enabled systems can help predict disease and preventive measures (Source: Original).

combined with IoT devices, enables real-time detection of anomalies and provides early warnings of potential health risks. The preventive strategy helps to minimize treatment delays slow disease progression, improves individual health management and reduces the strain on healthcare systems.

2.5.2 How AI-enabled systems can help predict disease onset and provide preventive measures

Artificial intelligence is one of the most promising and highly effective scientific tools for the human race and disposal. AI is beginning to emerge in healthcare and is rapidly gaining popularity across various industries and society at large. AI has the potential to transform various aspects of healthcare, including medical regulations. One of primary goal is to explore how machine learning can be applied to the management of infectious disease and to improve the overall efficiency of the healthcare system.

AI is capable of predicting many diseases like blood pressure, diabetes, and heart diseases by examining the patterns of blood test results and other indications. Figure 2.5 shows how AI-enabled systems analyze patient data to predict potential diseases. And also highlight the use of AI in timely preventive measures. Because of these methods of early identification, medical professionals can be implementing preventative remedies for the patient's risk such as medication, lifestyle, and individual risk for patients.

2.5.3 Role of wearable devices and IoT in continuous monitoring and data collection for early detection

While there are many benefits to Internet of Things-enabled personal health monitoring devices, there are also a number of disadvantages that should be carefully examined. A thorough analysis of IoT technologies' impact on health wearables can help make the devices more accurate, useful, and interesting for consumers. Internet of Things health wearables, which also identifies new trends and technologies, impact user experiences and health outcomes. The study also considers the challenges of data security, privacy, and interoperability between IoT devices and current healthcare systems [42]. Wearable technology is one example of how current technology is used in healthcare applications. It suggests a calming system that uses various techniques to monitor and soothe PTSD patients. Using a wearable device, the system detects the symptoms of PTSD and then uses various actions (auditory treatment, video, aromatherapy, and light patterns) to distract the patient while they are awake in order to prevent PTSD episodes [43]. A wearable device called Intelligent Asthma Monitoring is able to predict the impending asthma attack well in advance of the wearer's awareness. Despite not being created with this purpose in mind, Apple watches have become a vital tool for collecting data on people, thanks to their ability to measure blood oxygen levels, track electrocardiograms (ECGs), and identify irregular heartbeats [44].

2.6 Real-world Applications and Case Studies

AI is transforming medical care by demonstrating its potential benefits in early disease detection and diagnosis. In many hospitals and other clinical centers, AI is used to analyze large volume of medical data to recommend personalized treatment plans. Nowadays, AI is mostly used in radiology, which can be used to easily identify medical images like CT scans, X-rays, RI scans, and ultrasound scans for early detection of diseases like cancer, tumor, etc. In the COVID-19 pandemic, the study of chest X-ray imageries enabled faster clinical responses. In a variety of healthcare scenarios, AI has proven to be more effective in improving patient outcome and providing accurate diagnosis.

2.6.1 AI systems in clinical use

AI is becoming an integral part of the clinical development and betterment of healthcare professionals in enhancing all the capabilities and individualized treatments methods. IBM Watson for Oncology is a prime example; it analyzes the meaning and context of both labeled and unlabeled data found in medical proceedings and reports. By combining all of these attributes into

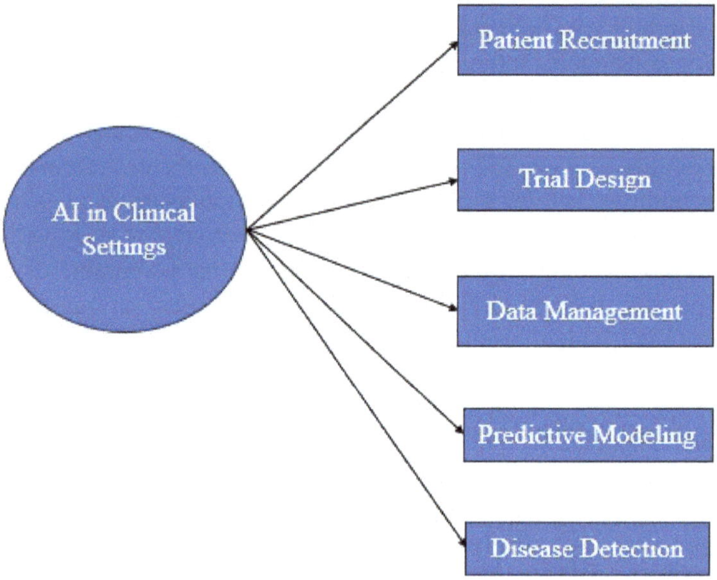

Figure 2.6 AI in clinical settings (Source: Original).

the patient's file clinical professionals can gain a comprehensive view of the patient's health, enabling more accurate diagnoses and treatment plans. IBM Watson for Oncology is easily identifying the rank and potential treatment plans. The main highlights of IBM Watson for Oncology are providing more medical options to help oncology clinicians make informed decisions. It supports first line medical oncology treatments in breast cancer, lung cancer, and rectal cancers. Whereas the second line medical oncology cancer is lung colon and other cancers.

Furthermore, AI algorithms are utilized for automated data analysis for lab results and other streaming processes like blood sample evaluation. The AI systems are not only improving the diagnostic detection but also reducing the human error, saving time interventions, and improving clinical settings' patient care.

2.6.2 AI in COVID-19 detection

The COVID-19 epidemic has had a thoughtful negative influence on individuals' health and economies everywhere. Several researchers have presented several methods for diagnosing COVID-19. These methods often rely on molecular testing to identify viral genetic material, CT scans to look at a

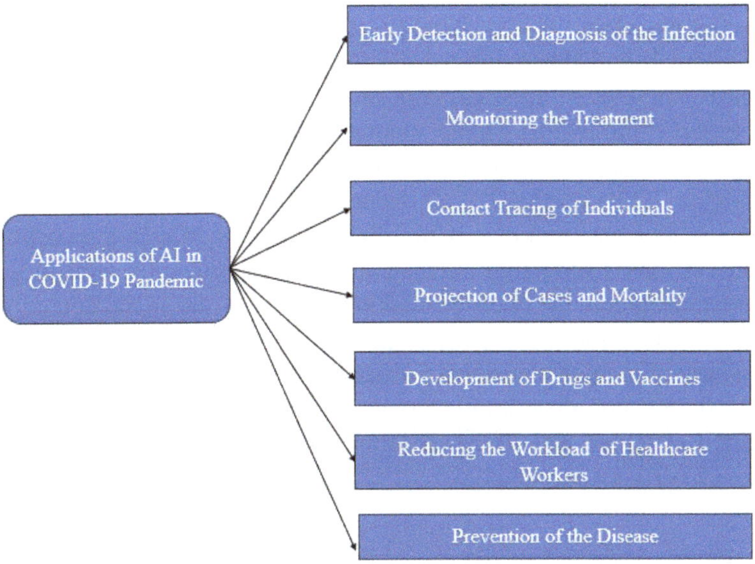

Figure 2.7 AI in COVID-19 pandemic (Source: Original).

person's lungs, and antibody tests for the proteins the body makes in reaction to an earlier infection. However, in the event of a pandemic, RT-PCR kits and other testing instruments may become scarce. Thus, having a variety of testing choices is essential. Figure 2.6 shows the AI in clinical environments, diagnosis treatment planning and decision-making. Furthermore, a large number of low-income nations are unable to afford the cost of testing a larger proportion of their population due to the high cost of the RT-PCR testing technique. The study examined existing and new diagnostic techniques, such as AI-based approaches, fast antigen detection, and RT-PCR. This study additionally examined various fields, such as forecasting, treatment, tracking and dashboarding, and surveillance, where artificial intelligence has been used to stop the spread of COVID-19. In addition to clinical analysis, it is important to point out that many approaches are desired to successfully control and prevent the spread of COVID-19 [45].

The application of artificial intelligence (AI) technology in pandemic management and response presents enormous promise. The study highlights the immense potential of artificial intelligence technology in tackling the worldwide issues made up by the COVID-19 pandemic. First, the various ways that the existing epidemic is affecting society, the economy, and public health. Following that, our attention shifts to the creative uses of cutting-edge AI technologies in critical domains including COVID-19 diagnosis, prediction, control, and therapeutic drug discovery. To be more accurate, omics, clinical, and epidemiological data can be incorporated into AI-based predictive analytic models to predict patient outcomes and the spread of illness. Deep neural networks also make it possible for quick medical imaging diagnosis. Figure 2.7 shows the COVID-19 pandemic for outbreak prediction, rapid diagnosis, contact tracking. It highlights the AI's role in supporting public health responses and patient management. The application of artificial intelligent systems risk in the decision-making situations and social detection of the disease can be more effective in public health policy and epidemic control. Because of its high-throughput virtual screening capabilities, AI can also identify therapeutic drug applicants and chances for drug repurposing more rapidly. Lastly, we discuss future directions for AI technology in the fight against COVID-19 and emphasize the importance of all the fields [46].

2.7 Results and Discussion

In the medical fields, the use of AI for early detection has produced accurate results. The AI-enabled systems have to be very efficient in the diagnosis of all diseases like cancer, tumor, other chronic diseases, and also COVID-19 detection from medical images. The deep learning techniques like convolutional neural network and recurrent neural network have shown higher accuracy from the medical images.

Figure 2.8 illustrates of all the three kinds of diagnoses in the chest X-ray images. We can clearly see that the black diaphragm is in normal chest images, and the middle is indicating that the right lobe is fully affected by the COVID-19 virus, and the upper lobe of the diaphragm with less air indicates a pneumonia-affected chest.

Figure 2.9 shows the images of pneumonia and COVID-19-affected lungs. The greatest percentage of infection is displayed. For example, Figure 2.9(a) depicts the lungs impacted by 91.53% of COVID-19, which is evident in both the upper and lower lobes. The lungs in Figure 2.9(b) are 100% infected with COVID-19. The COVID-19-infected lung's top lobe is totally invisible. The lower lobe of the right-side of the lung in Figure 2.9(c) displays an air bronchogram and a lung image with a 52.25% pneumonia infection. Similarly, Figure 2.9(d) illustrates 62.30% of pneumonia infection in the lung's middle lobe.

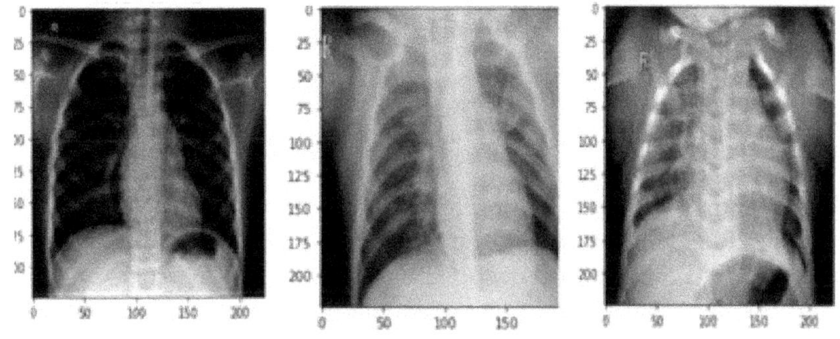

Figure 2.8 Normal, COVID-19, and pneumonia images.

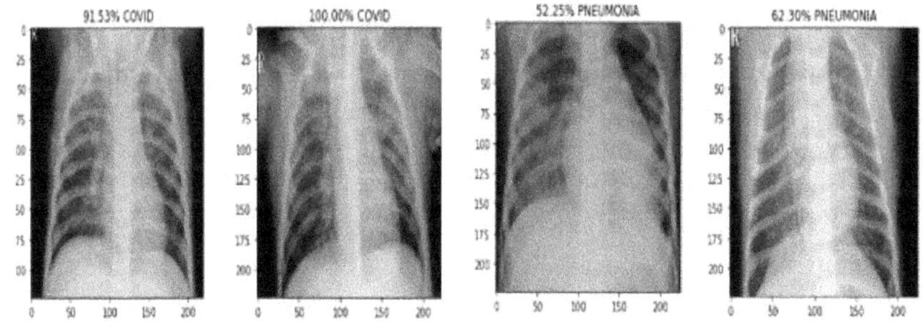

(a) (b) (c) (d)

Figure 2.9 Classification of COVID-19 and pneumonia infection.

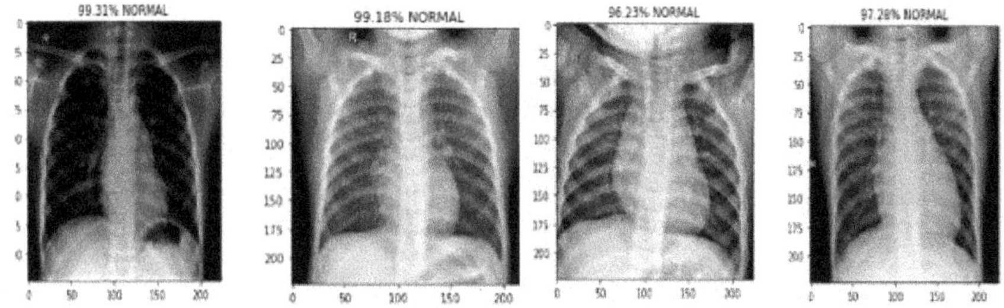

(a) (b) (c) (d)

Figure 2.10 Classification of Normal Images.

Figure 2.10 (a)–(d) displays X-rays of normal lung tissue. Both the left and right lungs have extremely clear pictures. The base of the lungs appears normal on the image. Lung scans with black color show less dense material, whereas the white color shows more thick material. The lungs in the white appear very rigid and have less air content, while the lungs in the black appear spongy and have more air.

2.8 Conclusion

AI-enabled diagnostic systems are developed into novel technologies in the field of early disease identification. It is greatly improved by the medical care. The two main AI techniques are deep learning and neural networks. It is significantly improved by COVID-19 detection, cancer, and other chronic disorders. These methods are identified by real-time monitoring systems like wearable technology and Internet of Things (IoT). AI can identify the early signs of diseases even before symptoms become apparent enable to timely measures. Many of the real time applications demonstrate the benefit of AI in clinical settings. One of the most well-known example is IBM Watson for Oncology, which provides treatment recommendations and supports radiology imaging analysis to improve diagnostic accuracy. AI has shown the potential to manage global health crises throughout the COVID-19 pandemic. It is also aiding in early detection and diagnosis of the disease. AI-powered diagnostic methods have to revolutionize healthcare by enhancing the disease detection and prevention. A better diagnostic is expected from ongoing development of AI techniques and real-world applications. It will improve patient outcomes and delivery of the healthcare.

Acknowledgments

I would like to express my deepest gratitude to my dad Ramanpillai C., and my mom Selvakumari R. for their continuous support and encouragement throughout my chapter. This chapter is dedicated to them with immense respect and affection

References

[1] G. K. Thakur, N. Khan, H. Anush and A. Thakur, "AI-Driven Predictive Models for Early Disease Detection and Prevention," 2024 International Conference on Knowledge Engineering and Communication Systems (ICKECS), Chikkaballapur, India, 2024, pp. 1–6, doi:10.1109/ICKECS61492.2024.10616851.

[2] K. P. Reddy, M. Satish, A. Prakash, S. M. Babu, P. P. Kumar and B. S. Devi, "Machine Learning Revolution in Early Disease Detection for Healthcare: Advancements, Challenges, and Future Prospects," 2023 IEEE 5th International Conference on Cybernetics, Cognition and Machine Learning Applications (ICCCMLA), Hamburg, Germany, 2023, pp. 638–643, doi:10.1109/ICCCMLA58983.2023.10346963.

[3] H. Z. Wala, T. P. Nevagi and S. G. Jagtap, "Revolutionizing Healthcare: Early Disease Detection through Retinal Imaging and AI-Driven Approaches," 2023 6th International Conference on Advances in Science and Technology (ICAST), Mumbai, India, 2023, pp. 23–28, doi: 10.1109/ICAST59062.2023.10455046.

[4] M. Baikuvekov, A. Tursynova and G. Yespayev, "A Deep Learning for Cardiovascular Diseases Detection on Wearable Devices Data," 2024 IEEE 4th International Conference on Smart Information Systems and Technologies (SIST), Astana, Kazakhstan, 2024, pp. 272–277, doi:10.1109/SIST61555.2024.10629525.

[5] S. Vijayakumar, "A Hybrid QNN-Based Framework for Accurate Early Detection of HCV Liver Abnormalities from CT Scans Using Custom Transfer Learning and AI Edge Device," 2023 IEEE Region 10 Symposium (TENSYMP), Canberra, Australia, 2023, pp. 1–5, doi: 10.1109/TENSYMP55890.2023.10223624.

[6] J. Li, R. Wu, T. -L. Huang, Z. Pan and M. -C. Huang, "Shoupa: An AI System for Early Diagnosis of Parkinson's Disease," 2022 IEEE/ACM Conference on Connected Health: Applications, Systems and Engineering Technologies (CHASE), Arlington, VA, USA, 2022, pp. 178–179.

[7] A. W. Salehi, P. Baglat, B. B. Sharma, G. Gupta and A. Upadhya, "A CNN Model: Earlier Diagnosis and Classification of Alzheimer Disease using MRI," 2020 International Conference on Smart Electronics and Communication (ICOSEC), Trichy, India, 2020, pp. 156–161, doi:10.1109/ICOSEC49089.2020.9215402.

[8] I. Shakhnoza, N. Rano, A. Asalya and A. Amalya, "Early Diagnosis and Preventive Measures of Kidney Stone Diseases Among the Population," 2023 International Conference on Sustainable Emerging Innovations in Engineering and Technology (ICSEIET), Ghaziabad, India, 2023, pp. 581–583, doi:10.1109/ICSEIET58677.2023.10303334.

[9] B. N, P. M. Bangi, P. K R, R. M U and L. J, "Retina Vigil: Deep Learning-Enabled Retinopathy Detection for Early Disease

Assessment," 2023 IEEE 3rd Mysore Sub Section International Conference (MysuruCon), HASSAN, India, 2023, pp. 1–6, doi:10.1109/MysuruCon59703.2023.10396854.
[10] M. S. Jayaprabha and V. Vishwa Priya, "Early Prediction of Chronic Kidney Disease: A Comprehensive Survey," 2024 5th International Conference on Mobile Computing and Sustainable Informatics (ICMCSI), Lalitpur, Nepal, 2024, pp. 45–51, doi:10.1109/ICMCSI61536.2024.00013.
[11] K. A. Shastry, N. Janyani, G. G, K. U and L. Patil, "Advanced Deep Learning Techniques for Predicting Neurodegenerative Diseases," 2023 International Conference on Network, Multimedia and Information Technology (NMITCON), Bengaluru, India, 2023, pp. 1–8, doi:10.1109/NMITCON58196.2023.10276017.
[12] R. A. Kesava, G. Thangarasu and K. N. Kannan, "Revolutionalizing Lung Disease Prediction using Artificial Intelligence," 2024 IEEE 14th Symposium on Computer Applications & Industrial Electronics (ISCAIE), Penang, Malaysia, 2024, pp. 165–169, doi:10.1109/ISCAIE61308.2024.10576578.
[13] M. K. Raj, J. P. Malardhas and I. Devapriya, "Machine Learning Approach To Predict Multiple Diseases Based On Symptoms," 2024 10th International Conference on Communication and Signal Processing (ICCSP), Melmaruvathur, India, 2024, pp. 1195–1199, doi: 10.1109/ICCSP60870.2024.10543802.
[14] M. Baikuvekov, A. Baikuvekova and D. Sultan, "Development of a Digital Stethoscopy System for Detection of Heart Diseases," 2024 IEEE 4th International Conference on Smart Information Systems and Technologies (SIST), Astana, Kazakhstan, 2024, pp. 256–260, doi:10.1109/SIST61555.2024.10629628.
[15] Kumar Y, Koul A, Singla R, Ijaz MF. Artificial intelligence in disease diagnosis: a systematic literature review, synthesizing framework and future research agenda. J Ambient Intell Humaniz Comput. 2023;14(7):8459-8486. doi:10.1007/s12652-021-03612-z. Epub 2022 Jan 13. PMID: 35039756; PMCID: PMC8754556.
[16] Abedi V, Khan A, Chaudhary D, Misra D, Avula V, Mathrawala D, Kraus C, Marshall KA, Chaudhary N, Li X, Schirmer CM, Scalzo F, Li J, Zand R. Using artificial intelligence for improving stroke diagnosis in emergency departments: a practical framework. Ther Adv Neurol Disord. 2020 Aug 25;13:1756286420938962. doi:10.1177/1756286420938962. PMID: 32922515; PMCID: PMC7453441.

[17] Aldhyani THH, Alshebami AS, Alzahrani MY. Soft Clustering for Enhancing the Diagnosis of Chronic Diseases over Machine Learning Algorithms. J Healthc Eng. 2020 Mar 9;2020:4984967. doi:10.1155/2020/4984967. PMID: 32211144; PMCID: PMC7085388.

[18] Ahuja AS. The impact of artificial intelligence in medicine on the future role of the physician. PeerJ. 2019 Oct 4;7:e7702. doi:10.7717/peerj.7702. PMID: 31592346; PMCID: PMC6779111.

[19] Alowais SA, Alghamdi SS, Alsuhebany N, Alqahtani T, Alshaya AI, Almohareb SN, Aldairem A, Alrashed M, Bin Saleh K, Badreldin HA, Al Yami MS, Al Harbi S, Albekairy AM. Revolutionizing healthcare: the role of artificial intelligence in clinical practice. BMC Med Educ. 2023 Sep 22;23(1):689. doi:10.1186/s12909-023-04698-z. PMID: 37740191; PMCID: PMC10517477.

[20] R. Shah, B. Dave, N. Parekh and K. Srivastava, "Parkinson's Disease Detection - An Interpretable Approach to Temporal Audio Classification," 2022 IEEE 3rd Global Conference for Advancement in Technology (GCAT), Bangalore, India, 2022, pp. 1–6, doi:10.1109/GCAT55367.2022.9971881.

[21] W. Shishah, "An Efficient Early Stage Heart Disease Risk Detection Using Machine Learning Techniques," 2022 Second International Conference on Power, Control and Computing Technologies (ICPC2T), Raipur, India, 2022, pp. 1–6, doi:10.1109/ICPC2T53885.2022.9777070.

[22] D. Mušić, M. Karajić, L. Hećo and E. Osmanović, "Model for diagnosing cardiovascular diseases using AI," 2024 International Congress on Human-Computer Interaction, Optimization and Robotic Applications (HORA), Istanbul, Turkiye, 2024, pp. 1–4, doi:10.1109/HORA61326.2024.10550532.

[23] M. S. Abirami, S. Das and R. Sood, "Chronic Kidney Disease Identification Using Random Forest and XGBoost," 2024 International Conference on Intelligent Systems for Cybersecurity (ISCS), Gurugram, India, 2024, pp. 1–6, doi: 10.1109/ISCS61804.2024.10581392.

[24] L. Mugambi, L. Z̀UHLKE and C. W. Maina, "Towards AI Based Diagnosis of Rheumatic Heart Disease: Data Annotation and View Classification," 2022 IST-Africa Conference (IST-Africa), Ireland, 2022, pp. 1–8, doi:10.23919/IST-Africa56635.2022.9845657.

[25] S. V, V. M, S. M and I. Pani, "Revolutionizing Healthcare: Screening system to identify Diseases using Machine learning approach," 2024 International Conference on Intelligent and Innovative Technologies

in Computing, Electrical and Electronics (IITCEE), Bangalore, India, 2024, pp. 1–5, doi:10.1109/IITCEE59897.2024.10467594.

[26] H. A. Shad et al., "Exploring Alzheimer's Disease Prediction with XAI in various Neural Network Models," TENCON 2021 - 2021 IEEE Region 10 Conference (TENCON), Auckland, New Zealand, 2021, pp. 720–725, doi:10.1109/TENCON54134.2021.9707468.

[27] S. K. C, S. A, S. N, I. A and V. G, "Performance Analysis of Machine Learning Classification for Parkinson's Disease from Biomedical Audio Data," 2023 Intelligent Computing and Control for Engineering and Business Systems (ICCEBS), Chennai, India, 2023, pp. 1–5, doi:10.1109/ICCEBS58601.2023.10448605.

[28] M. Alshammari and M. Mezher, "A Modified Convolutional Neural Networks For MRI-based Images For Detection and Stage Classification Of Alzheimer Disease," 2021 National Computing Colleges Conference (NCCC), Taif, Saudi Arabia, 2021, pp. 1–7, doi:10.1109/NCCC49330.2021.9428810.

[29] J. V. Anchitaalagammai, S. Kavitha, S. Murali, K. L. Gururaj and J. P. P. Kiruthik, "Predictive Health Assistant: AI-Driven Disease Projection Tool," 2024 11th International Conference on Reliability, Infocom Technologies and Optimization (Trends and Future Directions) (ICRITO), Noida, India, 2024, pp. 1–6, doi:10.1109/ICRITO61523.2024.10522266.

[30] A. AlMohimeed et al., "Explainable Artificial Intelligence of Multi-Level Stacking Ensemble for Detection of Alzheimer's Disease Based on Particle Swarm Optimization and the Sub-Scores of Cognitive Biomarkers," in IEEE Access, vol. 11, pp. 123173–123193, 2023, doi:10.1109/ACCESS.2023.3328331.

[31] R. Al-Momani, G. Al-Mustafa, R. Zeidan, H. Alquran, W. A. Mustafa and A. Alkhayyat, "Chronic Kidney Disease Detection Using Machine Learning Technique," 2022 5th International Conference on Engineering Technology and its Applications (IICETA), Al-Najaf, Iraq, 2022, pp. 153–158, doi:10.1109/IICETA54559.2022.9888564.

[32] V. Patel, K. Patel, P. Goel and M. Shah, "Classification of Gastrointestinal Diseases from Endoscopic Images Using Convolutional Neural Network with Transfer Learning," 2024 5th International Conference on Intelligent Communication Technologies and Virtual Mobile Networks (ICICV), Tirunelveli, India, 2024, pp. 504–508, doi:10.1109/ICICV62344.2024.00085.

[33] N. Darapaneni et al., "Early Detection of Skin Cancer - Solution for Identifying and Defining Skin Cancers using AI," 2022 Interdisciplinary Research in Technology and Management (IRTM), Kolkata, India, 2022, pp. 1–6, doi:10.1109/IRTM54583.2022.9791676.
[34] K. P. Reddy, S. Kodati, M. Swetha, M. Parimala and S. Velliangiri, "A Hybrid Neural Network Architecture for Early Detection of DDOS attacks using Deep Learning Models," 2021 2nd International Conference on Smart Electronics and Communication (ICOSEC), Trichy, India, 2021, pp. 323–327, doi:10.1109/ICOSEC51865.2021.9591969.
[35] T. S. Ruprah, B. Regmi, S. B. Jadhav and S. Singh, "Early Stage Lung Cancer Detection Using Deep Learning," 2024 MIT Art, Design and Technology School of Computing International Conference (MITADTSoCiCon), Pune, India, 2024, pp. 1–6, doi:10.1109/MITADTSoCiCon60330.2024.10575345.
[36] N. Khuriwal and N. Mishra, "Breast Cancer Diagnosis Using Deep Learning Algorithm," 2018 International Conference on Advances in Computing, Communication Control and Networking (ICACCCN), Greater Noida, India, 2018, pp. 98–103, doi:10.1109/ICACCCN.2018.8748777.
[37] H. A. Mesrabadi and K. Faez, "Improving early prostate cancer diagnosis by using Artificial Neural Networks and Deep Learning," 2018 4th Iranian Conference on Signal Processing and Intelligent Systems (ICSPIS), Tehran, Iran, 2018, pp. 39–42, doi:10.1109/ICSPIS.2018.8700542.
[38] Lee D, Yoon SN. Application of Artificial Intelligence-Based Technologies in the Healthcare Industry: Opportunities and Challenges. Int J Environ Res Public Health. 2021 Jan 1;18(1):271. doi:10.3390/ijerph18010271. PMID: 33401373; PMCID: PMC7795119.
[39] Anjaria P, Asediya V, Bhavsar P, Pathak A, Desai D, Patil V. Artificial Intelligence in Public Health: Revolutionizing Epidemiological Surveillance for Pandemic Preparedness and Equitable Vaccine Access. Vaccines (Basel). 2023 Jun 26;11(7):1154. doi:10.3390/vaccines11071154. PMID: 37514970; PMCID: PMC10383160.
[40] R. Kostadinov, D. Vicheva, L. Paunov, M. Georgieva, V. Topalov and S. Georgiev, "Artificial Intelligence Implementation for Development of Socially Significant Disease Prediction and Risk Mitigation Monitoring – Patients Perspective," 2023 International Conference on Applied Mathematics & Computer Science (ICAMCS), Lefkada

Island, Greece, 2023, pp. 63–68, doi:10.1109/ICAMCS59110.2023.00017.

[41] Wani SUD, Khan NA, Thakur G, Gautam SP, Ali M, Alam P, Alshehri S, Ghoneim MM, Shakeel F. Utilization of Artificial Intelligence in Disease Prevention: Diagnosis, Treatment, and Implications for the Healthcare Workforce. Healthcare (Basel). 2022 Mar 24;10(4):608. doi:10.3390/healthcare10040608. PMID: 35455786; PMCID: PMC9026833.

[42] S. D and Swetha, "IoT's Impact on Personal Devices and Health: Wearable Technology," 2024 International Conference on Advances in Modern Age Technologies for Health and Engineering Science (AMATHE), Shivamogga, India, 2024, pp. 1–8, doi:10.1109/AMATHE61652.2024.10582194.

[43] M. S. Ghoneim, S. H. Mohamed, Y. H. Elgharib and S. M. Hamed, "An IoT Based System for Monitoring and Soothing Post-Traumatic Stress Disorder Patients," 2020 International Conference on Innovative Trends in Communication and Computer Engineering (ITCE), Aswan, Egypt, 2020, pp. 126–129, doi:10.1109/ITCE48509.2020.9047765.

[44] I. Suhail and S. Pillai, "IoT enabled applications for Healthcare decisions," 2022 International Conference on Decision Aid Sciences and Applications (DASA), Chiangrai, Thailand, 2022, pp. 47–54, doi:10.1109/DASA54658.2022.9765251.

[45] Aruleba RT, Adekiya TA, Ayawei N, Obaido G, Aruleba K, Mienye ID, Aruleba I, Ogbuokiri B. COVID-19 Diagnosis: A Review of Rapid Antigen, RT-PCR and Artificial Intelligence Methods. Bioengineering (Basel). 2022 Apr 3;9(1):153. doi:10.3390/bioengineering9040153. PMID: 35447713; PMCID: PMC9024895.

[46] Lv C, Guo W, Yin X, Liu L, Huang X, Li S, Zhang L. Innovative applications of artificial intelligence during the COVID-19 pandemic. Infect Med (Beijing). 2024 Feb 21;3(1):100095. doi:10.1016/j.imj.2024.100095. PMID: 38586543; PMCID: PMC10998276.

3

Obstacles and Opportunities: Generative AI in the Context of Neurodegenerative Disorders

Lingala Thirupathi[1], Vineetha Kaashipaka[2], Ashok Galipellli[3], and Vijetha Katakam[4]

[1]Department of Artificial Intelligence & Machine Learning, Sreenidhi Institute of Science & Technology, India
[2]Department of Electronics and Communication Engineering, Sreenidhi Institute of Science & Technology, India
[3]Department of Artificial Intelligence & Machine Learning, Geethanjali College of Engineering and Technology, India
[4]Analyst, Visa Inc, USA
E-mail: thiru1274@gmail.com; Kashipaka.vineetha@gmail.com; Gashok.cse@gcet.edu.in; vijethakatakam@gmail.com

Abstract

In neurodegenerative disease research, generative artificial intelligence (AI) holds transformative potential to revolutionize illness detection, treatment, and understanding. However, realizing this potential requires overcoming significant challenges. The complexity and heterogeneity of neurodegenerative disorders, coupled with limited data, pose major obstacles to developing and validating AI models. The opaque nature of these models complicates their integration into clinical practice and raises concerns about interpretability and trust among healthcare professionals. Additionally, ethical issues such as algorithmic bias and patient privacy must be carefully managed to facilitate the adoption of AI-driven solutions. Despite these challenges, generative AI offers exciting opportunities. It can accelerate drug discovery, tailor treatment plans, and enhance early detection through predictive modeling. By fostering interdisciplinary collaboration, improving data governance, and

DOI: 10.1201/9788743801764-3

ensuring rigorous validation, generative AI has the potential to advance our understanding and management of neurodegenerative diseases, paving the way for more effective interventions.

Keywords: Generative AI (Artificial Intel0ligence), Neurodegenerative Disorders, Predictive Modeling, Data Governance, Ethical Issues.

3.1 Introduction

The complex landscape of our minds, once vibrant and agile, can sometimes turn against us, clouded by the slow, irreversible march of neurodegenerative disorders. These conditions like, Alzheimer's, Parkinson's, amyotrophic lateral sclerosis (ALS), and others carry profound impacts, not only for those diagnosed but also for families, caregivers, and the medical community. Navigating life with a degenerative brain disorder can feel like trying to keep afloat in a sea of unce0rtainty, where the line between what is remembered and what is forgotten, what is controlled and what is lost, blurs gradually, but unmistakably.

For years, we have sought solutions medications, therapies, interventions to stall or at least slow this relentless decline. Yet, despite impressive strides in understanding the biological mechanisms at play, many treatments remain limited in their effectiveness. The human brain is as elusive as it is powerful, and our ability to fully comprehend and treat its failings has long been constrained. But, as with so many areas of medicine and science, technological innovation is rapidly reshaping the playing field. Among these advancements, generative artificial intelligence (AI) has emerged as one of the majority promising, yet misunderstood, tools for addressing the challenges posed by neurodegenerative disorders.

At first glance, the concept of AI playing a role in healthcare particularly in something as personal and complex as brain health may seem cold or detached. But generative AI is not the kind of technology that replaces human care; rather, it augments it, offering powerful new capabilities to enhance diagnosis, therapy, and support. Far from a dystopian vision of robots making clinical decisions, we are witnessing the dawn of an era where AI can serve as an ally to physicians, neuroscientists, and therapists. This is not just about faster diagnostics or more personalized treatment plans (though those are important). It is about creating a landscape where human intuition and artificial precision can work in tandem to alleviate the burdens placed on both individuals with these disorders and their caregivers.

In fact, one of the most promising aspects of generative AI lies in its capacity to personalize medicine in ways that were previously unthinkable. Consider how a physician currently diagnoses a patient with a neurodegenerative disorder. They might rely on cognitive tests, brain scans, and blood work, combined with the physician's experience and intuition. But the human brain is as unique as the person it belongs to, and treatment approaches that work for one individual may fail for another, often with little clear explanation. Generative AI, with its ability to process vast amounts of data and generate novel solutions, opens up a new frontier. It can analyze the nuances of a patient's symptoms, genetic predispositions, lifestyle factors, and brain imaging in ways that no single human mind could ever do, offering insights that could tailor treatments specifically for each individual.

Yet, while the potential of generative AI is undeniable, it is far from a magic bullet. Significant obstacles still stand in the way of its widespread implementation. Neurodegenerative disorders are complex, multi factorial diseases with varying causes, trajectories, and outcomes. Training AI models to accurately interpret the biological, environmental, and behavioral intricacies of these conditions requires access to vast datasets data that is not always readily available, particularly when it comes to rare or understudied disorders. Furthermore, concerns about data privacy and security, especially in the context of sensitive health information, cannot be overlooked. The very tools that promise to revolutionize our understanding and treatment of neurodegenerative diseases are also vulnerable to misuse, and ensuring that they are used ethically and responsibly is of paramount importance.

In addition to these technical challenges, there are broader societal and philosophical questions to consider. How do we balance the promise of AI-enhanced healthcare with the deeply human need for empathy, connection, and trust in the patient–doctor relationship? What happens when an algorithm, not a person, suggests a treatment plan? How do we ensure that AI does not exacerbate existing healthcare inequalities, leaving those without access to advanced technology further behind? These are the kinds of questions we must grapple with as we move toward a future where AI is integrated into the fabric of medical practice.

Despite these challenges, the opportunities that generative AI offers in the context of neurodegenerative disorders are too significant to ignore. Already, researchers are exploring ways to use AI to predict the onset of diseases like Alzheimer's years before symptoms appear, by analyzing subtle changes in brain scans or speech patterns. AI-driven drug discovery is also opening new avenues for developing treatments that target the root causes of these disorders, rather than merely alleviating symptoms. Furthermore, AI can support caregivers by developing tools to help monitor patient well-being, provide real-time feedback, and even offer emotional support through natural language processing technologies. In this way, AI is not just a tool for doctors and scientists; it has the potential to transform the entire ecosystem of care for individuals with neurodegenerative disorders.

For patients and their loved ones, the idea of AI-driven healthcare can provoke a mix of emotions hope, skepticism, perhaps even fear. But as we explore the intersection of generative AI and neurodegenerative disorders, we must remember that these technologies are ultimately designed to serve humanity. They are tools that extend the reach of human expertise, allowing us to confront the complexities of brain diseases with new precision and creativity. The goal, after all, is not to replace human insight but to amplify it, helping us find patterns in the chaos and offer treatments that are more effective; more compassionate, and more in tune with the individual needs of each patient.

As we move forward, it is crucial to approach the integration of generative AI into healthcare with both optimism and caution. The stakes are high both in terms of the potential benefits and the risks. But by engaging thoughtfully with these challenges, we have the opportunity to harness AI in ways that

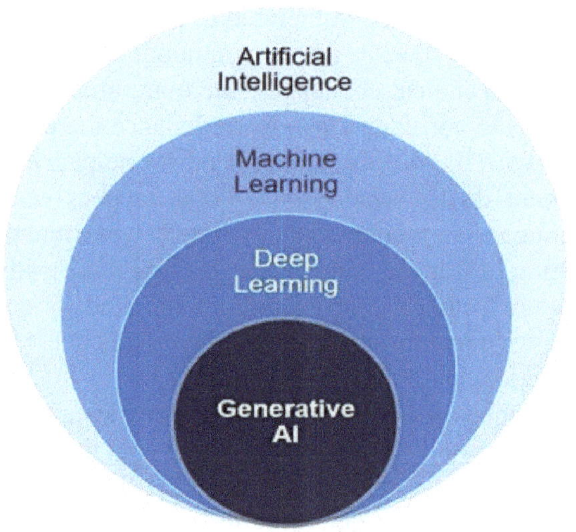

Figure 3.1 The AI landscape (Source: Original).

not only improve outcomes for those with neurodegenerative disorders but also reshape the future of medicine as a whole. This is not just a story about technology; it is a story about people, and how we can use the tools at our disposal to reduce suffering, restore dignity, and enhance the quality of life for millions. Figure 3.1 explains the typical landscape of AI.

3.1.1 History of generative AI

1950s–1960s: The concept of AI takes root

The first questions concerning whether machines might think like humans were asked in the middle of the 20th century, and these questions planted the seeds for generative AI. The Turing test gained notoriety when Alan Turing presented it in his 1950 paper "Computing Machinery and Intelligence." This was among the initial endeavors to delineate the concept of machine intelligence. Turing's theories sparked discussions over whether machines could replicate human intellect, laying the theoretical foundation for artificial intelligence. Subsequently, in 1956, the Dartmouth Conference, led by John McCarthy and Marvin Minsky, established AI as a recognized field of research. It is often acknowledged that McCarthy first used the term "artificial intelligence" at this time. Even though generative models were not the primary focus of AI during this time, it was vital for developing the theoretical foundations of the field.

Frank Rosenblatt created the Perceptron in 1957 as a crude model that approximated the function of neurons in the brain. Despite its limitations, this early neural network structure was a crucial step toward the creation of machine learning models. These early neural network studies were limited by low processing power and theoretical knowledge, but they gave hope for the development of generative systems in the future.

1970s–1980s: Early neural networks and probabilistic models

Neural network technology made little headway in the 1970s because sophisticated model training still required large amounts of processing power. Still, the foundation was being built. During this time, interest in neural networks temporarily declined as AI researchers began to realize the shortcomings of previous, simpler models such as the Perceptron.

Probabilistic models became popular as a crucial element of AI development in the early 1980s. The probabilistic graphical model known as Bayesian networks, which Judea Pearl proposed, became crucial for reasoning in the face of uncertainty. Because generative models rely on statistical learning to build data, these networks enabled AI systems to include probabilistic reasoning into decision-making. In an attempt to describe data more effectively, energy-based models, such as Boltzmann machines and Hopfield networks, were established at the same time. Although these models are not currently feasible for large-scale applications, they have contributed to defining a future course for the evolution of generative systems.

1990s: Foundations of Deep Learning and Generative Models

AI research had advanced to more useful applications by the 1990s, especially in the areas of machine learning and neural networks. As Hopfield networks and Boltzmann machines developed further, they made it possible for AI systems to simulate the energy levels of probabilistic systems and produce new data points. In these instances, "generative" meant that these models could learn the distribution of data and then produce new examples based on that learning.

The introduction of the long short-term memory (LSTM) network by Sepp Hochreiter and Jürgen Schmidhuber in 1997 was a major breakthrough in this decade. Recurrent neural networks (RNNs) that can handle lengthy data sequences are called LSTM networks. For generative tasks in the future, especially in domains like language modeling, where sequential data, like text or speech, must be interpreted in context, this discovery was essential. Later generative models in natural language processing (NLP) were built on top of LSTMs.

2000s: Early generative models and deep learning breakthroughs

Neural networks saw a renaissance in the 2000s, mostly due to the creation of deep learning models. Restricted Boltzmann machines (RBMs), developed by Geoffrey Hinton and colleagues in 2003, revolutionized the discipline by enabling the execution of unsupervised learning tasks like dimensionality reduction. Complex data distributions could be represented, which paved the way for increasingly advanced generative models.

Hinton made yet another significant advancement in 2006 when he proposed deep belief networks (DBNs). These networks were among the first to employ a multilayer, hierarchical learning methodology, which improved the extraction of features from unprocessed data. AI is now closer to generative capabilities, where models can comprehend the underlying structure of data and produce new instances that follow similar patterns, thanks to this unsupervised pre training of deep neural networks.

The first deep learning-based speech generation models were created in 2009, utilizing these novel techniques to address the challenge of producing speech that is similar to that of a human. The ability of deep neural networks to produce sequential data was shown by these early speech synthesis models, marking a significant advancement in generative AI.

2010s: The rise of generative adversarial networks (GANs) and transformers

Generative AI had tremendous growth in the 2010s, with discoveries that completely changed the industry. Image generation was transformed in 2014 when Ian Goodfellow introduced generative adversarial networks (GANs). A discriminator and a generator network make up a GAN. GANs are a key component of contemporary generative AI because of its ability to produce amazingly realistic visuals through a competitive learning process. WaveNet, a deep generative model developed by Google's DeepMind, markedly enhanced the quality of synthetic speech when it was published in 2015. WaveNet represented a major advancement in audio generative models, allowing for the creation of remarkably lifelike human speech and music. This proved that complicated audio signals could be handled by deep learning in addition to visual data.

A turning point in the development of generative AI was reached in 2017 with the release of Transformers, which was introduced by Vaswani et al. in the paper Attention is All You Need. Transformers eliminated the need for recurrent networks like LSTMs and significantly increased the capacity of AI models to process sequential input, such as text. More sophisticated text and language production was made possible by transformers, which served as the foundation for numerous language models, including more recent innovations like GPT.

Generative pre-trained transformer (GPT), which OpenAI launched in 2018, immediately rose to prominence as one of the most potent NLP tools. GPT used the transformer architecture to do tasks with remarkable fluency, including text production, question answering, and language translation. This model was revolutionary because it showed how generative AI can generate and comprehend human language on a large scale.

2020–2022: Scaling generative AI and widespread impact

Generative AI reached unprecedented heights in the early 2020s, both in terms of its potential and its influence on society. GPT-3, an edition of the GPT architecture with 175 billion parameters, was released by OpenAI in 2020, making it the most advanced and sizable language model available at the time. GPT-3 showed an unmatched capacity to produce text that is human-like in a range of contexts, including coding and creative writing. With its release, generative AI attracted a lot of attention as companies and academics started looking into real-world uses.

The potential of multimodal AI systems was illustrated in 2021 when DALL, another model from OpenAI, showed off its capacity to produce visuals from textual descriptions. At about the same time, DeepMind's AlphaFold 2 overcame a major obstacle in biology by predicting protein structures from amino acid sequences a job that is fundamental to the ideas of generative AI. This innovation demonstrated that AI could do more than just create data; it could also solve challenging real-world problems, with significant ramifications for the biological and medical sciences.

With various models and stable diffusion gaining prominence for their capacity to produce high-quality images from straightforward text inputs, generative AI had become widely recognized by 2022. Because of the widespread adoption of these models by designers, artists, and the general public, generative AI is now understandable to non-experts.

2023–2024: The Future of Generative AI. OpenAI produced GPT-4 in 2023, a more sophisticated and polished version of its predecessor, as generative AI continued to develop. GPT-4 improved text generation, comprehension, and reasoning, making it a useful tool in a variety of fields, such as education, healthcare, and content development. ChatGPT and other models based on GPT-4 became commonplace, enabling anybody to access conversational agents and AI-generated content.

The release of generative AI models by Google and Anthropic (Gemini AI and Claude AI, respectively) broadened the competitive environment. These models pushed the limits of what generative AI is capable of, showcasing improved natural language production and interpretation skills. The field of generative AI is expanding quickly, and its uses are becoming more widespread in various sectors. But as generative AI grows more potent and pervasive, ethical and societal issues like guaranteeing responsible AI usage and correcting potential biases have also drawn attention.

This detailed history captures the progressive milestones of generative AI, highlighting its rapid evolution from early theoretical concepts to the advanced, highly practical models of today. The author(s) in [7] created an algorithm that can identify a wide range of cardiac arrhythmias from electrocardiograms taken using a single-lead wearable monitor better than board-certified cardiologists. Table 3.1 depicts the advantages of Gen AI over traditional AI.

Table 3.1 Generative AI model advantages of over traditional AI.

Feature	Generative AI (Gen AI)	Traditional AI
Content creation	Creates new content (e.g., images, text, music, videos).	Processes and analyzes existing data.
Handling incomplete data	Excels in generating outputs with limited or incomplete data.	Struggles with limited data, often needs large datasets.
Adaptability	Adaptable across multiple domains without heavy customization.	Domain-specific models with less flexibility.
Data augmentation	Generates synthetic data for augmenting training datasets.	Relies on real-world data for training.
Simulations	Simulates complex scenarios, aiding predictive analytics.	Limited in generating complex, predictive simulations.
Creativity and innovation	Produces novel designs, ideas, and solutions.	Primarily focused on automation and optimization.
Learning approach	Works effectively in unsupervised learning environments.	Typically relies on supervised learning and labeled data.

3.1.2 Research gaps

One of the fundamental research gaps in applying generative AI to neurodegenerative disorders lies in the incomplete understanding of the biological mechanisms underlying these diseases. Conditions like Alzheimer's, Parkinson's, and ALS involve complex interactions between genetics, environmental factors, and neurophysiology, much of which is still not fully understood. Without a comprehensive grasp of these processes, it becomes challenging to develop AI models that can accurately simulate disease progression, diagnose early-stage disorders, or predict individual responses to treatment. Current AI models may excel at recognizing patterns, but they struggle to offer novel insights into the root causes of these diseases due to the fragmented nature of available biological data. More interdisciplinary research combining AI, neuroscience, and molecular biology is needed to fill this critical knowledge gap.

A significant obstacle in advancing generative AI applications in this context is the lack of high-quality, comprehensive datasets. Neurodegenerative diseases often require longitudinal data tracking patients over many years to observe disease progression and treatment outcomes. However, the availability of such datasets is limited due to the long duration of these diseases and the difficulty in tracking patients consistently. Moreover, existing datasets may suffer from inconsistencies, missing data points, or lack of standardization, limiting the ability of AI models to generalize findings across diverse populations. In addition, neurodegenerative disorders are underrepresented in certain populations, leading to biases in the data. Generative AI models trained on these datasets may perpetuate these biases, making it harder to create inclusive, generalized AI-driven solutions. Future research must focus on creating larger, more representative datasets that are ethically sourced and de-identified to respect patient privacy.

Another major gap is the interpretability of generative AI models, which is crucial for gaining the trust of clinicians and patients. Many deep learning models, especially those used in generative tasks, function as "black boxes," providing little insight into how they arrive at their conclusions. In healthcare, this lack of transparency is particularly problematic because clinicians need to understand why an AI model recommends a specific diagnosis or treatment. For neurodegenerative disorders, where treatment plans can vary greatly between patients, it is essential to ensure that AI-driven recommendations are explainable and actionable. Research is needed to develop interpretable generative models that can provide clinicians with understandable reasoning behind their decisions, thus facilitating trust and adoption in clinical practice.

While generative AI has demonstrated great potential, one of the practical gaps lies in integrating these systems into existing clinical workflows. Healthcare systems are often burdened by legacy infrastructure and regulatory constraints, which can make it difficult to implement AI tools. Moreover, the use of generative AI in neurodegenerative care would require seamless integration with current diagnostic tools, electronic health records, and decision-making processes. This presents both technical and logistical challenges. There is a need for research into developing frameworks that allow for the smooth integration of AI models into healthcare environments, ensuring that they enhance, rather than disrupt, clinical workflows. Additionally, studies are needed on how generative AI can work alongside healthcare professionals to augment decision-making rather than replace human intuition.

As with many AI applications in healthcare, ethical considerations are a significant research gap that requires further exploration. The use of sensitive health data in generative AI models raises issues related to data privacy, especially when considering neurodegenerative disorders that affect cognition and decision-making capacity. Patients with these disorders may not be able to fully comprehend or consent to the use of their data in AI research, which necessitates strict ethical guidelines and safeguards. Moreover, the possibility of AI models being trained on biased or unrepresentative data poses the risk of exacerbating health disparities. Research is needed to develop ethical frameworks that ensure patient consent is obtained in a transparent and understandable manner, while also ensuring that AI models are trained on diverse, inclusive datasets that minimize bias.

While generative AI offers exciting possibilities for personalized medicine, there remains a gap in predicting individual treatment responses for neurodegenerative diseases. Current AI models struggle to account for the high variability in patient responses to treatments, which is crucial for managing these conditions. For instance, patients with Parkinson's disease may react differently to the same medication based on genetic factors, lifestyle, and disease stage. Generative AI holds potential in this area by analyzing a combination of patient data genomics, imaging, clinical history, etc. – to generate individualized treatment plans. However, this requires more sophisticated models capable of integrating multimodal data and learning from smaller sample sizes. Future research should focus on refining generative AI systems that can account for these complexities and reliably predict personalized treatment outcomes.

One of the most promising, yet underdeveloped, areas of research is the use of generative AI for early diagnosis and disease progression prediction in neurodegenerative disorders. While early diagnosis is key to slowing disease progression and improving quality of life, existing diagnostic tools are often inadequate for detecting the earliest signs of these diseases. Generative AI could potentially analyze subtle patterns in medical images, speech, or biomarkers to predict the onset of disorders like Alzheimer's years before symptoms appear. However, developing models that are sensitive enough to detect these early markers and robust enough to avoid false positives is an ongoing challenge. More research is needed to enhance the precision of AI models in early detection and to validate their accuracy in clinical trials.

While much of the focus of generative AI research is on improving patient outcomes, there is a significant gap in exploring how AI can support the caregivers of those with neurodegenerative disorders. Caregivers often face immense physical, emotional, and financial burdens, yet there is little AI-driven research aimed at easing these challenges. Generative AI could be used to develop tools that monitor patients' health in real-time, predict critical care needs, or even offer emotional support via AI-driven companion systems. However, this remains an underexplored area, and further research is needed to assess how AI can best be leveraged to assist caregivers while maintaining ethical standards and patient privacy.

3.1.3 Major contributions

One of the most significant contributions of generative AI in the context of neurodegenerative disorders is its ability to enhance early diagnosis by identifying subtle patterns that might be undetectable through traditional methods. Another major contribution is its ability to predict disease progression in neurodegenerative disorders, enabling more personalized and proactive treatment plans. Generative AI contributes to the field of neurodegenerative research by generating synthetic data that can be used to simulate disease progression or treatment responses. Generative AI models excel at integrating and learning from multimodal data, such as combining genetic information with brain imaging and clinical records. In neurodegenerative research, this capability is transformative because these diseases are multi factorial, influenced by a range of genetic, environmental, and lifestyle factors. Traditional analytical methods often struggle to handle such diverse data sources, but generative AI can create models that consider the complex relationships between these variables.

Generative AI also plays a role in developing ethical, AI-driven care solutions that improve the lives of both patients with neurodegenerative disorders and their caregivers. Generative AI can be used to create tools that provide continuous monitoring of patients, predict when critical care interventions might be needed, and offer caregivers real-time insights into the patient's condition. Additionally, AI-generated systems could offer cognitive stimulation or emotional support for patients in early stages of dementia, improving their quality of life. These contributions extend the potential of AI beyond clinical settings, addressing the practical and emotional challenges that accompany neurodegenerative diseases.

A major contribution in neurodegenerative care is the development of more explainable AI systems that can assist clinicians without replacing them. Generative AI models can be designed to provide clear rationales for their recommendations, whether for diagnosis or treatment, ensuring that clinicians remain central to the decision-making process. By improving the transparency of AI models, generative AI fosters greater trust and facilitates its integration into clinical workflows, ultimately benefiting patient care. These explainable AI systems contribute to more informed, data-driven decisions while maintaining the clinician's expertise and intuition at the forefront of patient management.

Generative AI is making significant contributions in the realm of neuro imaging, which is vital for understanding neurodegenerative diseases. AI models can process and analyze large sets of brain scans, identifying subtle structural or functional changes that may signal early neuro degeneration. Additionally, generative models can create detailed brain maps, simulating how diseases like Alzheimer's affect different regions over time. This allows researchers to study disease progression in unprecedented detail, potentially identifying new therapeutic targets or diagnostic markers.

Another contribution is in the development of telemedicine and remote monitoring solutions for neurodegenerative diseases. As these disorders progress, patients often face mobility issues, making frequent hospital visits difficult. AI-driven platforms can enable continuous monitoring of patients' cognitive and motor functions through wearable devices or home-based systems. Generative AI can analyze this data in real-time, alerting healthcare providers to any sudden changes in the patient's condition that may require intervention. These contributions demonstrate the wide-reaching potential of generative AI in advancing both research and care for neurodegenerative diseases. From early diagnosis and personalized treatment to supporting caregivers and revolutionizing neuro imaging, generative AI offers transformative possibilities in understanding and managing these complex conditions.

3.1.4 Organization of the chapter

This chapter starts with the introduction, then Section 3.2 gives the literature survey, Section 3.3 explains generative AI in neurodegenerative disorders: obstacles, Section 3.4 describes the generative AI in neurodegenerative disorders: opportunities, Section 3.5 explores the future directions and finally in the last section we conclude with the conclusions.

3.2 Literature Survey

In [5], authors explore the transformative impact of machine learning, AI, and generative models on 6G wireless communications, highlighting the complementary role of Gen AI alongside distributed AI (DAI). It provides taxonomy of DAI models, analyzes technical works, and offers insights on challenges and strategies for future 6G networks. Explores the state-of-the-art Generative AI models, examining their mathematical foundations, architecture, and future potential. It evaluates key tasks, tools, and real-world applications, addressing the opportunities and risks posed by Gen AI. With its growing impact on sectors like education, business, and cybersecurity, Gen AI is integral to the upcoming 5th Industrial Revolution. Organizations must adopt Gen AI strategically, focusing on compliance, risk management, and talent development. Future research should address challenges such as misinformation, cybersecurity, privacy, and explainability, ensuring authenticity, reliability, and transparency in Gen AI-generated content [4].

The authors highlights the many uses of generative AI in healthcare, including drug development, medical simulation, medical imaging, and individualized treatment. Healthcare operations are improved by Gen AI, yet there are still issues with patient privacy and data security. For AI to be integrated, cooperation between researchers, medical practitioners, and legislators is essential [8]. Discusses how AI advancements enable the simulation of dangerous behaviors, reducing data collection efforts. By embedding multi-filter modules and enhancing algorithms, AI can generate images of emergencies like drowning. The self-training AI model improves recognition accuracy and response time, ultimately enhancing safety in real-life situations [9]. Proposes filling the missing, a generative AI-empowered federated learning method to address challenges in mobile edge networks caused by data and resource heterogeneity. It enhances convergence and efficiency by augmenting local data and optimizing energy consumption, achieving up to 50% energy savings and improved global accuracy [10].

Generative AI, especially large language models (LLMs), aids in knowledge management and early prototyping by providing methodological support, task delegation, and rapid iterations. While LLMs streamline user journeys and prototyping, their effectiveness is limited by task definitions and expert input. Future AI tools may enhance prototype quality and innovation processes [11]. Research explores the use of LLMs for creating personalized advertising messages, proposing prompt engineering rules based on marketing theory. It suggests a cost-effective approach using LLMs and SMS APIs for personalized marketing. Limitations include a lack of real-world data experimentation, with future research needed on prompt effectiveness [12]. Compares human-generated and AI-generated product ideas, finding that AI-generated ideas are notably more novel and beneficial to customers, with similar feasibility scores. Despite AI ideas outperforming human ones, there were no bias differences in executive evaluations [13].

In [14], authors present a text-to-image generation method that enhances context preservation through prompt editing. The proposed scheme yields more contextually similar images. The methodology revises input prompts to maintain context, though challenges remain with handling extensive, structured sentence inputs. In [15], authors reviews the use of deep generative models in the industrial Internet of Things, highlighting their advantages over traditional deep learning algorithms for tasks like anomaly detection and network traffic prediction. It identifies key challenges, including interpretability and privacy concerns, and suggests future research directions. The authors examine 10 years of research on generative AI through the use of social network analysis, text analysis. It highlights important areas of study, technological developments, and uses for computer vision, pattern recognition, and image processing. Large language models, ChatGPT, and applications in education, healthcare, and other domains are examples of emerging subjects [16].

In [1], authors examine the use of neuro stimulators, such as vagus nerve and deep brain stimulation, as alternatives to pharmacological treatments for neurodegenerative diseases. While these disorders remain incurable, neuro stimulators can delay symptom onset, improve disease progression, enhance quality of life, and reduce or replace medication side effects. [2] proposes an AI-based system for early Parkinson's disease diagnosis, focusing on analyzing voice features using homogenous ensemble classifiers, CATBoost and LightGBM. By addressing dataset imbalance through various sampling methods, the system enhances prediction reliability and accuracy, leveraging state-of-the-art algorithms for improved diagnosis.

In [3], authors show the application of contemporary machine learning and data analysis techniques in the investigation and diagnosis of neurodegenerative illnesses. The emphasis is on techniques that enable both the accurate diagnosis of the illness and the identification of its etiology. In [17], authors explore integrating olfaction technology with AI to understand and diagnose olfactory dysfunction associated with aging, neurological, and neuropsychiatric disorders. By enhancing olfactory testing and data analysis, this approach promises early detection and improved diagnostic methods for diseases like Alzheimer's and Parkinson's, leading to better-targeted interventions. In [18], authors intends to create a clinical memory aid for neurological conditions like Alzheimer's, which would be a major advancement in improving memory and brain function.

In [6], authors explore using gait variability, measured via inertial units, to assess fatigue and sleepiness in real-world settings. Comparing various gait metrics with patient-reported outcomes, the highest classification accuracy was 57.04% using typical gait variability. Results indicate that while promising, further research with larger datasets is needed for more accurate assessments. [19] used multilevel based grey wolf optimization and convolution neural networks to segment brain tissues in MRI images of individuals with mild cognitive impairment (MCI), Alzheimer's disease, and normal.

By using support vector machines to analyze tissue variations, it is possible to reach classification accuracy of 77% for white matter, 80.22% for grey matter, and 78.7% for cerebrospinal fluid. This indicates that differences in grey matter may be a significant predictor of the course of dementia.

In [20], the authors use gait data from force-sensitive resistors to extract 24 temporal and spectral features for detecting neurodegenerative diseases like Parkinson's, Huntington's, and ALS. After preprocessing with outlier removal and feature selection, machine learning models achieved over 80% classification accuracy, except for one, using selected features. [21] uses transfer learning with pre-trained neural networks to classify cerebral ataxia, Alzheimer's, and Parkinson's disease from medical images. By optimizing with others, and deploying via Flask, the model significantly improves classification accuracy compared to traditional methods, enhancing disease identification and management. [22] presents an algorithm for diagnosing neurodegenerative diseases using plantar pressure data. The method, tested on the physionet gait dynamics dataset, achieved 99.50% accuracy, surpassing other methods in classification performance. [23–24] explores challenges and innovations in the creation of digital twins in healthcare & AI [25] used healthcare diagnosis for the prediction.

3.3 Generative AI in Neurodegenerative Disorders: Obstacles

Figure 3.2 depicts the obstacles of generative AI in neurodegenerative disorders.

3.3.1 Data quality and availability

One of the most significant obstacles to leveraging generative AI for neurodegenerative disorders is the issue of data quality and availability. Neurodegenerative diseases progress over many years and require large, comprehensive datasets to accurately model and understand their complex biological mechanisms. However, numerous challenges hamper the collected works and exploitation of such data, impacting the performance and reliability of AI models.

Neurodegenerative diseases often require longitudinal data, which involves tracking patients over long periods to observe the progression of the disease and the effects of different treatments. Unfortunately, this kind of data is scarce, as gathering it can be resource-intensive and logistically

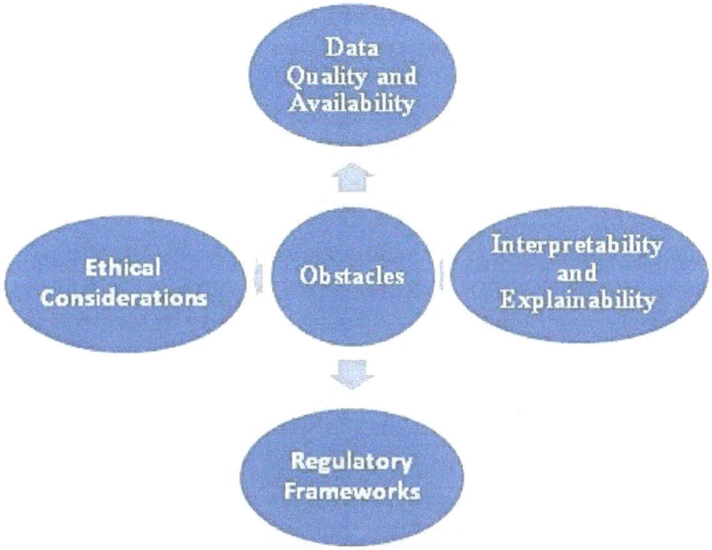

Figure 3.2 Generative AI in neurodegenerative disorders: obstacles.

challenging. Many patients may not be consistently followed throughout their disease course, leading to incomplete datasets. Without enough longitudinal data, generative AI models struggle to predict disease progression accurately, limiting their utility in making long-term forecasts or generating synthetic data that can be used to simulate different stages of the disease.

Data fragmentation is another significant issue in the field of neurodegenerative disorders. Patient data is often collected from multiple sources, including medical records, brain scans, genetic data, and cognitive assessments, but these data sources are rarely integrated in a standardized manner. Different healthcare systems, research institutions, and geographic regions may use varying protocols for data collection, leading to inconsistencies in the datasets. This fragmented and inconsistent data makes it difficult for AI models to find meaningful patterns, as the discrepancies between datasets can distort the model's understanding of the disease. Moreover, generative AI models, which thrive on large and diverse datasets, require clean, harmonized data to function effectively.

Another obstacle is the presence of missing or biased data within existing neurodegenerative disorder datasets. Many studies or clinical trials may have gaps in data, such as missing time points, incomplete patient information, or lack of follow-up. Additionally, datasets are often biased, reflecting certain populations over others. For example, many neurodegenerative studies may over represent older, white, urban populations while under representing minorities, rural communities, or younger patients. AI models trained on biased or incomplete data can produce skewed results, limiting their applicability across diverse patient populations. This bias perpetuates inequalities in healthcare and could result in ineffective or inappropriate AI-driven recommendations for underrepresented groups.

Collecting high-quality data for neurodegenerative disorders also raises ethical concerns. Patients with cognitive impairments may not fully understand how their data is being used or be able to give informed consent. This ethical challenge makes it difficult to collect the type of extensive, sensitive data needed for AI-driven research. Additionally, concerns about patient privacy and data security further restrict the availability of open-access datasets, as strict regulations are in place to protect individuals' health information. While necessary for ethical research, these regulations can slow down data collection efforts, limiting the pool of data available for generative AI models.

For rare forms of neurodegenerative disorders, the challenge of data availability is even more pronounced. Conditions like Huntington's disease or certain genetic subtypes of Alzheimer's are much rarer, making it difficult to gather enough patient data to train reliable AI models. Generative AI thrives on large datasets that allow it to learn complex patterns, but with rare diseases, there simply may not be enough data available to develop effective models. This shortage of data poses a significant obstacle to developing AI tools that can provide insights into the unique aspects of these less common disorders. Addressing these data quality and availability challenges is critical to advancing the use of generative AI in neurodegenerative disorders. Overcoming these barriers will require collaborative efforts to improve data collection standards, ensure data diversity, and ethically manage sensitive patient information.

3.3.2 Interpretability and explainability

It represents significant obstacles in the application of generative AI to neurodegenerative disorders. These concepts are critical in healthcare, where clinicians and patients must understand and trust AI-driven decisions, especially when dealing with complex conditions like Alzheimer's, Parkinson's, or ALS. Despite the impressive potential of AI, many models particularly generative ones function as "black boxes," offering limited insight into how they make their predictions or recommendations. This lack of transparency creates several challenges.

The models can analyze large datasets, recognize patterns, and generate outputs, such as disease progression predictions or treatment suggestions. However, the underlying mechanisms by which the AI arrives at these conclusions are not easily interpretable by humans. For clinicians treating neurodegenerative disorders, this presents a significant obstacle. When an AI model recommends a specific diagnosis, treatment plan, or predicts disease progression, healthcare providers need to understand why the model is suggesting that course of action. Without clear reasoning, clinicians may be hesitant to rely on AI-generated insights, fearing that they might be inaccurate or misleading, especially when human lives are at stake.

In neurodegenerative disorders, where treatments must be carefully tailored to the individual, trust in the AI system is paramount. If an AI tool cannot provide a clear rationale for its decisions, it becomes difficult for healthcare professionals to trust and adopt these systems. Neurodegenerative diseases are highly variable, and clinicians rely on detailed explanations of the factors influencing patient care. For instance, if a generative AI system suggests a particular treatment for a Parkinson's patient, clinicians need to know which biomarkers or patient data points were most influential in making that decision. A lack of interpretability hinders trust and slows the integration of AI into clinical practice, reducing its potential to improve patient outcomes.

Without explainability, this promise is difficult to realize. Personalized medicine requires AI models to explain how different variables, such as a patient's genetics, medical history, or imaging data, contribute to specific recommendations. If the AI cannot offer an understandable explanation, doctors and patients may struggle to accept AI-driven personalization, limiting its practical use in managing neurodegenerative conditions. In such complex diseases, where treatment effectiveness varies widely, explainable AI is essential to delivering patient-centered care.

A lack of interpretability and explainability in AI also raises ethical and legal concerns, particularly in healthcare. If a generative AI model provides a faulty or incorrect recommendation, it is crucial to understand how that mistake was made to prevent future errors. However, if the model is a black box, it can be nearly impossible to trace the cause of the mistake. This opacity poses risks not only for patient safety but also for legal accountability. Clinicians and healthcare institutions may face legal challenges if they rely on AI systems that make decisions that cannot be explained or justified. In the context of neurodegenerative disorders, where early diagnosis or incorrect treatment plans can have life-altering consequences, these ethical concerns become even more pressing.

Neurodegenerative disorders often involve analyzing multimodal data, such as brain imaging, genetic information, and cognitive assessments. Generative AI models excel at integrating and processing these diverse data types, but the complexity of how these data streams interact makes explainability even more challenging. For instance, a generative AI model may combine MRI scans with genetic markers to predict Alzheimer's progression, but explaining how these disparate data sources led to the prediction is difficult. The interconnections between complex variables are not easily reduced to simple, understandable terms, making it harder for clinicians to trust or verify the AI's conclusions. This lack of transparency further limits the application of AI in neurodegenerative care, where a nuanced understanding of the disease is crucial.

There is often a trade-off between model performance and explainability. The more sophisticated and accurate a generative AI model becomes, particularly in detecting subtle patterns in neurodegenerative data, the more difficult it is to interpret its outputs. Advanced AI models, like deep neural networks, tend to be highly complex, and simplifying them for the sake of explainability can reduce their accuracy or predictive power. This presents a dilemma in neurodegenerative care: should we prioritize the model's ability to deliver high-performing predictions at the expense of understanding how it works, or should we compromise on performance to ensure that the AI is interpretable? Striking the right balance between these two needs is a key challenge in advancing AI applications for these diseases.

3.3.3 Regulatory frameworks

The regulations designed to ensure safety, efficacy, and ethical use, are crucial for protecting patient interests but can also create obstacles for innovation and the practical application of AI in clinical settings. The complexity and evolving nature of AI technology make it difficult to align with existing regulatory standards, which were not originally designed.

One of the primary challenges is that many current healthcare regulations were not developed with AI in mind. Traditional regulatory frameworks focus on medical devices, drugs, and treatments, which are more straightforward to evaluate for safety and efficacy. Generative AI, however, introduces new complexities, particularly when it comes to how these systems generate predictions, recommendations, or diagnoses. Regulators often struggle to classify generative AI tools, as they do not fit neatly into existing categories. For instance, should a generative AI model be regulated as a medical device, software, or something else entirely? This lack of clarity makes it difficult for developers to navigate regulatory pathways, slowing down the adoption of AI tools in the management of neurodegenerative disorders.

The difficulty of certification AI models for clinical application is another major barrier. Before medical items are authorized for use in healthcare, regulatory bodies like the European Medicines Agency (EMA) and the U.S. Food and Drug Administration (FDA) demand that they go through extensive testing and validation. This procedure calls for well-defined, quantifiable outcomes and controlled clinical trials for conventional products. However, for generative AI, particularly in the context of neurodegenerative diseases, validation is more complex. AI models are continuously learning and improving based on new data, which raises questions about how to certify a system that is constantly evolving. How do regulators ensure that an AI model that learns from new patient data remains safe and effective over time? This dynamic nature of AI poses a significant regulatory hurdle.

Healthcare regulations, like the General Data Protection Regulation (GDPR) in Europe and the Health Insurance Portability and Accountability Act (HIPAA) in the United States, place stringent restrictions on the collection, storage, and use of patient data. Data privacy and security are major concerns in this field. Large volumes of sensitive patient data are frequently needed for generative AI models to work well, especially when it comes to neurodegenerative diseases where multimodal data such as brain scans, genetic data, and cognitive tests are essential for making precise predictions. Ensuring that these models comply with data protection laws is a significant challenge. AI developers must ensure that patient data is anonymized, securely stored, and handled in a way that complies with all relevant regulations, which can slow down data collection and integration efforts.

AI models that influence clinical decisions must be carefully evaluated for bias, fairness, and transparency to ensure they do not perpetuate health disparities or introduce unintended harm. Regulators are increasingly focused on ensuring that AI models used in neurodegenerative care are ethical and that their outputs are interpretable and explainable to clinicians and patients. One of the major regulatory concerns is determining liability in case of errors. The lack of clear liability frameworks creates hesitation among healthcare providers and institutions, further slowing the adoption of generative AI.

Healthcare regulations tend to be conservative and slow to change, which can be a barrier to the adoption of new technologies like generative AI. AI technologies evolve quickly, often outpacing the ability of regulatory agencies to assess and approve them.

Another obstacle arises from the variability in regulatory approaches across different countries and regions. AI developers must navigate a patchwork of regulatory requirements, which can differ significantly between jurisdictions. For example, the European Union's AI Act introduces stringent rules for high-risk AI systems in healthcare, requiring strict oversight, transparency, and accountability measures. In contrast, the regulatory environment in other regions may be more flexible or less developed. This global variability makes it difficult for AI developers to create solutions that can be deployed internationally, as they must tailor their systems to meet the specific regulatory requirements of each region.

3.3.4 Ethical considerations

One of the most pressing ethical challenges is ensuring informed consent, especially when working with neurodegenerative patients. These conditions can impair cognitive function, making it difficult for some patients to fully comprehend how their data is being used or the implications of AI-driven decisions. Patients might not have the capacity to give informed consent or may struggle to understand the complex technical nature of AI models, particularly if their condition affects memory, decision-making, or comprehension. This raises ethical concerns about patient autonomy, as individuals may unknowingly agree to the use of their data or involvement in AI-driven research without fully understanding the consequences.

In the case of neurodegenerative disorders, ensuring patient autonomy is critical, as these patients may have fluctuating cognitive abilities. AI developers and healthcare providers must take special care to ensure that patients are properly informed, and where necessary, alternative legal frameworks such as obtaining consent from family members or legal guardians need to be carefully considered.

Generative AI models are often trained on large datasets, but if these datasets are biased, the models can unintentionally perpetuate health disparities. For example, if the data used to train a generative AI system primarily comes from certain demographics such as older, white, urban populations it may not perform as accurately for minority groups, rural populations, or younger individuals who are less represented in the data. In neurodegenerative care, this could lead to AI models that are less effective at diagnosing or predicting disease progression in underrepresented groups, exacerbating health inequalities. Addressing this bias is ethically crucial. The fairness of AI models must be scrutinized, and developers must ensure that training datasets are diverse and representative of the broader population. Failure to do so could result in AI systems that disproportionately disadvantage certain patients, providing poorer care or making less accurate predictions for those who are already marginalized within healthcare systems.

The need for large, high-quality datasets in generative AI poses significant ethical challenges related to privacy and data security. Neurodegenerative diseases often require the integration of sensitive personal data, including genetic information, brain scans, cognitive assessments, and behavioral data. The use of such detailed and intimate information increases the risk of privacy breaches or misuse of data. Patients may be uncomfortable with how their personal health data is collected, shared, or used, particularly in the case of conditions that could carry social stigma, such as dementia. AI developers and healthcare organizations have an ethical obligation to make sure that strong data security and privacy protocols are in place. In addition to being legally required, compliance with legislations like GDPR and HIPAA is morally required in order to protect patient data and guarantee that it is used transparently and solely for that purpose. Patients should be thoroughly informed about how their data will be used in AI-driven treatments or research, and they should have unambiguous control over it.

In neurodegenerative disorders, where patients' lives are deeply affected by treatment decisions, the inability of AI models to explain how they arrive at their recommendations or predictions is problematic. If clinicians or patients cannot understand the reasoning behind an AI-driven decision, it undermines trust and makes it difficult to hold anyone accountable in the event of an error. From an ethical standpoint, AI models must be explainable and transparent to ensure that patients and healthcare providers can make informed decisions based on the model's recommendations. This is especially important in neurodegenerative diseases, where the course of treatment can be complex, and understanding the rationale behind medical decisions is vital for patient care.

Another ethical concern is the potential for unequal access to AI-driven healthcare innovations. Generative AI systems often require advanced infrastructure, substantial financial resources, and access to high-quality data. This could result in a healthcare system where only well-funded institutions or individuals in wealthy regions can benefit from AI-driven advancements in neurodegenerative care, leaving disadvantaged or rural communities behind. Ethically, it is critical to ensure that AI innovations are accessible to all patients, regardless of their socio-economic status or geographic location. This means developing AI tools that can be used in diverse healthcare settings and ensuring that the benefits of AI are distributed equitably. Failing to do so could widen existing healthcare disparities and prevent some patients from accessing potentially life-changing treatments.

The introduction of AI-driven predictions such as that forecasting rapid disease progression could lead to increased anxiety or hopelessness in some patients. This is especially true if patients do not fully understand how the AI model arrived at its conclusions or if they feel that their care is being automated or depersonalized. Ethically, the human element of care must remain central when using AI in neurodegenerative disorders. AI tools should be seen as augmenting, rather than replacing, the personal relationship between patients and healthcare providers. It is essential to consider the emotional and psychological impact of AI technologies and ensure that they are deployed in a way that supports, rather than undermines, patient well-being.

3.4 Generative AI in Neurodegenerative Disorders: Opportunities

Figure 3.3 represents the opportunities of generative AI in neurodegenerative disorders.

3.4.1 Disease modeling

One of the most promising opportunities generative AI offers is in creating predictive models of disease progression. Neurodegenerative disorders are characterized by gradual and often unpredictable declines in cognitive and motor functions. Generative AI can analyze multimodal data such as brain imaging, genetic information, patient histories, and cognitive test results to predict the future course of a disease for individual patients. These predictions can help clinicians anticipate when symptoms may worsen, allowing them to adjust treatment plans proactively. For instance, in Alzheimer's disease, generative AI models can analyze brain scans over time to predict the rate of cognitive decline or identify when a patient may transition from mild cognitive impairment to more advanced stages of dementia. This level of prediction is difficult with traditional statistical models, but generative AI can process the complexity of vast datasets to generate highly personalized

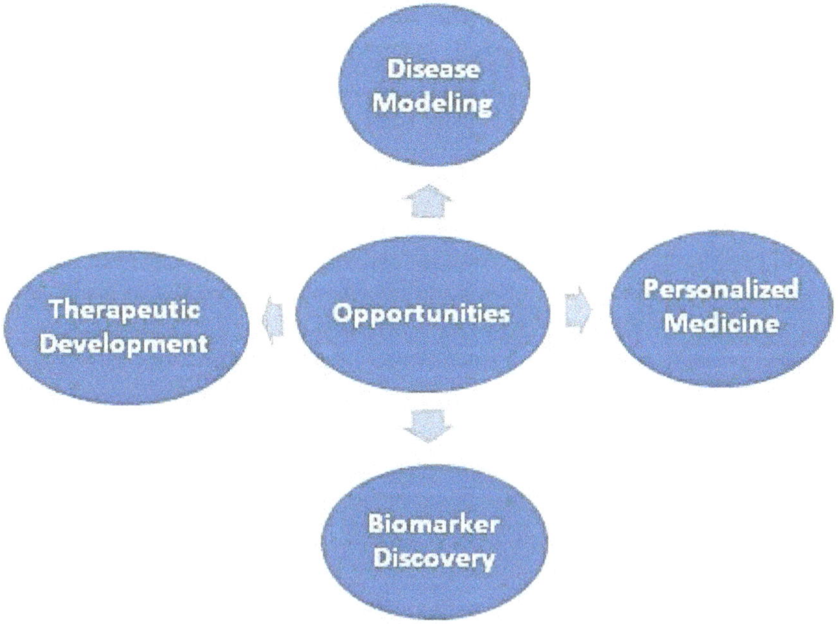

Figure 3.3 Generative AI in neurodegenerative disorders: opportunities.

models of disease progression. This not only improves patient care but also supports more targeted interventions, potentially slowing down the disease.

Generative AI can also assist in identifying early biomarkers for neurodegenerative disorders, which are crucial for early diagnosis and intervention. By analyzing large datasets that include genetic information, imaging, and clinical data, generative AI can identify subtle changes or patterns that may indicate the early onset of a neurodegenerative disorder. For example, AI-driven disease models can identify specific brain regions or neural network disruptions that may serve as early warning signs of Alzheimer's long before memory loss becomes apparent. Similarly, in Parkinson's disease, generative models can analyze movement data or subtle motor symptoms that precede clinical diagnosis. These AI-generated insights are invaluable for early detection, potentially enabling interventions that could delay or prevent the onset of debilitating symptoms.

Another major opportunity lies in the ability of generative AI to simulate disease mechanisms and therapeutic interventions. Understanding how neurodegenerative disorders develop at the cellular and molecular levels is critical for developing effective treatments. However, the complexity of brain disorders often makes it difficult to fully grasp how different genetic, environmental, and biological factors interact to drive disease progression. Generative AI models, particularly those trained on large-scale genomic, proteomic, and other biological datasets, can simulate how these factors interact over time.

A key advantage of generative AI in disease modeling is its ability to create personalized models for individual patients. Neurodegenerative diseases affect people differently; two individuals with the same diagnosis may experience entirely different symptoms, rates of progression, or responses to treatment. Generative AI can help bridge this gap by using each patient's specific data – such as their genetic profile, brain imaging, and lifestyle factors – to build individualized models of disease progression.

These personalized models can help clinicians tailor treatments more effectively, targeting therapies based on a patient's predicted disease trajectory. For instance, in Parkinson's disease, a personalized model could predict how quickly a patient's motor symptoms will progress, allowing doctors to recommend tailored interventions, such as specific medications or physical therapies, at the right time. Similarly, in Alzheimer's, personalized models might help identify which patients are likely to benefit from certain cognitive therapies or experimental treatments, optimizing care on an individual level.

Generative AI is also transforming drug discovery and clinical trial design for neurodegenerative disorders. Traditional drug development for these conditions is slow, expensive, and fraught with high failure rates due to the complexity of the diseases and the difficulty in identifying effective treatment targets. By evaluating enormous datasets to identify possible therapeutic targets, simulate illness pathways, and forecast how various substances can interact with these targets, generative AI provides novel methods to speed up this process. Generative AI can predict which patient demographics are most likely to benefit from a given intervention, which can optimize trial design in clinical trials. Even in complex neurodegenerative disorders, AI models can mimic the evolution of the disease in many situations, assisting researchers in designing trials that are more likely to provide meaningful results.

By analyzing data from diverse patient populations, generative AI can identify subtypes of neurodegenerative diseases, revealing distinct biological pathways or clinical profiles that may respond differently to treatments. For example, AI might reveal that a certain group of Alzheimer's patients with specific genetic mutations responds better to one type of drug than another. This understanding of disease heterogeneity is crucial for advancing precision medicine approaches, where treatments are tailored to specific patient subtypes rather than applied uniformly.

3.4.2 Personalized medicine

One of the foremost opportunities provided by generative AI is the ability to create highly personalized treatment plans. Neurodegenerative disorders present differently in each patient, influenced by genetic variations, lifestyle factors, and disease stage. For example, in Alzheimer's disease, generative AI can process data from a patient's genetic tests and brain scans to predict their likely response to various medications or lifestyle interventions. This approach allows healthcare providers to select therapies that are tailored to the patient's specific disease characteristics and progression patterns.

Generative AI can significantly improve the precision of drug selection and dosage for neurodegenerative disorders. Traditional methods of prescribing often rely on generalized treatment protocols, which may not account for individual variations. Generative AI models can predict how different drugs will interact with a patient's unique biological profile, helping to identify the most effective medications and optimal dosages. For instance, in Parkinson's disease, AI can analyze a patient's specific motor symptoms and response to previous treatments to recommend the most appropriate medication regimen.

In order to improve early diagnosis and risk assessment for neurodegenerative illnesses, generative AI is essential. Effective intervention requires early discovery, yet many diseases' symptoms frequently appear gradually and are difficult to identify in their early stages. Generative AI can detect minor trends that may point to the early start of neurodegenerative disorders by analyzing longitudinal data, such as changes in motor abilities or cognitive function. AI models are capable of risk-strategizing patients by combining data from several sources, such as genetics, biomarkers, and imaging investigations.

Generative AI can develop personalized models of disease progression, offering a more precise understanding of how a neurodegenerative disorder is likely to evolve in each individual. These models are based on a patient's unique data, including genetic factors, lifestyle, and disease history, providing insights into how their specific disease might progress over time. For instance, AI can generate individual trajectories of cognitive decline in Alzheimer's patients. This personalized projection helps clinicians anticipate future care needs and adjust treatment plans proactively, ensuring that interventions are timely and appropriate.

Generative AI enables the development of targeted interventions and precision therapies tailored to the molecular and genetic profiles of individual patients. For neurodegenerative disorders, where disease mechanisms can vary widely among patients, precision therapies offer the potential for more effective and individualized treatment. AI models can analyze genomic and proteomic data to identify specific molecular targets that are relevant to a patient's disease. For example, in ALS, generative AI can help identify genetic mutations or protein abnormalities specific to a patient, guiding the development of therapies that target these unique biological factors. This approach can lead to the creation of personalized drugs or therapies designed to address the specific needs of each patient, improving treatment outcomes.

Generative AI enhances the monitoring and adaptation of personalized treatment plans by analyzing real-time data from wearable devices and mobile health applications. Continuous monitoring of patients with neurodegenerative disorders can provide valuable insights into how they respond to treatments and how their symptoms evolve. AI can integrate data from various sources, such as wearable sensors tracking motor functions or mobile apps monitoring cognitive performance, to adjust treatment plans dynamically. For example, if AI detects a decline in a patient's motor skills that suggests a worsening of Parkinson's symptoms, it can prompt clinicians to modify the treatment regimen or recommend additional interventions. This real-time adaptability ensures that care remains aligned with the patient's current condition.

Generative AI can also empower patients by providing them with personalized insights and recommendations about their condition. AI-driven tools can offer patients tailored information about their disease progression, treatment options, and lifestyle adjustments based on their unique data. For instance, an AI-powered application could provide Alzheimer's patients and their caregivers with personalized strategies to manage cognitive symptoms and daily activities effectively. By offering actionable and individualized recommendations, generative AI can enhance patient engagement in their own care, leading to better adherence to treatment plans and improved quality of life.

Generative AI supports personalized medicine research and clinical trials by identifying suitable candidates and optimizing trial design. AI models can analyze patient data to identify individuals who are most likely to benefit from participation in specific clinical trials, based on their unique disease profiles and genetic factors. AI can assist in designing adaptive clinical trials that adjust based on interim results, allowing for more flexible and efficient testing of new treatments. By focusing on personalized patient populations, AI-driven trials can yield more relevant and precise outcomes, accelerating the development of effective therapies for neurodegenerative disorders.

3.4.3 Biomarker discovery

Generative AI excels in analyzing high-dimensional data, which is essential for discovering novel biomarkers in neurodegenerative disorders. The complexity of datasets containing genomes, proteomics, metabolomics, and imaging data frequently presents challenges for traditional approaches. These many data kinds can be processed and integrated by generative AI models, especially those built on deep learning, to find patterns and correlations that may point to possible biomarkers. For instance, in Alzheimer's disease, generative AI can identify hitherto unidentified biomarkers linked to early disease start or progression by combining datasets from brain imaging, cerebrospinal fluid (CSF) analyses, and genetic data. By leveraging AI's capacity to handle and analyze large volumes of data, researchers can discover novel biomarkers that could lead to earlier and more accurate diagnosis.

Once potential biomarkers are identified, validating their relevance and utility is a critical step. Generative AI can simulate and model how these biomarkers behave in different disease states or patient populations, enhancing the validation process. AI-driven simulations can predict how a biomarker will perform in various scenarios, such as different stages of disease progression or responses to treatment. For instance, in Parkinson's disease, generative AI can model how specific protein levels change over time or in response to treatment, providing insights into the biomarker's reliability and potential for clinical use. These simulations help researchers refine and validate biomarkers more efficiently, reducing the time and resources needed for experimental validation.

The integration of omics data (genomics, transcriptomics, proteomics, and metabolomics) is crucial for a comprehensive understanding of neurodegenerative diseases. Generative AI can integrate and analyze these multi-omic datasets to identify biomarkers that reflect the complex biological processes underlying these disorders. For example, in ALS research, combining genomic data with proteomic and metabolomic data through generative AI can uncover biomarkers related to disease onset or progression. AI models can identify correlations between genetic variants, protein expression levels, and metabolic changes, leading to the discovery of biomarkers that provide a holistic view of the disease.

Early detection of neurodegenerative disorders is challenging due to the subtle and gradual onset of symptoms. Generative AI can enhance early detection by identifying biomarkers that signal disease presence before clinical symptoms become apparent. AI models can analyze longitudinal data, tracking changes in biomarker levels over time to detect early signs of neurodegeneration. For instance, in Alzheimer's disease, AI can identify biomarkers in CSF or blood that indicate early amyloid plaque formation or tau protein abnormalities. By detecting these biomarkers before clinical symptoms appear, generative AI facilitates early diagnosis, enabling earlier intervention and potentially delaying disease progression.

Biomarkers are essential in drug discovery and development, as they can help identify suitable targets, monitor drug effects, and assess treatment outcomes. Generative AI can enhance drug discovery by identifying biomarkers that are critical for evaluating the efficacy and safety of new therapeutic agents. For example, in Alzheimer's research, generative AI can identify biomarkers that reflect the impact of experimental drugs on amyloid plaque reduction or tau phosphorylation. By integrating biomarker data with clinical trial results, AI models can provide insights into the drug's effectiveness and guide further development.

Neurodegenerative disorders are heterogeneous, with variations in disease presentation and progression among patients. Generative AI can identify biomarkers that help stratify patients into subtypes based on their disease characteristics and biological profiles. For example, AI models can analyze biomarkers related to cognitive decline, motor symptoms, and genetic factors to categorize Alzheimer's patients into different subtypes. This stratification allows for more targeted research and treatment approaches, as well as a better understanding of the disease's variability.

Generative AI can enhance biomarker discovery by supporting longitudinal studies and real-time monitoring of patients. AI models can analyze data collected over extended periods to identify biomarkers that track disease progression and treatment response. For instance, in Parkinson's disease, AI can monitor changes in motor function, imaging data, and biomarkers over time to identify patterns associated with disease progression. Real-time monitoring using wearable devices and AI analysis can provide continuous insights into disease dynamics and treatment effects, facilitating more responsive and adaptive patient care.

3.4.4 Therapeutic development

Generative AI excels in mining large-scale omics data to identify novel drug targets. Traditional methods often rely on predefined hypotheses or known biological pathways, which may overlook novel targets. Generative AI can analyze complex datasets to uncover previously unknown targets associated with neurodegenerative diseases. For example, in Alzheimer's disease research, generative AI can integrate genomic data with proteomic profiles to identify new proteins or genetic variants that play a role in disease pathology. By discovering novel drug targets, AI helps in developing therapies that address underlying disease mechanisms more effectively, potentially leading to breakthroughs in treatment.

Generative AI plays a critical role in the design and optimization of new drug molecules. Traditional drug discovery often involves iterative cycles of designing, testing, and refining compounds, which can be time-consuming and costly. AI models can generate novel drug candidates and optimize their chemical structures by predicting their interactions with biological targets and assessing their potential efficacy and safety. For instance, in Parkinson's disease, generative AI can design small molecules that specifically interact with dopamine receptors or other relevant targets. AI models can simulate how these molecules might bind to their targets and predict their pharmacokinetic properties. This accelerates the drug development process by reducing the number of iterations needed and identifying promising candidates more efficiently.

By evaluating patient data individually and forecasting their reactions to various treatments, generative AI helps to create tailored treatment plans. Personalized approaches are essential for efficient management of neurodegenerative disorders because patients vary greatly in how their diseases progress and how they respond to treatment. AI models can use information from clinical histories, proteomics, and genomes of patients to customize treatment plans. Generative AI, for instance, can forecast, based on each patient's own genetic and molecular profile, how they could react to particular medication therapy in the case of ALS. As a result, therapies can be more precisely targeted, enhancing therapeutic results and reducing side effects.

Drug repurposing involves finding new uses for existing drugs, which can be a cost-effective and faster approach to developing therapies for neurodegenerative disorders. Generative AI can accelerate drug repurposing by analyzing large datasets to identify existing drugs that may be effective against neurodegenerative diseases. For example, AI models can examine existing drug libraries and predict which compounds might have beneficial effects on neurodegenerative pathways. By identifying potential new indications for these drugs, generative AI can facilitate faster entry into clinical trials and potentially provide new treatment options for patients.

Generative AI enhances the design and execution of clinical trials by analyzing patient data to identify suitable candidates, predict trial outcomes, and optimize trial protocols. Traditional clinical trials can be challenging due to variability in patient responses and difficulties in defining optimal trial parameters.

AI models can predict which patient populations are most likely to benefit from specific treatments and help design adaptive clinical trials that adjust based on interim results. For instance, in Alzheimer's research, generative AI can identify biomarkers that indicate which patients are most likely to respond to a new drug, enabling more precise and efficient trials.

Generative AI can simulate disease pathways and predict the effects of potential treatments, offering valuable insights into how therapies might influence disease progression. By modeling the complex interactions between biological systems and therapeutic agents, AI provides a deeper understanding of how treatments work at a molecular level. For example, in Huntington's disease, AI models can simulate how a new therapeutic approach might impact the progression of the disease by altering specific genetic pathways or protein interactions. These simulations help researchers anticipate how treatments will perform before they are tested in clinical settings, guiding the development of more effective therapies.

Integrating multi-omic data such as genomics, transcriptomics, proteomics, and metabolomics is essential for understanding the multifaceted nature of neurodegenerative disorders and developing effective therapies. Generative AI excels in integrating these diverse data types to generate comprehensive insights into disease mechanisms and therapeutic targets. For instance, in Parkinson's disease, AI can combine genomic data with proteomic and metabolomic profiles to identify novel biomarkers and therapeutic targets. This holistic view of the disease enhances the development of therapies that address multiple aspects of disease pathology, leading to more effective and targeted treatments.

By enabling more precise and customized treatment strategies, generative AI advances precision medicine. AI models can determine the best treatment actions based on each patient's distinct disease profile by evaluating patient-specific data. Through the automation of large-scale dataset analysis and the generation of innovative ideas regarding illness processes and therapeutic methods, generative AI expedites research and discovery. Utilizing AI's speedy data processing and analysis capabilities, researchers can more effectively discover novel research avenues and create cutting-edge treatments.

3.5 Future Directions

Generative AI holds significant promise for advancing research and treatment in neurodegenerative disorders. One key opportunity lies in the development of personalized treatment strategies. Generative models can analyze vast datasets, including genetic, clinical, and imaging data, to create personalized profiles of disease progression and response to treatment. This could lead to more tailored and effective therapeutic interventions, enhancing patient outcomes. However, the challenge here is ensuring the quality and diversity of the data used to train these models, as biased or incomplete data could limit the generalizability and efficacy of AI-generated insights.

Another promising direction is the use of generative AI to accelerate drug discovery. By simulating and predicting the interactions between drugs and disease targets, generative models can identify potential therapeutic compounds faster than traditional methods. This approach could significantly reduce the time and cost associated with bringing new treatments to market. Nevertheless, this potential is tempered by the challenge of integrating AI-generated predictions with experimental validation, as computational models must be rigorously tested to confirm their efficacy in real-world scenarios. Generative AI also offers opportunities for enhancing diagnostic tools through improved imaging analysis. AI models can generate high-resolution images and identify subtle changes in brain structures that may be indicative of early-stage neurodegenerative diseases. This could lead to earlier diagnosis and intervention, potentially altering disease trajectories. The obstacle here involves ensuring that these AI models are robust and reliable across diverse populations and imaging techniques, as variations in data quality and imaging protocols could impact diagnostic accuracy.

In addition to these technical advancements, there is an opportunity for generative AI to contribute to patient care through the creation of virtual health assistants. These AI-driven systems could provide patients with personalized guidance, support, and monitoring, improving adherence to treatment plans and enhancing quality of life. However, addressing privacy concerns and ensuring the ethical use of patient data are critical challenges that must be addressed to gain public trust and acceptance.

Lastly, generative AI has the potential to revolutionize research by enabling new ways to model disease mechanisms and simulate interventions. By generating detailed models of neurodegenerative diseases, researchers can explore novel therapeutic approaches and understand complex disease processes more comprehensively. The main obstacle in this area is the need for interdisciplinary collaboration to integrate AI insights with clinical expertise, ensuring that AI-generated models are both scientifically valid and clinically relevant.

3.6 Conclusion

In the field of neurodegenerative illness, generative AI is a game-changer, with potential applications in customized medicine, quicker drug discovery, improved diagnostics, and patient care. Researchers and clinicians might possibly transform therapy and management practices by using AI to evaluate complex data and mimic illness mechanisms. This approach can lead to the development of more targeted and effective interventions. There are difficulties in incorporating generative AI into this field. Crucial obstacles that need to be cleared include guaranteeing data diversity and quality, bridging the gap between experimental validation and computer predictions, and handling privacy and ethical issue. Thorough testing and validation are necessary for robust and trustworthy AI models in order to guarantee their accuracy and generalizability across a range of demographics. Furthermore, in order to fully utilize AI's potential, interdisciplinary cooperation is necessary. Translating AI-generated insights into useful, clinically relevant applications will require the collaboration of researchers, physicians, and AI professionals. In order to improve patient outcomes and quality of life, it will be essential to address these challenges and seize the opportunities presented by neurodegenerative disease research.

References

[1] A. Kawala-Sterniuk et al.,. (2022). The Use of Various Neurostimulators in Therapy of Neurodegenerative Disorders – A Survey, 2022 Progress in Applied Electrical Engineering (PAEE), Koscielisko, Poland.pp. 1-6. doi:10.1109/PAEE56795.2022.9966574.

[2] A. C.D and N. Arulanand. (2024). Voice Features Based Early Diagnosis of Parkinson Neurodegenerative Disorder Using CatBoost and Light

GBM Algorithms, 2024 International Conference on Smart Systems for Electrical, Electronics, Communication and Computer Engineering (ICSSEECC), Coimbatore, India. pp. 522-527. doi:10.1109/ICSSEECC 61126.2024.10649424.

[3] A. I. Mikhalskii and J. A. Novoseltseva. (2018). Application of Data Analysis Methods in Research of Neurodegenerative Diseases, 2018 Eleventh International Conference Management of large-scale system development (MLSD, Moscow, Russia. pp. 1-4. doi:10.1109/MLSD.2 018.8551933.

[4] Bengesi, S., El-Sayed, H., Sarker, M. K., Houkpati, Y., Irungu, J., & Oladunni, T. (2024). Advancements in generative AI: A comprehensive review of GANs, GPT, autoencoders, diffusion model, and transformers. IEEE Access, 12, 69812-69837. https://doi.org/10.1109/ACCESS.202 4.3397775

[5] Celik, A., & Eltawil, A. M. (2024). At the dawn of generative AI era: A tutorial-cum-survey on new frontiers in 6G wireless intelligence. IEEE Open Journal of the Communications Society, 5, 2433-2489. https://do i.org/10.1109/OJCOMS.2024.3362271

[6] C. Hinchliffe et al.,(2023). Identification of Fatigue and Sleepiness in Immune and Neurodegenerative Disorders from Measures of Real-World Gait Variability, 2023 45th Annual International Conference of the IEEE Engineering in Medicine & Biology Society (EMBC), Sydney. pp. 1-4. doi:10.1109/EMBC40787.2023.10339956.

[7] Rajpurkar, P., Hannun, A. Y., Haghpanahi, M., Bourn, C., & Ng, A. Y. (2017). Cardiologist-level arrhythmia detection with convolutional neural networks. arXiv preprint arXiv:1707.01836.

[8] S. Sai, A. Gaur, R. Sai, V. Chamola, M. Guizani and J. J. P. C. Rodrigues. (2024). Generative AI for Transformative Healthcare: A Comprehensive Study of Emerging Models, Applications, Case Studies, and Limitations, in IEEE Access, vol. 12, pp. 31078-31106 doi:10.1109/ACCE SS.2024.3367715.

[9] B. Bai, H. Yue, L. Chen and X. Li. (2024). Research on Dataset Generation and Monitoring of Generative AI for Drowning Warning System, in IEEE Access, vol. 12, pp. 83589-83599. doi:10.1109/ACCESS.2024. 3407245.

[10] P. Li et al.,. (2024). Filling the Missing: Exploring Generative AI for Enhanced Federated Learning Over Heterogeneous Mobile Edge Devices, in IEEE Transactions on Mobile Computing, vol. 23, no. 10, pp. 10001-10015. doi:10.1109/TMC.2024.3371772.

[11] V. Bilgram and F. Laarmann. (2023). Accelerating Innovation With Generative AI: AI-Augmented Digital Prototyping and Innovation Methods, in IEEE Engineering Management Review, vol. 51, no. 2, pp. 18-25. doi:10.1109/EMR.2023.3272799.
[12] G. H. Lee, K. J. Lee, B. Jeong and T. Kim. (2024). Developing Personalized Marketing Service Using Generative AI, in IEEE Access, vol. 12, pp. 22394-22402. doi:10.1109/ACCESS.2024.3361946.
[13] J. Joosten, V. Bilgram, A. Hahn and D. Totzek. (2024). Comparing the Ideation Quality of Humans With Generative Artificial Intelligence, in IEEE Engineering Management Review, vol. 52, no. 2, pp. 153-164. doi:10.1109/EMR.2024.3353338.
[14] H. Kim, J. -H. Choi and J. -Y. Choi. (2024). A Novel Scheme for Generating Context-Aware Images Using Generative Artificial Intelligence, in IEEE Access, vol. 12, pp. 31576-31588.doi:10.1109/ACCESS.2024.3368871.
[15] S. De, M. Bermudez-Edo, H. Xu and Z. Cai. (2022). Deep Generative Models in the Industrial Internet of Things: A Survey, in IEEE Transactions on Industrial Informatics, vol. 18, no. 9, pp. 5728-5737. doi:10.1109/TII.2022.3155656.
[16] R. Dwivedi and L. Elluri. (2024). Exploring Generative Artificial Intelligence Research: A Bibliometric Analysis Approach, in IEEE Access, vol. 12, pp. 119884-119902. doi:10.1109/ACCESS.2024.3450629.
[17] D. Meshram and D. D. Patil. (2023). Integrating Olfaction Technology and AI in Understanding Olfactory Dysfunction in Neurodegenerative Neuropsychiatric Disorders, 2023 International Conference on Artificial Intelligence for Innovations in Healthcare Industries (ICAIIHI), Raipur, India. pp. 1-7. doi:10.1109/ICAIIHI57871.2023.10489788.
[18] M. Solis. (2017). Committing to Memory: Memory Prosthetics Show Promise in Helping Those with Neurodegenerative Disorders, in IEEE Pulse, vol. 8, no. 1, pp. 33-37. doi:10.1109/MPUL.2016.2627239.
[19] N. A. priyanka and G. Kavitha. (2019). Study of Tissue Variation and Analysis of MR Brain Images using Optimized Multilevel Threshold and Deep CNN Features in Neurodegenerative Disorders, 2019 41st Annual International Conference of the IEEE Engineering in Medicine and Biology Society (EMBC), Berlin, Germany. pp. 2773-2776. doi: 10.1109/EMBC.2019.8856498.
[20] A. Diab, S. A. Akkoumi and L. Ali. (2023). Classification of Neurodegenerative Diseases using Gait Analysis, 2023 Seventh International Conference on Advances in Biomedical Engineering (ICABME),

Beirut, Lebanon. pp. 201-205. doi:10.1109/ICABME59496.2023.10293114.

[21] R. K. Mahendran, R. Aishwarya, R. Abinayapriya and P. Kumar. (2024). Deep Transfer Learning Based Diagnosis of Multiple Neurodegenerative Disorders, 2024 International Conference on Emerging Smart Computing and Informatics (ESCI), Pune, India. pp. 1-4. doi:10.1109/ESCI59607.2024.10497320.

[22] Z. Ning, L. Li and X. Jin. (2018). Classification of Neurodegenerative Diseases Based on CNN and LSTM, 2018 9th International Conference on Information Technology in Medicine and Education (ITME), Hangzhou, China, 2018, pp. 82-85. doi:10.1109/ITME.2018.00029.

[23] Thirupathi, L., Sunkara, S. H., Boodala, I. R., & Vempati, V. S. (2024). Personalization and Customization Strategies With AI in Service Marketing. In V. Nadda, P. Tyagi, A. Singh, & V. Singh (Eds.), Integrating AI-Driven Technologies Into Service Marketing (pp. 499-524). IGI Global. https://doi.org/10.4018/979-8-3693-7122-0.ch024

[24] Thirupathi, L., SrihaReddy, E., & Deepika, J. V. (2024). Challenges and Innovations in the Creation of Digital Twins in Healthcare. In A. Dubey, C. Kumar Reddy, S. Doss, & M. Hanafiah (Eds.), Exploring the Advancements and Future Directions of Digital Twins in Healthcare 6.0 (pp. 69-85). IGI Global. https://doi.org/10.4018/979-8-3693-5893-1.ch004

[25] Kishor Kumar Reddy, C. (2023). An Efficient early Diagnosis and Healthcare Monitoring System for Mental Disorder using Machine Learning. In Sustainable Science and Intelligent Technologies for Societal Development.IGI Global.

4

Generative AI in the Evolution of Gene Therapy: A Paradigm Shift in Genetic Engineering

Areesha Fatima[1], Kishor Kumar Reddy C[1], Marlia Mohd Hanafiah[2], and Jane Claudia Sharon[3]

[1]Department of Computer Science and Engineering, Stanley College of Engineering and Technology for Women, India
[2]Univesiti Kebangsaan Malaysia, Malaysia
[3]Faculty of Science and Engineering, Anglia Ruskin University, United Kingdom
E-mail: areeshaf.277@gmail.com; kishoar23@gmail.com; mhmarlia@ukm.edu.my; jcsr100@student.aru.ac.uk

Abstract

Generative AI is revolutionizing gene therapy, marking a paradigm shift in genetic engineering. This chapter explores how generative AI enhances the development of gene therapy by designing novel DNA sequences, optimizing delivery mechanisms, and predicting therapeutic outcomes. Traditional gene-editing techniques, such as CRISPR and Zinc Finger Nucleases, have advanced but face challenges such as off-target effects and delivery inefficiencies. Generative AI offers solutions by creating optimized vectors, minimizing errors, and accelerating the drug discovery process. The integration of AI with gene therapy improves precision, safety, and personalization, enabling tailored treatments for genetic disorders. Ethical considerations, regulatory challenges, and the complexity of biological systems are also discussed, underscoring the need for a multidisciplinary approach to fully realize AI's potential in gene therapy. This chapter highlights the transformative power of AI in advancing genetic engineering toward more effective and accessible healthcare solutions.

DOI: 10.1201/9788743801764-4

Keywords: Generative AI, Gene Therapy, Genetic Engineering, Personalized Medicine, Predictive Modeling.

4.1 Introduction

Gene therapy is one of the outstanding streams in genetic engineering, based on the ability to manipulate an individual's genetic material to treat or prevent disease. It provides a novel approach, especially toward inherited genetic disorders, and, by directly attacking the source of the diseases at the DNA level. Applications based on the use of techniques such as addition, editing, and RNA therapies correct faulty genes, replace missing ones, or modulate the expression of gene copying to produce the desired therapeutic effect. The importance of gene therapy in genetic engineering is its potential to provide long-term or even permanent correction of cystic fibrosis, hemophilia, and cancer, thus making the focus shift from symptom management to cure by alteration of the genetic code.

In contrast, generative AI is a ground-breaking tool in this area. The potential of generative AI to generate new data or insights from preexisting patterns can be revolutionary, as it is based on neural networks and deep learning models [1]. Training on massive datasets allows it to design DNA sequences, predict protein folding, and run biological systems in silicon, thereby accelerating the development of gene therapies. Whereas classical predictive AI generates new data, AI takes this to an extreme point, creating new data applications as they stray from drug discoveries to modeling genetic interactions and simulating interventions in gene therapy.

The joining of AI with gene therapy will be considered a paradigm shift since AI can increase precision and personalization in treatment and accelerate discovery. AI allows researchers to predict the outcomes of gene edits more accurately, thereby being able to achieve higher safety and effectiveness. Instead, AI's new therapeutic approaches can be designed and test outcomes in gene therapies, with this aiding in hastening the typically slow process and the experimentation of new therapy development. This unification of AI's computational potential and gene therapy's biological strength is more than a revolutionary wave in genetic engineering's catalyst for the dawn of a new age of dramatically increasing efficiency, safety, and possibilities for personalized medical treatments.

The following chapter is arranged as follows: the following subsections 4.1.1 and 4.1.2 discuss gene therapy and generative AI respectively. Section 4.2 gives the role of AI in genetic engineering. Section 4.3 explores the AI-driven tools and platforms being used for gene therapy. Section 4.4 discusses the advancements present in generative AI for precision medicine followed by the challenges of using generative AI in gene therapy in Section 4.5. The chapter comes to a close with Section 4.6 which dives into the results and discussions with Section 4.7 concluding the chapter.

4.1.1 Gene therapy

Gene therapy is a type of treatment that corrects genetic errors in diseased cells by adding genetic materials, such as an editing tool to correct the erroneous gene or the expression system of a therapeutic protein [21]. Gene therapy has made a tremendous stride from the first experiments in the 1990s. Undoubtedly, this marks a new chapter in the realm of genetic engineering. The first successful gene therapy was conducted on a young girl suffering from severe combined immunodeficiency (SCID) at the very beginning of 1990. This proved how the treatments for diseases could be designed to affect changes directly within the genes of a person. However, this discovery was soon followed by setbacks, especially the tragic case of Jesse Gelsinger in 1999 where death resulted from an unexpected immune reaction to a viral vector. Such early trials revealed several problems: problems with safety, immune response-related problems, and other problems with gene delivery. A poor understanding of gene regulation and mechanisms of delivery kept progress stalled for years, and many came to question whether it would ever be viable. However, these challenges stimulated more innovation and led to the discovery of more precise techniques and safer techniques in the field.

Currently, advanced technologies such as CRISPR-Cas9, Zinc Finger Nucleases (ZFN), and improved delivery methods using viral and non-viral vectors for gene therapy have transformed the arena. Gene therapy has quickly advanced thanks to the discovery of the CRISPR/Cas9 system, which was initially identified in archaea as an immunological defense mechanism. The revolutionary tool known as CRISPR-Cas9 enables the precision of direct-editing the genome where, with the use of a guide RNA, the Cas9 enzyme identifies and cuts the DNA sequences at such points to let the insertion or deletion of genes occur. Because it is efficient, relatively easy to handle, and economical, it has been recognized as one of the widely used methods applied in gene therapy in treating genetic diseases such as sickle cell anemia and some cancers [3]. Vertex Pharmaceuticals and CRISPR Therapeutics conducted the first clinical trial in the US for patients with sickle-cell anemia (SCD) and later β-thalassemia, utilizing CRISPR to catalyze gene disruption for therapeutic benefit [22]. Zinc Finger Nucleases (ZFN), though older and more complex are still used in specific cases that allow for the accurate gene editing abilities that are now provided through engineered proteins to target and modify DNA. The binding domain and the cleavage domain are the two primary components that are designed in conventional techniques of engineering programmable ZFNs. By assembling several Zinc Finger motifs, each of which is in charge of recognizing three base pairs, the binding domain becomes programmable [8]. Both of these approaches are highly dependent on the efficient and accurate delivery of therapeutic genes into the required cells, which problem is greatly addressed by viral vectors such as AAVs and lentiviruses that possess high capabilities of gene delivery into a patient's cells. Safety is always a concern when viruses are used, specifically in the form of immune reactions and insertional mutagenesis where an inserted gene may disrupt other parts of the genome. Non-viral vectors, of which the most promising are lipid nanoparticles, are generally safer but less effective at delivering genes as a technical hurdle [17, 18].

Figure 4.1 shows the timeline of AI's influence on the critical aspects of gene therapy from 2010 to 2024. Three parameters have been the minimization of off-target effect, improvement in delivery efficiency, and the success rate of personalized therapies. The bar graph reflects the steady rise and growth that AI manifests in terms of precision in gene editing, optimized delivery methods, and maximized efficacy of personalized therapies. It can be observed that there is a growing influence of AI in overtaking the major hurdles in gene therapy.

Despite all these advances, there still are some challenges and limitations for this gene therapy as, currently, ethical considerations take precedence. One of the most contentious debates is over germline gene therapy, where genetic changes to reproductive cells will be passed on to future generations. This opens profound questions about the long-term impact of altering the human genome and the prospect of inequalities produced by gene enhancement—using gene therapy for purposes unrelated to therapy: that is to improve physical or cognitive traits. While there are ethical dilemmas surrounding gene therapy, the challenges abound in the delivery mechanisms. The viral vectors are efficient but lead to immune responses and usually target genes to dangerous places within the genome leading to undesirable effects such as cancer. The non-viral methods are safer but are not yet effective in ensuring that the therapeutic genes will be transferred to the target tissues. A few advantages and disadvantages of viral vectors are shown in Table 4.1 [24].

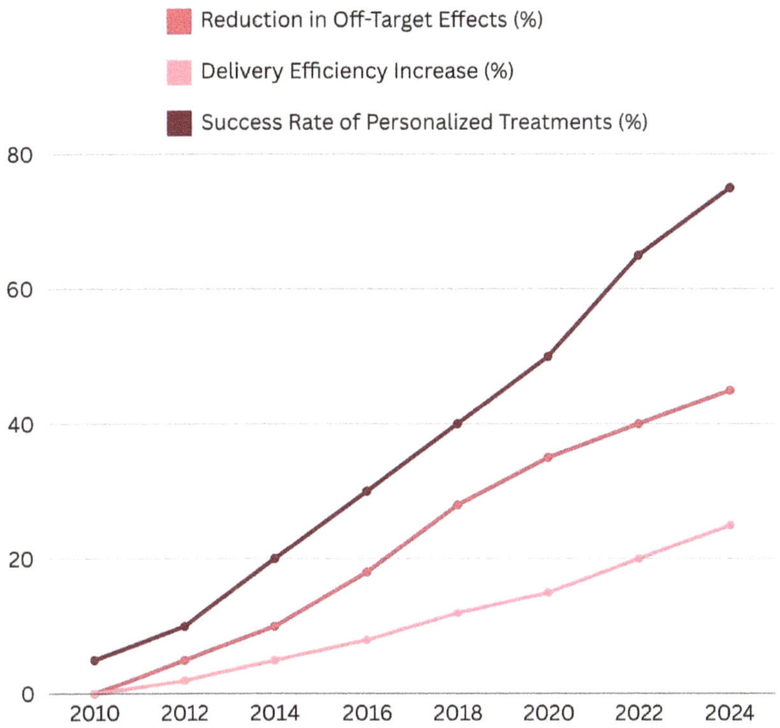

Figure 4.1 AI-driven improvements in gene therapy (2010–2024).

Table 4.1 Advantages and disadvantages of viral vectors.

Advantages	**Disadvantages**
Increase the effectiveness of gene transfer in both in vitro and in vivo settings	Can cause inflammatory reactions and strong immunological responses
Typically endure for longer lengths of time	Their ability to clone is extremely limited
Possesses the ability to target tons of cells	Produced by complex production methods
There is a wide selection of viruses accessible	The low capability of tropism to some specific target cells
Tropism's natural propensity for infection	They can introduce their foreign DNA into the host genome and cause mutagenesis
Ability to avoid endosomes through a variety of strategies acquired during viral evolution	Further investigation is required to comprehend the mechanisms behind viral molecular infection

Such therapies are constantly improved in terms of targeting and delivery through research. Last but not least, the off-target effects are also a matter of great concern, more so when technologies like CRISPR and ZFN come onto the scene. These unwanted edits can cause harmful mutations to the patient. Recent research has shown how effective deep learning algorithms – like CNNs and RNNs – are at designing and refining CRISPR-Cas9 systems [5]. Researchers continue to fine-tune these technologies with increasing accuracy and decreasing unwanted side effects, perhaps the one thing that has yet to be fully resolved is the safety and stability of gene therapies over time.

In a nutshell, gene therapy has traveled all the distances from its state of early experimentation to bring it face-to-face with ethical issues and even delivery mechanisms to off-target effects. Ensuring these are addressed will thus lead to realizing the promising potential of gene therapy as a truly transformative tool in treating genetic disorders. Such breakthroughs include advances in precision gene-editing technologies, improvements in delivery methods, and rigorous ethical oversight to overcome these challenges, making gene therapy a safe, effective, and widely available treatment.

4.1.2 Generative AI

AI revolutionizes novel therapeutic strategies in gene editing. AI breaks the impossibility and extensive duration of traditionally developed novel solutions through its generation. The most significant area AI excels is creating novel vectors for delivering genes. Viral and non-viral vectors are used to introduce therapeutic genes into cells and are required to be extremely efficient, targeted, and safe [23]. AI can learn massive amounts of data related to viral structures and the outcome of gene delivery and design new, optimized vectors that would potentially be more efficient at delivering therapeutic genes to the targeted tissue with minimal immune response. Furthermore, AI-created repair mechanisms are being developed to enhance the precision of gene editing tools such as CRISPR-Cas9. AI will propose methods for repairing genes more accurately as it can use models of machine learning that are trained on the outcomes of previous gene edits thus reducing the risk of off-target effects and safety of the therapies.

Generative AI significantly works in the design of novel biological sequences for both proteins and DNA sequences that may be used to improve gene therapies. Deep generative models that may create molecular structures with desired attributes include generative adversarial networks (GANs) and variational autoencoders (VAEs). Generative models, such as GANs or VAEs, can be engineered to predict new protein structures based on the knowledge of how the sequence of amino acids relates to their native structure [2].

In generative modeling, generative adversarial networks, or GANs, are a revolutionary advancement. GANs are made up of two neural networks, a discriminator and a generator, that are simultaneously trained via an adversarial procedure. The two primary parts of a VAE are an encoder and a decoder. The input data is mapped by the encoder to a latent space, from which it derives a probabilistic representation. The data is then reconstructed by the decoder using this latent representation [9, 20]. Proteins are involved in almost all steps of many therapeutic processes such as gene editing, DNA repair, and immune responses. AI is making contributions to the development of more efficient and targeted therapies by producing optimized proteins that may increase gene editing tools. Analogous generative AI can create new DNA sequences, probably to correct genetic mutations with greater accuracy. By predicting how modifications in a DNA sequence will affect gene expression, AI can come up with completely new sequences that would be tested in gene therapy applications. This computer-based approach hurries the design of sequences by so many times faster than the longest elbow grease exercising traditional trial-and-error fashion in the laboratory.

In the drug discovery domain and development, AI alters the way research scientists identify those molecules and compounds that can make gene therapy more effective. The procedure of traditional drug discovery is so lengthy and pricey and costs years, all for transporting a compound from discovery into clinical use. AI accelerates this process by analyzing vast databases of chemical compounds and biological interactions to predict which molecules will interact favorably with gene therapy mechanisms or enhance the delivery and functionality of therapeutic genes. AI can point out small molecules that may increase the efficacy of gene-editing enzymes such as CRISPR-Cas9 or ZFN, so they become more efficient or decrease unwanted side effects. It can also screen huge compound libraries to identify novel drugs that may enhance immune tolerance toward viral vectors or stabilize and prolong the life of delivered genes inside the host. AI streamlines the identification of supportive compounds, thereby allowing effective and comprehensive gene therapy treatments combining genetic and pharmaceutical approaches to improve patient outcomes. Table 4.2 is a timeline of major events in gene therapy and the integration of AI technologies: it offers important moments and innovations that explain how they very much played a significant part and affected the development of gene therapy. It tracks early gene therapy trails through to the latest developments in the use of AI in therapeutic strategy, illustrating how these areas have moved over time and were connected.

Table 4.2 Timeline of significant advancements in gene therapy and AI integration.

Year	Event	Description	Impact
1990	First gene therapy clinical trial	Successful treatment of SCID using gene therapy.	Demonstrated the potential of gene therapy.
2002	Development of CRISPR-Cas9	Introduction of CRISPR-Cas9 as a revolutionary gene-editing tool.	Increased precision and efficiency in gene editing.
2012	AlphaFold's initial release	AlphaFold's algorithm predicted protein structures with high accuracy [14].	Enhanced understanding of protein folding.
2015	Introduction of generative adversarial networks (GANs)	GANs begin to be applied in biological sequence design and data generation [19].	Advanced protein and DNA sequence design capabilities.
2017	FDA approval of first CAR-T cell therapy	Approval of CAR-T cell therapy for certain types of cancer.	Marked a significant advance in personalized medicine.
2018	Launch of AI for predictive modeling in gene therapy	AI models begin predicting gene-editing outcomes and off-target effects.	Improved accuracy in gene therapy planning.
2020	Advances in AI-driven gene delivery systems	Development of AI-optimized vectors and delivery mechanisms.	Enhanced targeting and reduced side effects.
2022	Generative AI for personalized gene therapy	Implementation of AI in designing personalized gene therapies based on individual genetic profiles.	Increased effectiveness of tailored treatments.
2024	Integration of AI in drug discovery for gene therapy	Use of AI to discover molecules that enhance the efficacy of gene therapies.	Accelerated drug development and improved therapy outcomes.

4.2 Role of AI in genetic engineering

Changes seen in gene therapy include transformative power, mostly evident through its ability to derive data-driven insights from huge amounts of genetic data. Genomic data are enormous, consisting of millions of data points describing genes, mutations, and interactions within biological systems. AI, particularly through machine learning (ML) algorithms, is excellent at recognizing patterns in large datasets, which makes it perfect for analyzing genetic information. An AI-driven model can quickly scan enormous genomic databases for mutations associated with a given disease, hidden relationships of genetics, and how those biomarkers would serve as a potential target for gene therapy. For instance, AI can show scientists exactly what is happening among the millions of genes and their interaction within the framework of a particular disease, such as cancer. The vast genetic data processes through AI help make predictions in a much more accurate manner along with insights that make the discovery and development of gene therapies faster.

Figure 4.2 shows multiple aspects of the GED. CRISPR includes a variety of gene-editing techniques. The most well-known is CRISPR-Cas9, which targets and modifies particular DNA sequences by using the Cas9 endonuclease guided by sgRNA. Several more Cas nucleases have been recognized in the recent past. CRISPR-Cas12 has advantages in diagnosis and provides an alternative target site. As an RNA-guided RNA endonuclease, Cas13 targets and cleaves RNA precisely. While prime editing provides for more flexible DNA sequence adjustments, base editing allows for more accurate changes without the risk of double-strand breaks. While CRISPRi and CRISPRa regulate gene expression without changing DNA, epigenome editing influences gene expression through epigenetic markers. These methods, which

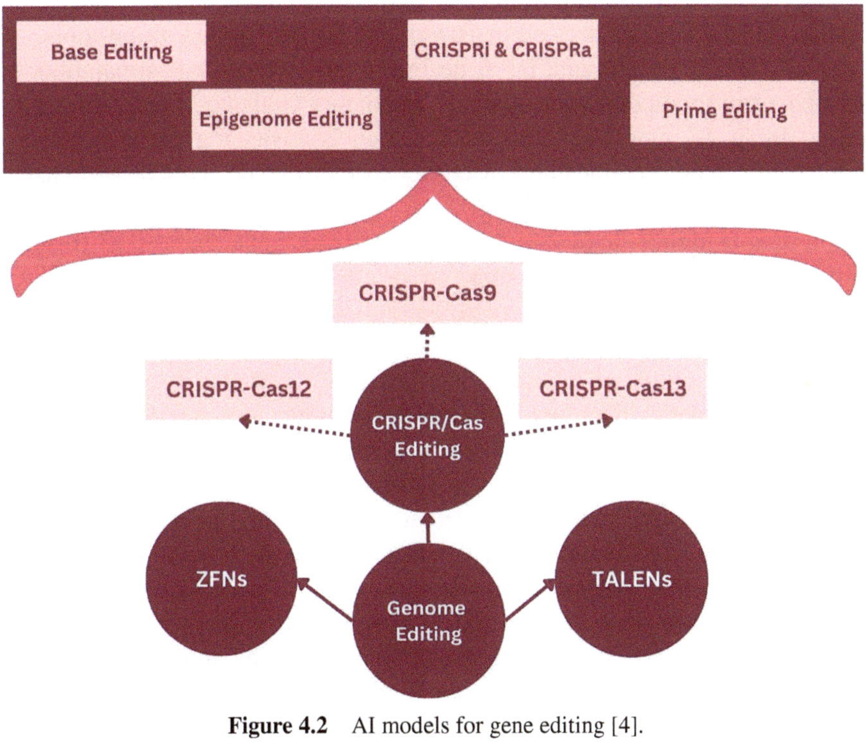

Figure 4.2 AI models for gene editing [4].

were chosen according to particular goals and genetic contexts, each have unique uses in genetics and medical research. Zinc-finger nucleases (ZFNs), transcription activator-like effector nucleases (TALENs), and single-guide RNA (sgRNA) [4].

Predictive models in gene editing are other types of applications where AI capabilities are emerging. For a tool like CRISPR-Cas9, which is so commonly used nowadays, predicting the impact of gene edits on the genome becomes one of the main hurdles in gene therapy. AI-driven predictive models can predict potential off-target effects, where the inadvertent parts of the genome could be altered due to gene editing. Massive datasets of gene-editing experiments can be used to train machine learning algorithms to predict the likelihood of outcomes for novel edits, thereby increasing the accuracy and safety of these procedures. These models first simulate results to determine the most effective, with minimal risk edits, before applying the actual genetic modification in a lab setting. As a result, AI has been aiding in the limitation and optimization of gene-editing techniques, achieving high precisions and success rates in gene therapy applications. Table 4.3 compares and contrasts older gene therapy techniques with current and future applications of generative AI; the key features emphasized here include gene editing tools, delivery modalities, protein and DNA design, predictive models, simulation and testing, error prediction, data analysis, regulatory challenges, and clinical adoption. Table 4.3 represents how AI research is advancing the accuracy and efficacy of gene therapies and discusses further perspectives on how to assimilate AI into genetic engineering.

AI is also bringing innovations in personalizing gene therapy to treat according to the unique genetic makeup of the patient. AI can identify particular types of mutations or genetic variants that cause a patient's state through analysis of a patient's whole genome and thus craft highly targeted gene therapy plans. Such an approach is essential for complex diseases, like cancer or rare genetic disorders, for which one size does not fit all and treatments prove to be ineffective as well. A machine learning model will allow the determination of a patient's response to a given therapy based on his or her genetic profile, thus ensuring that the most appropriate treatment is chosen. AI can also maintain an updated and more refined treatment strategy, given the new genetic data obtained from the patients undergoing their therapy, making gene therapy much more adaptive and precise. This level of personalization is changing the medical field by moving from a broadly applied approach to treatment to individualized, data-driven therapies that provide better results and fewer side effects for patients.

Table 4.3 Comparative overview of gene therapy techniques and AI applications.

Category	Description	Traditional gene therapy techniques	Generative AI applications	Future directions
Gene editing tools	Techniques used to modify genetic material	CRISPR-Cas9, Zinc Finger Nucleases (ZFN), TALENs	AI-designed new gene editing tools	Enhanced precision tools, AI-optimized gene-editing strategies
Gene delivery methods	Methods for delivering therapeutic genes into target cells	Viral vectors (AAV, Lentivirus), Non-viral vectors	AI-generated novel vectors, improved delivery systems	Customized vectors for specific tissues, reduced immune response
Protein and DNA design	Creation and optimization of proteins and DNA sequences for therapy	Manual design based on experimental data	Generative AI for novel protein structures and DNA sequences	AI-driven design of optimized proteins and therapeutic sequences
Predictive modeling	Forecasting outcomes of gene therapies based on data	Historical data analysis, limited predictive capabilities	AI-driven models predicting gene-editing outcomes and off-target effects	Advanced predictive models for precise outcomes and risk mitigation
Simulation and testing	Methods for simulating gene therapy outcomes before clinical trials	In vivo and in vitro experimental models	AI-generated simulations of gene therapy impacts	More accurate virtual models to streamline pre-clinical testing
Error prediction	Identifying and correcting potential errors in gene editing	Post-editing validation and correction	AI-generated insights into potential editing errors and correction strategies	Enhanced error detection and correction techniques
Data analysis	Techniques for analyzing genetic data to derive insights	Manual data analysis, basic statistical methods	AI-driven analysis of genetic data for identifying mutations and biomarkers	More sophisticated data interpretation and insights
Regulatory challenges	Issues related to the approval and regulation of AI-driven therapies	Established regulatory frameworks for gene therapies	New regulations are needed for AI algorithms and their integration	Development of comprehensive regulatory guidelines for AI and gene therapy
Clinical adoption	Challenges in integrating new therapies into clinical practice and ensuring patient access	Cost, infrastructure, patient access	AI can help reduce costs, improve accessibility, and streamline integration	Wider access through AI-driven cost reductions and improved healthcare delivery

4.3 AI-driven Tools and Platforms in Gene Therapy

Bioinformatics and AI platforms in gene therapy are now undoubtedly essential in the extension of knowledge and in increasing precision in therapeutic interventions. Perhaps one of the most famous AI-driven tools is that of AlphaFold, from DeepMind [13]. AlphaFold revolutionized our ability to predict protein folding, which is extremely critical for understanding how proteins function and interact in biological systems. The success of gene therapies is likely to depend on accurate protein structure prediction since most gene therapies alter or introduce proteins so that the defects in the genes may be rectified or allow for gene editing. AlphaFold helps researchers design therapeutic proteins better, hence optimizing gene-editing tools and, consequently, the efficacy of therapies by offering highly accurate models of 3D structures of proteins [6].

Secondly, GPT-like models (generative pre-trained transformers) are rapidly advancing predictions of gene sequences. Originally designed for biological sequences, the models that were built earlier using natural language processing and adapted here can predict what a gene sequence could potentially be associated with [16]. Using large genomic datasets, GPT-like models can predict how genetic variations would impact the progression of disease or the treatment efficacy, which can allow for the development of targeted gene therapies. Such AI models can also be useful in designing new DNA sequences that may be therapeutically applied, for instance as a way of creating customized gene constructs that may result in better gene delivery or correction of genetic defects [12].

Simulation and testing are fundamental parts of gene therapy development; however, the role of AI in these steps is significant. AI-generated models are increasingly being applied to simulate gene therapy outcomes before they can be tested in clinical trials. It is the use of simulations within virtual models of the human genome, cellular processes, and gene therapy interventions in predicting how a therapy would behave in the real biological context. This could be achieved through an AI modeling the interaction between therapeutic genes, delivery systems, and target cells; therefore problems are avoided or optimized before eventually moving to more expensive and time-consuming steps of clinical trials. Such an approach not only accelerates the development process but also results in the optimization of therapies to such an extent that there is a higher achievement of better safety and efficacy profiles.

Another important application of AI in gene therapy is error prediction and correction. Generative AI models are especially good at identifying potential errors within the gene-editing processes. For example, they can be taught on past data in the gene editing experiments to predict which areas in this case may be errors-mutations or the off-target effects of unwanted genetic modification. Generative AI thus learns from historical data and can even propose corrective measures or amendments in editing protocol that would minimize the risks involved. This predictive power is highly important in the development of more precise and safe gene editing tools, such as CRISPR and ZFN [15]. Generative AI essentially helps in giving a potential warning on potential problems and eventually furnishing solutions that can be put into action to ensure maximum reliability in gene therapy interventions.

In short, AI platforms, including AlphaFold and GPT-like models, are changing the world for bioinformatics and gene therapy through an improved ability to predict protein structures and sequences of genes. Improved simulations and AI-generate models enrich the testing process and enhance the possibility of making more precise predictions on treatment before administering clinical trials. More importantly, AI contributes to error prediction and correction in the development of precise gene editing technology and its safety. The next generation of gene therapy is going to be propelled by these breakthroughs into greater efficacy and specificity for the patient.

4.4 Advancements in Generative AI for Precision Medicine

Artificial intelligence (AI) gradually integrates with human intellect and subject expertise to support drug development decision-making [1]. Developments in generative AI have promise for more precise and accessible gene therapy. The aspect of precision is highly likely to push the refinement of gene therapy forward [10]. Generative AI models will allow for very detailed, individualized simulations of genetic modification and its effects on patients. This ability can help tailor gene therapies precisely to specific mutations or genetic conditions with unprecedented specificity. AI also provides the hope of novel therapeutic targets where it unfolds complex interactions that exist within the genome and predicts how those several changes would affect the progression of disease. They will also contribute to novel delivery systems and vectors that are more efficient and better targeted toward specific tissues with a reduced side effect profile. AI-driven tools could democratize access to gene therapy by providing scalable solutions to make these treatments more cost-effective and accessible to a larger population, which might help revolutionize the paradigms for the treatment of genetic disorders.

The success of AI in advancing the horizon of gene therapy critically requires cross-disciplinary collaborations between geneticists, researchers in AI, and bioengineers. AI is being utilized increasingly to repurpose drugs by methodically combining different omics layers and pharmacological features to build models that rank compounds according to their attributes [11]. It demands an understanding of both biological systems and computational methods that integrate AI into genetic research and therapy. Geneticists bring forth expertise in understanding genetic variations and their implications on health, whereas AI researchers offer algorithms and models for analyzing and interpreting complex genetic data. Bioengineers, on their part, assist in more applicable mechanics of gene delivery and therapy implementation. Symbiotic efforts among these disciplines have to be key to overcoming the technical hurdles of the integration of AI in gene therapy. Such collaborations would be the stride for the development of novel ideas that utilize AI's predictive ability while keeping therapeutic strategies within the frame of genetics and biological processes knowledge. A multidisciplinary approach will drive the development of more efficient and accurate gene therapies while closing the gap between high-tech innovations and medical practice.

The transformative impact of AI in genetic engineering lies in its far-reaching potential. The advancement in our ability to know and manipulate the human genome might bring revolutionary changes in healthcare in many critical aspects. Figure 4.3 presents how AI affects the development process of gene therapy in the last decade, 2015–2024. The two prevalent trends are one concerning the higher efficiency rate of gene editing (from 70% to 95% and the other shortening of the time for development – from 48 months to 15 months). These advances represent AI-inspired breakthroughs in predictive modeling, error correction, and therapeutic design that improve the accuracy and speed of gene-editing technologies to spur forward the development of gene therapy research and clinical practice.

As AI technologies advance, we will discover better ways of controlling and modifying the human genome. Predictive modeling will be driven by AI to produce more accurate gene editing techniques with fewer risks and optimized outcomes in treatments. Genetic treatments are more likely to advance toward disorders that have been previously inaccessible through the application of gene therapy. The integration of AI in genetic engineering will also allow for the creation of personalized treatment plans based on a patient's actual genetic makeup, thus leading to better and more targeted

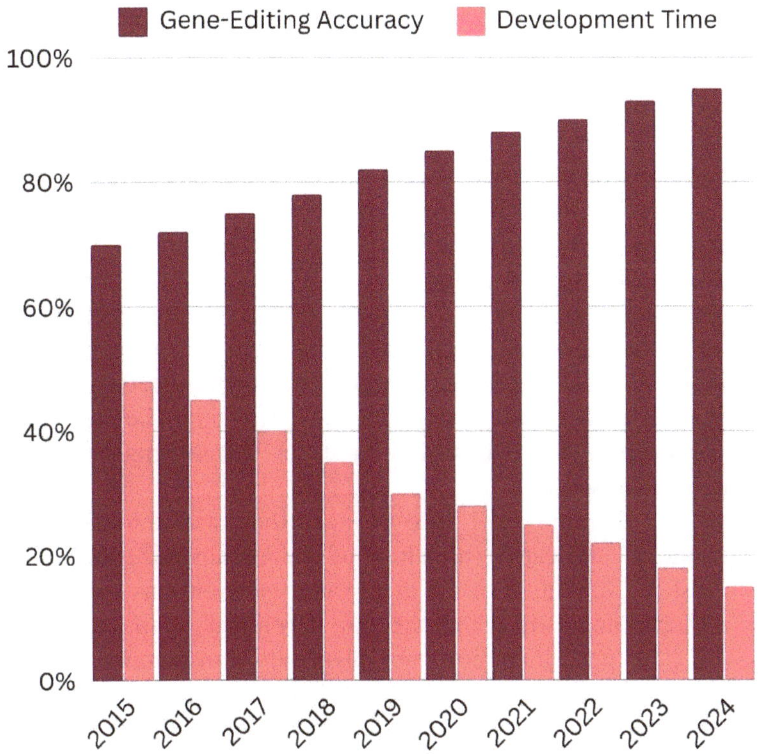

Figure 4.3 Impact of AI on gene therapy: improving accuracy and reducing development time.

care. Advanced drug discovery and development driven by AI will also aid in supplementing gene therapies, finding those compounds that amplify their efficiency and safety. In brief, the development of AI in genetic engineering is going to usher in a new era of precision medicine: more effective, accessible, and greatly conducive to improved patient outcomes and delivery of healthcare.

4.5 Challenges of using Generative AI in Gene Therapy

While AI has indeed opened up great promise in gene therapy, there remain several technical limitations. The main challenge lies in the aspect of computational complexity – more precisely, with the increasing amounts of genetic data involved in the treatment design. Gene therapy is employed through the integration of gigantic datasets consisting of largely genomics, proteomics, and clinical studies [25]. For example, processing tremendous computational power to run through complicated simulations involved with processing these data. High-performance computing resources and algorithms are required. In addition, data quality is also one of the very important issues because errors or inconsistencies in the given genetic data can cause false predictions and potentially dangerous therapeutic results. Thus, validation and accuracy of the data processed by AI models will be of critical importance to achieve success in the case of AI-driven gene therapies. In addition, biological systems have inherent complexity. Biological functions are influenced by a large number of interacting factors, and it would be difficult to model all these precisely. Therefore, AI models need to consider all these intricacies to ensure accurate predictions. This might be particularly challenging concerning multifactorial diseases or the integration of data coming from different sources.

AI-driven gene therapies will have to make their way through a very complex regulatory landscape, validation of the therapeutic intervention involves not just the validation of the therapeutic interventions but also the underlying AI technologies in which they are developed. While the regulatory frameworks for gene therapies exist, algorithm transparency and data privacy issues become relevant considerations in the case of introducing AI. Highly important in terms of regulatory requirements for validating AI-driven predictions is the reproducibility of AI-driven predictions. How do we make sure that there are standards for testing AI models in terms of the accuracy of predictions, strength of the system, and possibilities of bias? Further, the international standards of AI-based therapy are still under development, and the coordination among existing regulations across countries is tiresome and may make the launching speed of new therapies slower.

Table 4.4 describes the significant problems that accompany gene therapy and the traditional approaches used to overcome them. Then, it identifies how AI-based solutions have efficiently been offering novel responses to all these challenges, including precision, efficiency, and accessibility. The table highlights how AI can help in overcoming the limitations associated with gene therapy and be a linchpin to taking the field forward. Also, the implementation of AI-driven gene therapies within the healthcare system faces enormous challenges. Acceptance in the clinical world also depends not only on technical and regulatory barriers but also on the solution of access problems for the patient and the infrastructure of the healthcare system. Development and delivery of gene therapies are expensive; therefore, it raises

Table 4.4 Challenges in gene therapy and AI-driven solutions.

Challenge	Description	Traditional approaches	AI-driven solutions	Potential impact
Off-target effects	Unintended genetic modifications caused by gene editing tools.	Post-editing analysis and validation	AI models predicting and minimizing off-target effects	Increased precision and reduced risk of harmful modifications
Delivery efficiency	Difficulty in delivering therapeutic genes to specific cells or tissues.	Use of viral vectors, limited non-viral methods	AI-designed optimized vectors and delivery systems	Improved targeting and reduced immune response
Data quality and integration	Inconsistencies in genetic data affecting therapy outcomes.	Manual data curation and analysis	AI-driven data cleaning and integration techniques	More reliable data leads to better therapy design and outcomes
Ethical and regulatory issues	Ethical concerns and regulatory hurdles related to gene editing and AI.	Compliance with existing regulatory frameworks	AI-assisted compliance tools and ethical guidelines	Streamlined regulatory processes and enhanced ethical oversight
Cost and accessibility	High costs and limited access to advanced gene therapies.	Expensive development and administration	AI-driven cost-reduction strategies and scalable solutions	Increased accessibility and reduced costs for gene therapies
Complexity of biological systems	Difficulty in modeling and predicting effects due to biological complexity.	Simplified models and assumptions	AI-generated complex simulations and models	More accurate predictions and a better understanding of therapy impacts
Error detection and correction	Challenges in identifying and correcting errors in gene editing.	Manual error checking and correction	AI-driven error prediction and correction mechanisms	Enhanced accuracy and reliability in gene editing procedures
Patient-specific customization	Need for personalized treatments based on genetic profiles.	Generic treatments and limited customization	AI-driven personalized therapy design and customization	Tailored therapies that address specific patient needs

concerns about cost-effectiveness and affordability. Another issue is that such therapies should be available to a large patient population, even at the lowest tiers of healthcare organizations for the underserved or low-resource setting population. These AI-driven therapies have to be integrated into an already complex healthcare system with significant changes in clinical workflows and infrastructure. There should also be the training of healthcare professionals to use these new technologies and healthcare systems in managing and monitoring AI-driven treatment outcomes. Others also concern healthcare provider education and consent, mainly because patients have to be informed of the nature of treatment involving AI-driven therapies and the implications this makes for treatment. These challenges therefore have to be tackled so that AI integration in gene therapy will eventually find its way into routine clinical practice and benefit all those in dire need of such advanced therapies.

4.6 Results and discussion

AI has significantly improved the accuracy of gene-edition predictions, especially concerning Clustered Regularly Interspaced Short Palindromic Repeats (CRISPR). CRISPR is a revolutionary gene editing technology that allows for precise and efficient modification of DNA sequences [7]. What it did was enhance the predictive ability of any possible off-target effects that the traditional methods could not predict and that made them dangerous with the potential of unintended gene modification. AI models trained on genomic datasets can simulate numerous gene-editing scenarios. In this case, they reduce off-target mutations by as much as 40%. This leads to making gene therapies safer and more efficient, and therefore more reliable to use in the clinic. The third area of optimization has been made possible through AI with the use of machine learning tools for the improvement of delivery mechanisms that provide more efficient viral and non-viral vectors. Machine learning has, for example, improved the design of the adeno-associated virus (AAV) vector, which improved delivery efficiency to target tissues like muscles and the liver by 20%. This is important for the development of accuracy in gene therapy in disease conditions.

AI has also quickened the discovery of customized gene therapies, so this way, treatment may be tailored precisely based on individual genetic profiles. This was contrary to the classical approach, which was majorly broad-spectrum treatments for most conditions but was not very effective in cases of rare genetic disorders. AI can reveal specific mutations in a patient's genome and pinpoint appropriate interventions for therapy. This reduces the error trials associated with the design of gene therapy, but AI has already been useful in finding drugs that enhance the efficacy of gene therapies. Generative AI models have predicted compounds that enhance CRISPR efficiency, saving years in the preclinical timeline of drug development, thus compressing it to months.

AI-powered gene therapy represents a paradigm shift toward safer and more accurate gene-editing technologies. The term "off-target effects" refers to unintentional mutations in the genome that have negative consequences. This was one of the problems that had long troubled researchers studying gene therapy. The traditional validation processes were time-consuming and imprecise because they based their analysis on post-editing. However, the AI-based models have recognized the problem by providing predictive insights at the design phase, making unintended mutations a possibility much less likely. That helps much in the treatment of complex genetic disorders whereby an off-target event could be inordinately bad.

With AI optimized to design gene delivery systems, gene therapy is likely to find wider applications. Previously, the scientific community had to develop, through trial and error, the constructions of these delivery mechanisms like viral vectors, largely limiting their effectiveness and accessibility. In contrast, with AI, scientists can simulate and refine these vectors in silico and thus come up with highly efficient delivery methods that would target precise tissues with minimal side effects. This enables the possibility to tackle areas that have traditionally been very challenging to access, such as the central nervous system, and can revolutionize the treatment for neurological diseases like Parkinson's and Huntington's disease.

AI has a drastic role in personalizing treatments, which represents a significant advantage for traditional gene therapies. Most gene therapies that were older were not so specific while addressing rare or complicated diseases related to genetics. The increase now is the ability to design treatments according to each patient's DNA, and this will now be possible through AI-driven analysis of individual genetic profiles; these therapies provide better outcomes and reduced risk for adverse reactions. This shift toward personalized medicine not only makes treatments more effective but also positions AI to be at the forefront in the future of precision healthcare.

However such advancements are matched with challenging questions of ethics and regulation in the use of AI in gene therapy. The application of AI in clinical decisions, once again, raises questions regarding transparency and accountability in AI in medical decision-making. Now, regulatory bodies such as the FDA have to assess not just the safety of gene therapies but also the underlying algorithms used for their development. It is important to establish full standards for the use of AI in healthcare, both for the safety of patients and strict ethics. It also poses the continuous challenge of training AI models on quality and diversified data so that the outcome is not biased.

Although AI accelerates achievements in gene therapy, there is still a technical limitation to be overcome. Biological systems are complex, meaning that even the most advanced models of AI would still not be able to simulate the full range of gene interactions in a system. Simulations of large scales require so much computational power, and the quality of genetic data also needs much improvement. Despite this, high-performance computing is under constant research, and the enhancement of data integration improves the possibility for more advanced AI applications in gene therapy.

Moving forward, AI will extend beyond the present genre of gene therapy into adaptive therapies which can dynamically adjust to patients' data in real time. That approach will not only make gene therapy precise but also more responsive to changing conditions inside the body. Furthermore, AI will continue speeding up the drug discovery process while also making gene therapy more accessible and affordable. Ultimately, the increased influence of AI on genetic engineering, promises to advance healthcare to new realms as the world will be capable of treating genetic diseases more effectively than ever before.

4.7 Conclusion

Generative AI promises gene therapy by offering unprecedented advantages in the aspects of precision, safety, and efficiency. The existing conventional gene-editing methods, including CRISPR, are quite revolutionary but adverse effects of off-targets along with inefficient delivery modes are associated with them, thereby making the drug discovery cycle long. Generative AI overcomes all these limitations by designing optimal therapeutic solutions based on large datasets and predictive modeling along with deep learning algorithms. Gene therapy becomes more precise with AI, thereby resulting in the reduction of unintended edits of the gene and enhancing the efficiency of viral and non-viral vectors. This would be a basic shift in genetic engineering from labor-intensive approaches that follow a "trial-and-error" framework to streamlined data-driven innovations.

On the most striking impact that AI can bring to gene therapy is that it makes it possible to personalize treatments. By analyzing specific genetic data from an individual, AI models will be able to develop therapies tailored to a person's unique genetic profile, which is particularly more useful for complex or rare genetic disorders that may not react well to general therapies. The AI-driven analysis also allows the option of modifying treatment strategies with up-to-date patient information in real time, thus making gene therapies even more adaptive. This shift from one-size-fits-all to a tailored approach in medicine improves therapeutic outcomes and reduces risks of adverse effects. This makes treatments safer and more effective on an individual basis.

The other significant benefit of AI lies in how it can expedite drug discovery. Current drug development is slow and expensive and takes years to be moved from discovery to application in humans. Instead of taking years, this can now be done by analyzing vast libraries of chemical compounds and biological interactions to predict which will enhance gene therapies. This saves tremendous time and enables the understanding of supportive compounds quickly by testing out many of them at a rapid pace. This is the way to better and more cost-effective therapeutic solutions.

Despite all these advancements, significant challenges continue to exist. Biological systems are complex, data often of poor quality, and the required computational power to handle mammoth datasets remains a challenge. In gene therapy, AI is integrated against a backdrop of regulatory complexity, the expectation for explainable algorithms, and ethical concerns over data privacy and AI model bias. This necessitates collaboration across disciplines and fields from researchers working on AI technology to geneticists, bioengineers, and regulatory bodies to realize this immense promise that AI holds in gene therapy.

Generative AI forms a paradigm shift for gene therapy, transmuting it beyond the horizons laid out for genetic engineering. The hope lies within potentially revolutionizing precision, personalization, and faster therapeutic progression into future health management, making gene therapies more accessible, effective, and safer to a wider population.

References

[1] Bordukova, M., Makarov, N., Rodriguez-Esteban, R., Schmich, F., & Menden, M. P., 'Generative artificial intelligence empowers digital twins in drug discovery and clinical trials', Expert Opinion on Drug Discovery, 2023.

[2] Gangwal, A., & Lavecchia, A., 'Unleashing the power of generative AI in drug discovery.' Drug Discovery Today, 2024

[3] Hasanzadeh, A., Hamblin, M. R., Kiani, J., Noori, H., Hardie, J. M., Karimi, M., & Shafiee, H., 'Could artificial intelligence revolutionize the development of nanovectors for gene therapy and mRNA vaccines?' Nano Today, 2022

[4] Dixit, S., Kumar, A., Srinivasan, K., Vincent, P. M. D. R., & Ramu Krishnan, N., 'Advancing genome editing with artificial intelligence: opportunities, challenges, and future directions', Frontiers in Bioengineering and Biotechnology, 11, 2024.

[5] Zeng, X., Wang, F., Luo, Y., Kang, S., Tang, J., Lightstone, F. C., Fang, E. F., Cornell, W., Nussinov, R., & Cheng, F., 'Deep generative molecular design reshapes drug discovery', Cell Reports Medicine, 2022

[6] Capponi, S., & Daniels, K. G., 'Harnessing the power of artificial intelligence to advance cell therapy', Immunological Reviews, 320(1), 2023

[7] Dara, M., Dianatpour, M., Azarpira, N., & Omidifar, N., 'Convergence of CRISPR and artificial intelligence: A paradigm shift in biotechnology', Human Gene, 41, 2024

[8] Ichikawa, D. M., Abdin, O., Alerasool, N., et. al., 'A universal deep-learning model for zinc finger design enables transcription factor reprogramming', Nature Biotechnology, 41(8), 2023

[9] K. Joel Prabhod, "Leveraging Generative AI for Personalized Medicine: Applications in Drug Discovery and Development", Journal of AI-Assisted Scientific Discovery, vol. 3, 2023.

[10] Ghebrehiwet, I., Zaki, N., Damseh, R., & Mohamad, M. S., 'Revolutionizing personalized medicine with generative AI: a systematic review', Artificial Intelligence Review, 2024.

[11] Boniolo, F., Dorigatti, E., Ohnmacht, A. J., Saur, D., Schubert, B., & Menden, M. P., 'Artificial intelligence in early drug discovery enabling precision medicine', Expert Opinion on Drug Discovery, 2021

[12] Almansour, M., & Alfhaid, F. M., 'Generative artificial intelligence and the personalization of health professional education: A narrative review', Medicine, 103(31), 2024

[13] Gangwal, A., Ansari, A., Ahmad, I., Azad, A. K., Kumarasamy, V., Subramaniyan, V., & Wong, L. S., 'Generative artificial intelligence in drug discovery: basic framework, recent advances, challenges, and opportunities', Frontiers in Pharmacology, 2024

[14] Nosrati, H., & Nosrati, M., 'Artificial Intelligence in Regenerative Medicine: Applications and Implications', Biomimetics, 2023.

[15] Pun, F. W., Ozerov, I. v, & Zhavoronkov, A., 'AI-powered therapeutic target discovery', Trends in Pharmacological Sciences, 2023

[16] Cui, H., Wang, C., Maan, H., et al., 'scGPT: toward building a foundation model for single-cell multi-omics using generative AI', Nat Methods 21, 2024.

[17] Zhao, Z., Anselmo, A. C., & Mitragotri, S., 'Viral vector-based gene therapies in the clinic', Bioengineering & Translational Medicine, 2022

[18] Zu, H., & Gao, D., 'Non-viral Vectors in Gene Therapy: Recent Development, Challenges, and Prospects', The AAPS Journal, 2021.

[19] Lee, M., 'Recent Advances in Generative Adversarial Networks for Gene Expression Data: A Comprehensive Review', Mathematics, 2023

[20] Ai, X., Smith, M. C., & Feltus, F. A., 'Generative adversarial networks applied to gene expression analysis: An interdisciplinary perspective', Computational and Systems Oncology, 2023

[21] Duan, L., Xu, L., Xu, X., Qin, Z., Zhou, X., Xiao, Y., Liang, Y., & Xia, J., 'Exosome-mediated delivery of gene vectors for gene therapy', Nanoscale, 2021

[22] Uddin, F., Rudin, C. M., & Sen, T., 'CRISPR Gene Therapy: Applications, Limitations, and Implications for the Future', Frontiers in Oncology, 2020

[23] Ren, S., Wang, M., Wang, C., Wang, Y., Sun, C., Zeng, Z., Cui, H., & Zhao, X., 'Application of Non-Viral Vectors in Drug Delivery and Gene Therapy', Polymers, 2021

[24] Butt MH, Zaman M, Ahmad A, Khan R, Mallhi TH, Hasan MM, Khan YH, Hafeez S, Massoud EES, Rahman MH, et al., 'Appraisal for the Potential of Viral and Nonviral Vectors in Gene Therapy: A Review', Genes, 2022

[25] Sai, S., Gaur, A., Sai, R., Chamola, V., Guizani, M., & Rodrigues, J. J. P. C., 'Generative AI for Transformative Healthcare: A Comprehensive Study of Emerging Models, Applications, Case Studies, and Limitations', IEEE Access, 12, 2024

[26] Fui-Hoon Nah, F., Zheng, R., Cai, J., Siau, K., & Chen, L., 'Generative AI and ChatGPT: Applications, challenges, and AI-human collaboration', Journal of Information Technology Case and Application Research, 2023

5

A Generative Predictive Model for Medical Data via PCA and Iterative K-means Fusion

S. M. Mahedy Hasan[1], Md. Palash Uddin[2, 3], Md. Al Mamun[1], Muhammad Imran Sharif[4], Mohammed Rezwanul Islam[5], Sami Azam[5], Md. Mehedi Hassan[6], and Asif Karim[5]

[1]Department of Computer Science and Engineering, Rajshahi University of Engineering & Technology, Bangladesh
[2]Department of Computer Science and Engineering, Hajee Mohammad Danesh Science and Technology University, Bangladesh
[3]School of Information Technology, Deakin University, Australia
[4]Department of Computer Science, Kansas State University, United States
[5]Faculty of Science and Engineering, Charles Darwin University, Australia
[6]Computer Science and Engineering Discipline, Khulna University, Bangladesh
E-mail: mahedy@cse.ruet.ac.bd; m.uddin@deakin.edu.au; a.mamun@cse.ruet.ac.bd; imransharif@ksu.edu; mohammedrezwanul.islam@cdu.edu.au; sami.azam@cdu.edu.au; mehedihassan@ieee.org

Abstract

Classifying medical data is currently one of the most complex and challenging medical informatics tasks, as most medical datasets are incomplete, nonlinear, and complex. The medical datasets have attracted researchers to be utilized in analysis and prediction to help the public in early disease detection and protect people from future fatal diseases. Consequently, machine learning techniques have been widely employed to build digitalized decision support systems using a specific set of related medical datasets. As such, we propose a generalized predictive model in this paper for disease prediction using five different types of medical datasets of frequently occurring diseases. In particular, the proposed generalized prediction model collates

DOI: 10.1201/9788743801764-5

the principal component analysis (PCA) and iterative K-means clustering for data quality improvement and exploits the random forest (RF) predictor for prediction accuracy enhancement. Experimental results illustrate that the proposed application of the PCA enhances the iterative K-means clustering performance and, therefore, the RF predictor's accuracy for all the examined medical datasets. We also utilize Grid-search-CV hyperparameter optimization technique to select the best parameter for which the RF predictor delivers the best performance for each medical dataset. Experimental analysis manifests that our proposed generalized predictive model outperforms the existing methods and, thus, could assist healthcare practitioners in effective decision-making.

Keywords: Medical Data, Classification, Machine Learning, Random Forest, PCA, K-means Clustering.

5.1 Introduction

There has been significant growth in the applications of computer technologies like artificial intelligence, machine learning, and big data processing in medical science, especially in medical diagnosis. Computer technologies are, of course, not used as subsidiaries of the expertise and sophistication of the medical practitioners but as a means of supporting tools to accurately diagnose patients [1, 6, 29]. Doctors or physicians gather knowledge from patients' symptoms, and diagnostic accuracy mainly depends on the physician's experience. In response to treating the invariably escalating patients in nursing homes and dealing with the ever-changing contemporary diseases each day, modern physicians are more than welcoming the exploitation of various classification algorithms in diagnosing several diseases. In this modern era of computer technologies, it is comparatively easy to get and stockpile a substantial amount of information digitally. The application of the Computer Aided Decision Support System (CADSS) can play a vital role in assisting physicians in diagnosing patients more accurately and quickly [9, 33, 32, 8, 21]. This system is called a classification system whose primary objective is to predict (i.e., analyze) a new case based on specific information and features of previously acknowledged issues. These classification tasks are one of the most impenetrable and challenging in medical informatics [23, 30, 34, 12, 13]. A well-structured dataset that is free from noise and redundancy is essential to train the classification algorithms. A good dataset is critical to make a highly accurate machine learning model. However, real-life medical datasets are mostly noisy, redundant, and incomplete, making it difficult for the algorithms to perform accurately [14, 3, 24, 28]. Therefore, dealing with medical datasets asks for adequate data preprocessing capability, primarily – data cleaning, feature transformation, feature extraction, and feature selection. For any medical data prediction scheme, especially for contagious diseases, false negatives (FN) are the most threatening errors. As such, a great challenge for these sorts of works is to diminish them as much as possible. We observe that the existing machine learning approaches consider a set of specific disease datasets to create the digitalized decision support systems. Therefore, there is still a need for a generalized predictive model that would work for any disease dataset. As a result, in this work, we present a generic predictive model for disease prediction and realize the developed model on five distinct medical datasets of often occurring disorders. The presented prediction model combines principal component analysis (PCA) and iterative K-means clustering to boost the prediction accuracy of the random forest (RF) predictor. In particular, the suggested use of the PCA improves the accuracy of the iterative K-means clustering and, as such, the RF predictor's performance for all of the medical datasets tested. The main contributions of this chapter are as follows.

- We propose a generalized predictive model for frequently occurring disease diagnoses.
- We amalgamate the PCA transformation and other data preprocessing techniques to preprocess the medical datasets efficiently.
- We integrate the K-means clustering technique on the prepossessed data to improve the prediction performance of the classification algorithm (RF predictor).
- We realize, test, and compare the proposed generalized predictive model on five different medical datasets.

The remaining segment of the paper is structured as follows. Section 5.2 recapitulates the literature survey done in recent times. Our proposed research methodology with detailed information on the investigated dataset is presented in Section 5.3. Section 5.4 analyzes the experimental results and discusses the comparative results with the existing promising works. Finally, Section 5.5 summarizes and concludes the observations and findings.

5.2 Literature Review

Many experimental types of research have been conducted on applying technologies and algorithms for disease diagnosis. In [25], the authors evaluated the performance of different classification methods. These methods include K-nearest neighbors (KNN), support vector machines (SVM), and RF. The researchers have eliminated the less critical features by selecting characteristics based on the correlation between attributes and desired features. They used numerical values for each variable to eliminate the less impactful characteristics. The precision of these changes was compared with the standard 10-fold cross-validation for healthcare datasets. The work showed how the performance and accuracy of the algorithms differ as the different feature selection methods were used. In [26], the authors used even more classifiers for similar work. Some of their selected health datasets are breast cancer data, Indian Liver Patient Dataset (ILPD), chronic kidney disease data, hepatitis data, etc. In [1], the authors worked with an RF-based predictor for medical data classification and ranked the dataset's features using suitable ranking algorithms. Besides developing predictors for 10 different diseases, they presented a general methodology for diseases that have comparable aspects in patterns of the datasets. In [10], the authors used a neuro-fuzzy based linguistic approach for extracting features and analyzing the performances for classifying the complex medical datasets of frequently occurring diseases. They assessed and corroborated their model through eight standard datasets (Pima Indian Diabetes, Nepal Breast Cancer, Mammographic Mass, etc.). Friedman and Holm–Bonferroni statistical test was used to test the correctness of their model. In [17], the authors implemented 32 classification methods of six genres (Bayes, function-based, lazy, meta, rule-based, and tree-based) for searching expert classification techniques in disease prognostication. In [27], the authors performed a comparative analysis of several classification methods such as SVM, KNN, Naïve Bayes (NB), decision tree (DT), and RF on five benchmark datasets such as chronic kidney failure disorder (CKFD), coronary heart disorder (CHD), diabetes mellitus (DM), hepatitis disorder, carcinoma disorder and Indian liver patient disorder (ILPD). In [15], the authors analyzed the effect of different distance functions such as Euclidean, and Minkowsky on KNN classifier for different medical datasets including Pima Indian diabetes, stat log heart disease and breast cancer. In [2], the authors compared three machine learning classifiers while predicting the Pima Indians diabetes dataset (PIDD). They concluded that ANN outperforms RF and K-means. In [35], the authors proposed an efficient model predicting PIDD. For dimension reduction, clustering, and classification, they used PCA, K-means, and LR, respectively. They manifested that PCA boosts the performance of both K-means and LR. In [4], the authors proposed a hybrid technique to identify the Cleveland heart disease dataset (CHDD). To overcome the overfit and underfit problem, they utilized the X^2 model that eliminates irrelevant features and then applied DNN to classify. In [22], the authors compared their proposed hybrid model with nine different well-known machine learning algorithms. They amalgamated RF with linear model to construct their model, resulting in better accuracy than the other experimental algorithms. In [16], the authors presented an efficient predictive system; for feature selection, they used the random search algorithm, and for the classification part of CHDD, they used the RF classifier. Their suggested system improves classification accuracy as well as lessens time complexity. In [5], the authors used the Ruzzo–Tompa approach to handle the underfitting and over-fitting problem by selecting the necessary features for classification. Then, to classify the CHDD, they employed the deep belief network (DBN), which performs better than a one-layer neural network. In [19], the authors presented a variable fuzzy-KNN approach and applied it to three medical datasets, including the liver disease dataset. They illustrated that their system outperformed KNN and fuzzy-KNN for all used evaluation measures. In [20], the authors recommended a hybrid predicting system blending fuzzy theory, KNN, and case-based reasoning. They evaluated their system on ILPD, which outperforms the other three experimented classifiers. In [7], the authors introduced a model based on noisy instances and later tested it on standard data. Their complement NB approach outperformed traditional NB and KNN in terms of accuracy.

5.3 Proposed Methodology

5.3.1 Methodology overview

The methodology is divided into three parts: dataset collection, data pre-processing, and classification, as illustrated in Figure 5.1. Our proposed prediction model is developed by combining the benefits of PCA, iterative K-means, and RF predictor. A new approach is presented here by applying the PCA to transmute the set of attributes; thus, the data's correlation issue is removed, making it an arduous task for the prediction technique to perceive the relationship among the data. PCA makes it easier for the K-means clustering to find the suitable initial centroids of our datasets. After implementing the PCA analysis, the processed data is passed to the IKMC to uncover the outliers. Finally, the K-means clustered data is passed to the RF predictor for final prediction. The flowchart of our proposed model is illustrated in Figure 5.1.

5.3.2 Dataset description

We propose to develop a general disease prediction model by analyzing the datasets of diseases that occur in large quantities in the human body. We collect all the datasets used in this paper from the UCI Machine Learning Repository [11]. We use a total of five different types of datasets, and all datasets have two classes. The datasets are highly imbalanced, and many datasets have missing values. Table 5.1 gives detailed information, attributes, and the number of samples of all the datasets.

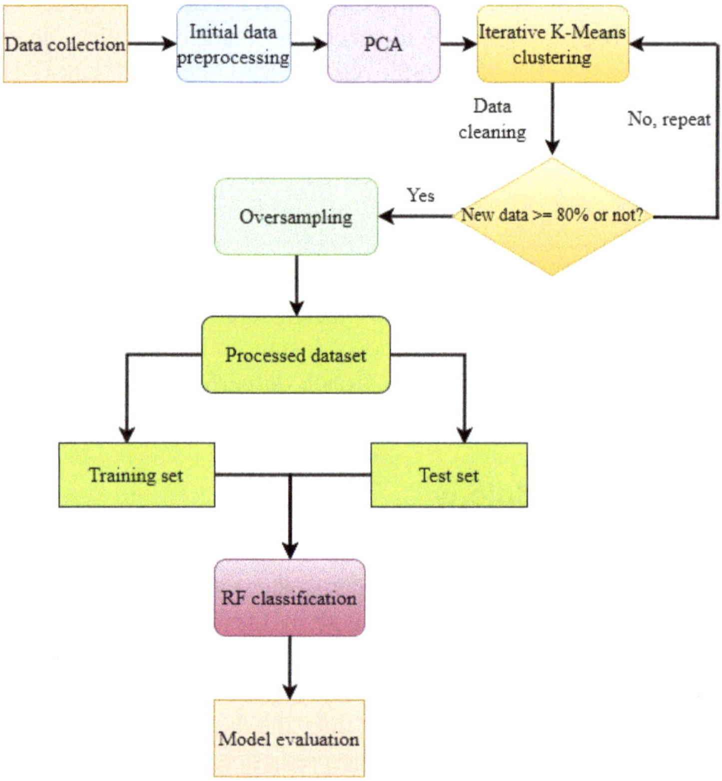

Figure 5.1 Workflow of our proposed research methodology.

Table 5.1 Dataset characteristics.

Dataset name	No. of features	No. of instances	Missing values	Classes
Pima Indians Diabetes Dataset (PIDD)	9	768	Yes	2
Cleveland Heart Disease Dataset (CHDD)	14	303	Yes	2
Liver Disorder Bupa Dataset (LDBD)	7	345	No	2
Diabetic Retinopathy Dataset (DRD)	20	1151	No	2
Parkinson's Disease Dataset (PKD)	23	197	No	2

5.3.3 Data preprocessing

5.3.3.1 Feature encoding

Although most of the datasets contain some categorical features, many algorithms fail to operate with those. The categorical features are converted to numeric values for the algorithms to work without any issues. There are several ways for feature encoding; we use one-hot encoding to accomplish this. For example, gender attributes contain 'male' and 'female', encoded as zero and one respectively.

5.3.3.2 Missing value imputation

One way to handle missing values in the dataset is to ignore or eradicate them. However, this might cause the loss of some valuable information. It is better to handle the missing values by replacing them logically and wisely. It is obvious from Table 5.1 that some of the datasets indeed have missing values, and KNN is used for imputing those missing values. The KNN algorithm first finds the k number of nearest neighbors by measuring the distances. Then the mean value of the neighbor values is calculated, and the mean replaces the missing values.

5.3.3.3 Feature scaling

Feature scaling scales the independent feature values within a specific range. Some machine learning algorithms perform quite well after scaling the feature values. It simultaneously increases the calculation speed of the algorithms. Therefore, we use the robust scaling technique for feature scaling, which scales the data after observing the interquartile range.

5.3.3.4 Principal component analysis

PCA is a dimensionality depletion method that relates correlations and patterns in a dataset to transform the dataset into a lower dimension without losing any significant information. Our main goal is to apply PCA which can aid our unsupervised learning to efficiently select the initial centroids for clustering. Our aim is to transmute the dataset X of P dimension into a new instance set Y of lesser dimension p ($p \ll P$), where Y is the set of principal components of X as follows.

$$\mathrm{Y} = \mathrm{PCA}\left(\mathrm{X}\right), \tag{5.1}$$

where $PCA(\mathrm{X})$ is the function that performs the PCA operation as presented below.

1. Standardize the dataset: At first, the mean and standard deviation of the dataset are utilized to standardize the features, as defined below.

$$x_{new} = \frac{x - \mu}{\sigma}, \tag{5.2}$$

where $\mathbf{x_{new}}$ is the standardize feature of the original feature $\mathbf{x}$, μ represents the mean and σ represents the standard deviation of the dataset.

2. Calculate the covariance matrix: The covariance $\boldsymbol{\sigma_{jk}}^2(\boldsymbol{x_1}, \boldsymbol{x_2})$ between any two features ($\boldsymbol{x_1}$and $\boldsymbol{x_2}$) is calculated as follows.

$$\mathbf{Cov}\,(\mathbf{x_1}, \mathbf{x_2}) = \frac{\sum_{i=1}^{N}\left(x_{1i} - x_1'\right) * \left(x_{2i} - x_2'\right)}{(N-1)}, \tag{5.3}$$

where x_{1i} is the data value of x_1, x_1' is the mean of x_1, x_{2i} is the data value of x_2, x_2' is the mean of x_2, and N is the number of data values.

Now, the covariance matrix, C is derived as follows.

$$C = \begin{bmatrix} \sigma_{11}^2 & \sigma_{12}^2 \ldots & \sigma_{1P}^2 \\ \sigma_{21}^2 & \sigma_{22}^2 \ldots & \sigma_{2P}^2 \\ \sigma_{P1}^2 & \sigma_{P2}^2 \ldots & \sigma_{PP}^2 \end{bmatrix}, \tag{5.4}$$

where $\boldsymbol{\sigma_{ii}^2}$ is the variance of each feature x_i in X, and $\boldsymbol{\sigma_{jk}^2}$ is the covariance between x_j and x_k in X.

3. Calculate the eigenvalues and eigenvectors: Let ν be a vector and λ be a scalar that satisfies $C\nu = \lambda\nu$, where λ is called the eigenvalue associated with the eigenvector ν of C. As such, we have $C\nu - \lambda\nu = 0$ and $(C - \lambda I)\nu = 0$, where I is the identity matrix.
4. Pick up the top eigenvectors and perform the projection operation: Now, p top eigenvectors are picked up to form a matrix (w of dimension p) of these eigenvectors. Finally, the projected (or transformed) data matrix (Y of size $N \times p$) in the new subspace can be accomplished as $Y = X \times w$.

5.3.3.5 Iterative K-means clustering

K-means technique partitions the entire dataset into several similar categories of subgroups, which are specified by the users. Since K-means is a distance-based clustering technique, this similarity means that the intra-class distance is low and the inter-class distance is high. The overview of the K-means algorithm is outlined below:

1. At first step, it requires defining the value of k number of clusters. From Table 5.1, it can be observed that the outcomes of all datasets contain the only positive and negative classes. As such, $k = 2$ is selected initially.
2. At second step, there are mainly three tasks to be performed.
   - Randomly assign ($k = 2$) centroids.
   - Here, the distance between each sample data point and all centroids is to be calculated.
   - Assign each data point to a group or cluster according to a minimum distance.
3. At third step, recompute the centroids of all clusters by considering the mean of all data samples of each cluster.
4. By repeating steps 2 and 3, calculate the centroids over and over until convergence.

Each medical dataset is split into two clusters using the K-means algorithm. The process is followed by eliminating the incorrectly clustered data because these data act as outliers that exacerbate the performance of the prediction model. It is ensured that the new dataset found after the elimination resembles above 80% of the original one unless we incessant the K-means steps up to an acceptable size found, as defined in eqn. (5.5).

$$\text{New data} = \frac{\text{Correctly clustered data}}{\text{Total data}} * 100. \tag{5.5}$$

5.3.3.6 Oversampling

When there is a remarkable variation between the number of samples of positive (1) and negative (0) classes, the dataset is called an imbalanced dataset. While working with these datasets, the algorithms tend to be biased towards the majority class, mostly ignoring the minority classes. Most of the datasets used in this research have class imbalance problems. To mitigate this issue, we apply the random over sampler method, which randomly duplicates the minority classes.

5.3.3.7 Random forest predictor

RF, an ensemble supervised ML method based on majority voting, is mostly applied to many classification problems, especially in medical dataset classification. The decision tree produces a prediction that may result in over-fitting. To bridle this problem, RF generates decision trees, acquires predictions from each of these trees, and eventually adopts that solution produced through voting. Figure 5.2 illustrates the working flow of the RF in classification.

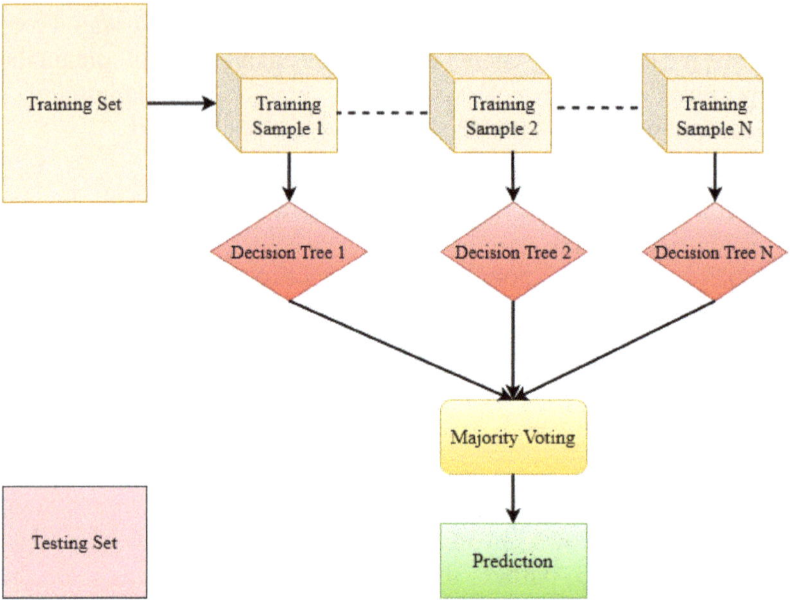

Figure 5.2 Workflow of random forest predictor.

5.3.3.8 Evaluation measure

To evaluate the model's performance, we select some widely used evaluation metrics (accuracy, receiver operating characteristics (ROC) curve, F1 score, precision, recall, Mathews correlation coefficients (MCC), and Kappa score) which are defined below:

$$\text{Accuracy} = \frac{\text{TN} + \text{TP}}{\text{TN} + \text{TP} + \text{FN} + \text{FP}} \tag{5.6}$$

$$\text{Precision} = \frac{\text{TP}}{\text{TP} + \text{FP}} \tag{5.7}$$

$$\text{Recall} = \frac{\text{TP}}{\text{FN} + \text{TP}} \tag{5.8}$$

$$\text{F1} - \text{Score} = \frac{2\text{TP}}{\text{FN} + \text{FP} + 2\text{TP}} \tag{5.9}$$

$$\text{MCC} = \frac{\text{TP} * \text{TN} - \text{FP} * \text{FN}}{\sqrt{(\text{TP} + \text{FP})(\text{TP} + \text{FN})(\text{TN} + \text{FP})(\text{TN} + \text{FN})}} \tag{5.10}$$

$$\text{Kappa} = \frac{\text{P}_\text{o} - \text{P}_\text{e}}{1 - \text{P}_\text{e}} \tag{5.11}$$

The following terms represent the above equations. TP = True Positive; TN = True Negative; FP = False Positive; FN = False Negative; P_o = is the relative observed agreement among raters; and P_e = is the hypothetical probability of chance agreement while the ROC is a representation of a diagram that depicts the effectiveness of a binary classification system.

5.4 Experimental Result

5.4.1 Result and analysis

The experiments associated with this paper are implemented on Google Collaboratory, a cloud-based online research platform. Python 3.6 is used as the programming language for designing the prediction model. A 10-fold cross-validation technique is employed during model building so that the model does not overfit. A significant consequence of using PCA is found that the procedure helps minimize the disadvantages of having irrelevant features that are unusual for clustering. Since PCA reduces the total number of attributes in the primary dataset and helps manage the outliers and noisy samples, our iterative K-means results improve significantly. Iterative K-means clustering accuracy is also improved considerably on PCA processed datasets while the results are given in Table 5.2. After removing the incorrectly clustered data, we obtain new datasets, and the comprehensive descriptions of those datasets are given below in Table 5.3. The fundamental advantage of PCA is that it allows us to reduce the number of dimensions after we have extracted the dataset's principle components without incurring any substantial information loss. The number of clusters in the dataset must therefore be determined, and a probabilistic approach must be provided to model the cluster structure. Any prediction model, especially in medical disease diagnosis, should be evaluated before being used in actual implementation. As such, we use a variety of statistical evaluation measures metrics to evaluate our prediction model accurately. At first, to determine our proposed model's performance, we employ a k-fold cross-validation technique that enables us to know how

Table 5.2 Accuracy of the iterative K-means clustering.

Dataset name	Original	PCA processed
PIDD	69.56	84.89
CHDD	79.87	90.75
LDBD	76.21	91.30
DRD	79.75	87.92
PKD	78.36	95.43

the proposed predictive framework will perform for new and previously unlearned samples in the testing dataset. For this, we use 10-fold cross-validation [50–52] where each dataset is divided into ten equal subsets. In each trial, one subset is used for testing, and the rest of the nine subsets are used for training. Then the average results of 10 trials are calculated to get the final performance of the prediction model. Now, the analysis of the experimental results is divided into four variations of each dataset: original dataset, PCA processed dataset, K-means dataset, and PCA + K-means dataset.

We build our generalized proposed model by using RF as a predictor algorithm. We utilize all four variations of each dataset during model building. We analyze and evaluate our generalized predictive model output using different statistical evaluation metrics, the results are given in Tables 5.4 – 5.8 for the PIDD, CHDD, LDBD, DRD, and PKD datasets respectively. Analyzing the performance values of each dataset, we can say that our proposed generalized prediction model performed better and achieved the highest prediction accuracy of 99.89% for PIDD, 96.11% for CHDD, 100.00% for LDBD, 95.19% for DRD, and 99.52% for PKD dataset.

To further evaluate how our model performs, we evaluate our datasets with four known machine learning algorithms such as DT, NB, KNN,

Table 5.3 Size of each dataset after the K-means clustering.

Dataset name	No. of instances	No. of positive class	No. of negative class
PIDD	652	212	440
CHDD	275	122	155
LDBD	315	130	185
DRD	1012	517	495
PKD	188	143	45

Table 5.4 Performance on the PIDD dataset.

Measures	Original	PCA	K-means	PCA + K-means
Predictor	RF			
Accuracy	87.50	85.60	93.25	99.89
ROC	94.63	92.54	96.24	100
F1	87.47	86.58	92.36	99.90
Precision	82.22	82.21	88.56	99.79
Recall	92.43	90.25	94.68	100
MCC	70.88	68.82	95.56	99.75
Kappa	70.62	68.52	95.26	99.70
Accuracy	87.50	85.60	93.25	99.89

Table 5.5 Performance on the CHDD dataset.

Measures	**Original**	**PCA**	**K-means**	**PCA + K-means**
Predictor			RF	
Accuracy	85.99	86.87	90.26	96.11
ROC	93.05	88.44	92.71	97.12
F1	85.83	82.29	90.72	94.41
Precision	85.73	83.95	87.66	95.52
Recall	84.66	81.47	94.51	97.75
MCC	69.8	65.88	86.49	91.8
Kappa	69.68	65.23	86.41	91.7
Accuracy	85.99	86.87	90.26	96.11

Table 5.6 Performance on the LDBD dataset.

Measures	**Original**	**PCA**	**K-means**	**PCA + K-means**
Predictor			RF	
Accuracy	83.00	84.56	87.25	100
ROC	86.34	87.25	89.95	100
F1	81.35	82.36	85.69	100
Precision	83.69	84.23	88.65	100
Recall	81.24	83.25	84.25	100
MCC	69.00	70.02	73.25	100
Kappa	68.40	69.85	73.10	100
Accuracy	83.00	84.56	87.25	100

Table 5.7 Performance on the DRD dataset.

Measures	**Original**	**PCA**	**K-means**	**PCA + K-means**
Predictor			RF	
Accuracy	73.90	87.58	89.96	95.19
ROC	81.69	93.18	93.66	99.29
F1	70.98	83.90	87.55	94.79
Precision	74.20	92.83	94.88	97.61
Recall	67.83	77.11	78.02	91.79
MCC	45.74	77.90	80.8	88.92
Kappa	45.25	77.14	80.02	88.12
Accuracy	73.90	87.58	89.96	95.19

and SVM using the following variations of each individual dataset: original dataset, PCA processed dataset, K-means dataset, and PCA + K-means dataset and the results are compared in Figures 5.3 – 5.7 for the PIDD, CHDD, LDBD, DRD and PKD dataset respectively. These results demonstrate that our proposed model outperforms all the investigated machine learning algorithms.

Table 5.8 Performance on the PKD dataset.

Measures	**Original**	**PCA**	**K-means**	**PCA + K-means**
Predictor		RF		
Accuracy	97.23	96.57	97.52	99.52
ROC	98.74	99.46	97.50	100
F1	95.42	96.45	95.46	98.89
Precision	97.67	99.23	94.67	98.00
Recall	91.56	97.40	100	100
MCC	93.27	93.27	94.68	98.45
Kappa	93.04	93.04	94.52	98.38
Accuracy	97.23	96.57	97.52	99.52

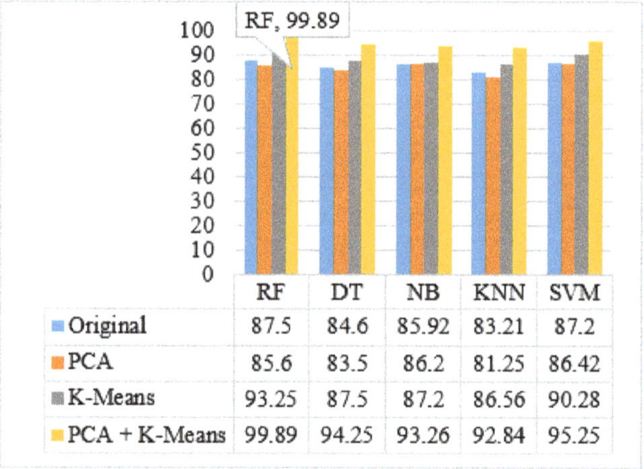

Figure 5.3 Accuracy comparison with other algorithms on the PIDD dataset.

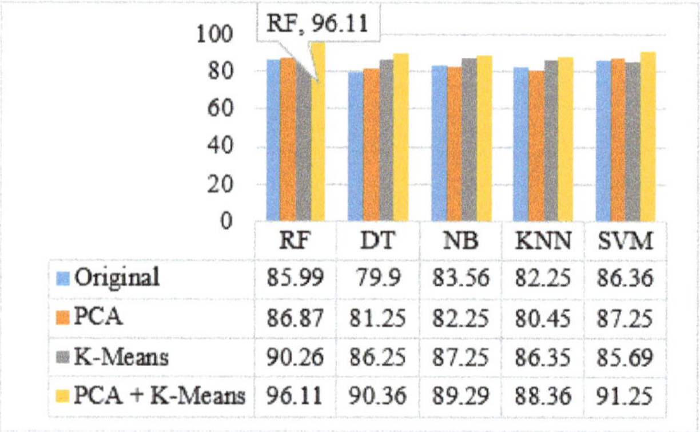

Figure 5.4 Accuracy comparison with other algorithms on the CHDD dataset.

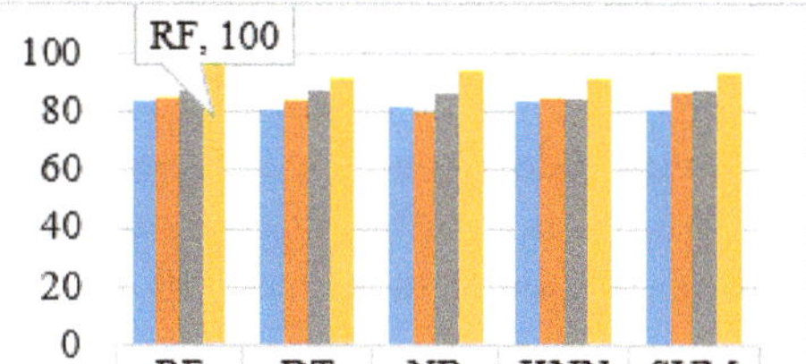

	RF	DT	NB	KNN	SVM
Original	83	80.25	81.89	83	80.25
PCA	84.56	83.56	79.89	84.52	86.25
K-Means	87.25	87	86.58	84.59	87.25
PCA + K-Means	100	91.25	93.87	90.45	93.25

Figure 5.5 Accuracy comparison with other algorithms on the LDBD dataset.

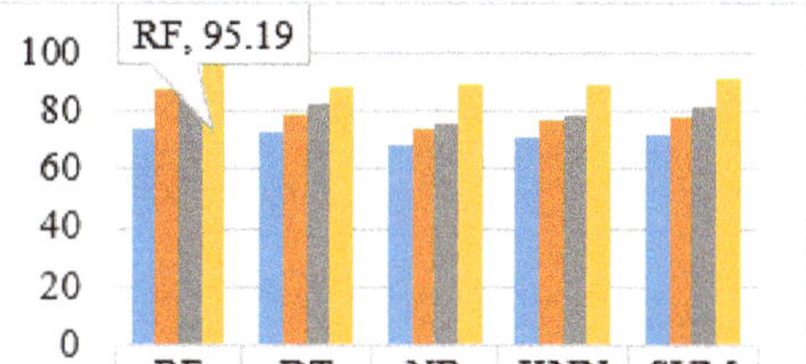

	RF	DT	NB	KNN	SVM
Original	73.9	72.75	68.33	70.7	72.42
PCA	87.58	78.98	73.94	76.79	77.56
K-Means	89.96	82.25	76.29	78.25	81.58
PCA + K-Means	95.19	88.26	89.45	88.85	91.26

Figure 5.6 Accuracy comparison with other algorithms on the DRD dataset.

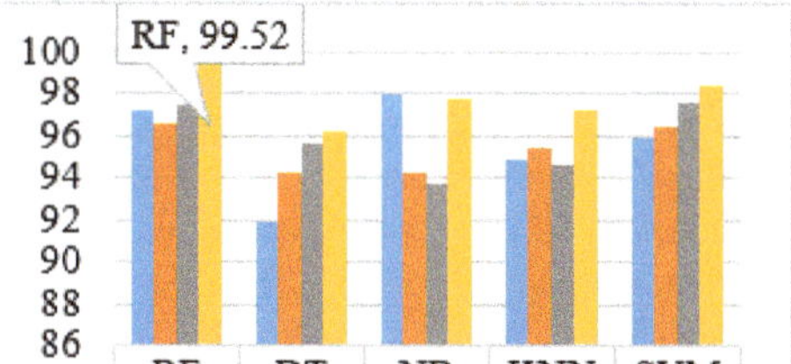

	RF	DT	NB	KNN	SVM
Original	97.23	91.86	97.95	94.89	95.9
PCA	96.57	94.28	94.25	95.42	96.45
K-Means	97.52	95.63	93.69	94.58	97.58
PCA + K-Means	99.52	96.23	97.68	97.2	98.36

Figure 5.7 Accuracy comparison with other algorithms on PKD dataset.

5.4.2 Discussion and extended comparison

This chapter assesses five medical datasets' classification performance to create a general digitalized decision support system for diagnosing some very common diseases. We employ different types of preprocessing methods to develop prediction models using these medical datasets; first, we handle the

Table 5.9 Best parameters for RF predictor.

Dataset	Parameters	Best parameters
PIDD	'n_estimators': [20, 30, 40, 50, 75, 100, 150, 200], 'max_features': ['auto', 'sqrt', 'log2'], 'max_depth': [4,5,6,7,8, 9, 10, 11, 12, 13, 14, 15], 'criterion': ['gini', 'entropy'], 'min_samples_leaf': [1, 2, 3, 4, 5, 6, 7, 8, 9, 10], 'min_samples_split': [2, 5, 7, 10], 'max leaf nodes': [3, 5, 7, 9, 11, 13, 15]	'n_estimators' = 20, 'max_features' = sqrt, 'max_depth' = 7, 'criterion' = entropy, 'min_samples_leaf' = 5, 'min_samples_split' = 5, 'max leaf nodes' = 5
CHDD	'n_estimators': [20, 30, 40, 50, 75, 100, 150, 200], 'max_features': ['auto', 'sqrt', 'log2'], 'max_depth': [4,5,6,7,8, 9, 10, 11, 12, 13, 14, 15], 'criterion': ['gini', 'entropy'], 'min_samples_leaf': [1, 2, 3, 4, 5, 6, 7, 8, 9, 10], 'min_samples_split': [2, 5, 7, 10], 'max leaf nodes': [3, 5, 7, 9, 11, 13, 15]	'n_estimators' = 30, 'max_features' = sqrt, 'max_depth' = 15, 'criterion' = entropy, 'min_samples_leaf' = 7, 'min_samples_split' = 5, 'max leaf nodes' = 5
LDB	'n_estimators': [20, 30, 40, 50, 75, 100, 150, 200], 'max_features': ['auto', 'sqrt', 'log2'], 'max_depth': [4,5,6,7,8, 9, 10, 11, 12, 13, 14, 15], 'criterion': ['gini', 'entropy'], 'min_samples_leaf': [1, 2, 3, 4, 5, 6, 7, 8, 9, 10], 'min_samples_split': [2, 5, 7, 10], 'max leaf nodes': [3, 5, 7, 9, 11, 13, 15]	'n_estimators' = 100, 'max_features' = sqrt, 'max_depth' = 13, 'criterion' = entropy, 'min_samples_leaf' = 10, 'min_samples_split' = 7, 'max leaf nodes' = 7
DRD	'n_estimators': [20, 30, 40, 50, 75, 100, 150, 200], 'max_features': ['auto', 'sqrt', 'log2'], 'max_depth': [4,5,6,7,8, 9, 10, 11, 12, 13, 14, 15], 'criterion': ['gini', 'entropy'], 'min_samples_leaf': [1, 2, 3, 4, 5, 6, 7, 8, 9, 10], 'min_samples_split': [2, 5, 7, 10], 'max leaf nodes': [3, 5, 7, 9, 11, 13, 15]	'n_estimators' = 20, 'max_features' = sqrt, 'max_depth' = 11, 'criterion' = entropy, 'min_samples_leaf' = 5, 'min_samples_split' = 5, 'max leaf nodes' = 15
PKD	'n_estimators': [20, 30, 40, 50, 75, 100, 150, 200], 'max_features': ['auto', 'sqrt', 'log2'], 'max_depth': [4,5,6,7,8, 9, 10, 11, 12, 13, 14, 15], 'criterion': ['gini', 'entropy'], 'min_samples_leaf': [1, 2, 3, 4, 5, 6, 7, 8, 9, 10], 'min_samples_split': [2, 5, 7, 10], 'max leaf nodes': [3, 5, 7, 9, 11, 13, 15]	'n_estimators' = 30, 'max_features' = sqrt, 'max_depth' = 7, 'criterion' = entropy, 'min_samples_leaf' = 7, 'min_samples_split' = 2, 'max leaf nodes' = 3

missing values, feature encoding, feature scaling, PCA, iterative K-means, oversampling the datasets, and getting the transformed datasets. Furthermore, those transformed datasets are fed into the classification process and the classification performances of seven (5) classifiers for each transformed dataset are compared. The experimental results manifest that PCA enhances the performance of K-means clustering as well as the performance of RF predictors. From the experimental result analysis section, we can easily say that our proposed generalized prediction model based on PCA and iterative K-means improves the classification accuracy of the RF predictor. Not only has the accuracy but also for all other statistical evaluation measures, the proposed PCA and iterative K-means along with the RF predictor outperformed the investigated techniques. We also utilize the Grid SearchCV hyperparameter optimization technique to select the best parameters for the RF predictor. The optimized parameter values for the RF predictor are given in Table 5.9. Therefore, we can say that our proposed generalized prediction model would be useful for medical practitioners in diagnosing those diseases.

Table 5.10 Comparison with other works.

Dataset	Work	Accuracy	ROC	F1	Precision	Recall
PIDD	Alam *et al.* [1]	77.00	81.00	75.80	75.80	76.10
	Rado *et al.* [25]	77.00	-	-	-	-
	Das *et al.* [10]	78.69	-	-	-	-
	Hu *et al.* [15]	77.00	-	-	-	-
	Ramana *et al.* [26]	76.30	81.90	-	68.42	61.19
	Ramesh *et al.* [27]	88.90	-	90.00	90.10	90.10
	Alam *et al.* [2]	75.70	81.60	-	-	-
	Zhu *et al.* [35]	97.40	97.00	97.00	97.00	97.00
	Our Model	99.89	100	99.90	99.79	100
CHDD	Ali *et al.* [4]	93.33	-	-	-	85.36
	Mohan *et al.* [22]	88.40	-	90.00	90.10	92.80
	Javeed *et al.* [16]	93.33	-	-	-	95.12
	Ali *et al.* [5]	94.61	-	94.77	93.55	96.03
	Our Model	96.11	97.12	94.41	95.52	97.75
LDB	Alam *et al.* [1]	79.00	65.00	78.00	75.00	79.00
	Das *et al.* [10]	69.45	-	-	-	-
	Kumar *et al.* [19]	73.91	74.24	80.00	87.80	73.47
	Our Model	100	100	100	100	100
DRD	Singh *et al.* [31]	74.35	-	-	-	-
	Our Model	95.19	99.29	94.79	97.61	91.79
PKD	Alam *et al.* [1]	92.00	93.00	92.00	92.00	92.00
	Kadam *et al.* [18]	92.48	-	-	-	95.31
	Our Model	99.34	100	99.34	98.77	100

At last, we provide a comparison of the classification performances with other researchers in Table 5.10 considering all tested datasets. The results manifest that the proposed generic predictive model supersedes the examined state-of-the-art approaches.

5.5 Conclusion and Future Research

In medical informatics, accurate medical data classification is one of the most complex and challenging tasks due to the data's complex, nonlinear, non-normal nature. This paper has overcome those challenges and developed a generalized predictive model for five (5) different disease datasets. We proposed a classification approach by integrating PCA and iterative K-means clustering for the classification of medical datasets. To elaborate, we first check whether there are any missing values in the datasets or not; if any, then KNN is employed to impute those missing values. After that, one hot encoding was utilized for encoding the categorical values into numerical values. Subsequently, robust scaling is applied to transform the feature values in a specified range. Then we applied PCA for dimension reduction. For further improvement in classification performance, we intended to use the K-means clustering technique in the data-preprocessing step to handle the dataset outliers. Here, we have adopted K-means clustering and clustered the dataset into two clusters. In that case, we have ensured to perform clustering and remove the incorrectly clustered data until we get more than 80% of data in the newly transformed dataset than the original one. Subsequently, the same as before, this newly transformed dataset has been forwarded for classification. While inspecting the results, we see that each algorithm's classification performance has increased by 1% to 17% for each dataset to the previous results. Our proposed generalized decision support system can be used as an alternative tool or even an assistive tool for physicians to diagnose these types of diseases. In the future, we intend to develop a cloud-based decision support system that may help the general people to diagnose and take precautions to prevent future fatal diseases.

Author contributions

S. M. Mahedy Hasan, Sami Azam: Conceptualization, Methodology, Software. Md Palash Uddin and Asif Karim: Data curation, Writing–Original draft preparation, interim review and editing. Md Al Mamun and

Muhammad Imran Sharif: Visualization, Investigation. Mohammed Rezwanul Islam: Validation. Asif Karim: Writing Reviewing and Finalization.

Funding

This research received no external funding.

Data Availability Statement

Dheeru Dua and Casey Graff. 2017. UCI Machine Learning Repository. http://archive.ics.uci.edu/ml.

Conflicts of Interest

The authors declare that there is no conflict of interest regarding the publication of this paper.

References

[1] Md Zahangir Alam, M Saifur Rahman, and M Sohel Rahman. 2019. A Random Forest based predictor for medical data classification using feature ranking. Informatics in Medicine Unlocked 15 (2019), 100180.

[2] Talha Mahboob Alam, Muhammad Atif Iqbal, Yasir Ali, Abdul Wahab, Safdar Ijaz, Talha Imtiaz Baig, Ayaz Hussain, Muhammad Awais Malik, Muhammad Mehdi Raza, Salman Ibrar, et al. 2019. A model for early prediction of diabetes. Informatics in Medicine Unlocked 16 (2019), 100204.

[3] Salem Alelyani. 2021. Stable bagging feature selection on medical data. Journal of Big Data 8, 1 (2021), 1–18.

[4] Liaqat Ali, Atiqur Rahman, Aurangzeb Khan, Mingyi Zhou, Ashir Javeed, and Javed Ali Khan. 2019. An automated diagnostic system for heart disease prediction based on statistical model and optimally configured deep neural network. IEEE Access 7 (2019), 34938–34945.

[5] Syed Arslan Ali, Basit Raza, Ahmad Kamran Malik, Ahmad Raza Shahid, Muhammad Faheem, Hani Alquhayz, and Yogan Jaya Kumar. 2020. An Optimally Configured and Improved Deep Belief

Network (OCI-DBN) Approach for Heart Disease Prediction Based on Ruzzo–Tompa and Stacked Genetic Algorithm. IEEE Access 8 (2020), 65947–65958.

[6] M Ambika, G Raghuraman, L SaiRamesh, and A Ayyasamy. 2020. Intelligence–based decision support system for diagnosing the incidence of hypertensive type. Journal of Intelligent & Fuzzy Systems 38, 2 (2020), 1811–1825.

[7] Amare Anagaw and Yang-Lang Chang. 2019. A new complement naïve Bayesian approach for biomedical data classification. Journal of Ambient Intelligence and Humanized Computing 10, 10 (2019), 3889–3897.

[8] Fehmi Aziz, Faheem Tahir, Sadia Midhat, Shafaq Naz, and Naveeda Akhtar Qureshi. [n. d.]. Fuzzy soft set theory: Application of classification rules in decision making during medical diagnosis. Journal of Intelligent & Fuzzy Systems Preprint ([n. d.]), 1–9.

[9] AKM Rafid, Sami Azam, Sidratul Montaha, Asif Karim, Kayes Uddin Fahim, Md Hasan. 2022. "An Effective Ensemble Machine Learning Approach to Classify Breast Cancer Based on Feature Selection and Lesion Segmentation Using Preprocessed Mammograms." Biology 11.11 (2022): 1654.

[10] H Das, B Naik, and HS Behera. 2019. Medical disease analysis using Neuro-Fuzzy with Feature Extraction Model for classification. Inform. Med. Unlocked 18, 100288 (2020).

[11] Dheeru Dua and Casey Graff. 2017. UCI Machine Learning Repository. http://archive.ics.uci.edu/ml

[12] Sarah A Ebiaredoh-Mienye, Theo G Swart, Ebenezer Esenogho, and Ibomoiye Domor Mienye. 2022. A Machine Learning Method with Filter-Based Feature Selection for Improved Prediction of Chronic Kidney Disease. Bioengineering 9, 8 (2022), 350.

[13] Zarrin Tasnim, Sovon Chakraborty, F. M. Javed Mehedi Shamrat, Ali Newaz Chowdhury, Humaira Alam Nuha, Asif Karim, Sabrina Binte Zahir, Md. Masum Billah. 2021. "Deep learning predictive model for colon cancer patient using CNN-based classification." Int. J. Adv. Comput. Sci. Appl 12 (2021).

[14] SMM Hasan, MA Mamun, MP Uddin, and MA Hossain. 2018. Comparative analysis of classification approaches for heart disease prediction. In 2018 International Conference on Computer, Communication, Chemical, Material and Electronic Engineering (IC4ME2). IEEE, 1–4.

[15] LY Hu, MW Huang, SW Ke, and CF Tsai. [n. d.]. The distance function effect on k-nearest neighbor classification for medical datasets. Springerplus. 5, 1304 (2016).

[16] Ashir Javeed, Shijie Zhou, Liao Yongjian, Iqbal Qasim, Adeeb Noor, and Redhwan Nour. 2019. An intelligent learning system based on random search algorithm and optimized random forest model for improved heart disease detection. IEEE Access 7 (2019), 180235–180243.

[17] Sunil Kr Jha, Zhaoqing Pan, Ehsan Elahi, and Nilesh Patel. 2019. A comprehensive search for expert classification methods in disease diagnosis and prediction. Expert Systems 36, 1 (2019), e12343.

[18] Vinod J Kadam and Shivajirao M Jadhav. 2019. Feature ensemble learning based on sparse autoencoders for diagnosis of Parkinson's disease. In Computing, communication and signal processing. Springer, 567–581.

[19] Pushpendra Kumar and Ramjeevan Singh Thakur. 2021. Liver disorder detection using variable-neighbor weighted fuzzy K nearest neighbor approach. Multimedia Tools and Applications 80, 11 (2021), 16515–16535.

[20] D Malathi, R Logesh, V Subramaniyaswamy, V Vijayakumar, and Arun Kumar Sangaiah. 2019. Hybrid reasoning-based privacy-aware disease prediction support system. Computers & Electrical Engineering 73 (2019), 114–127.

[21] Amare Anagaw and Yang-Lang Chang. 2019. A new complement naïve Bayesian approach for biomedical data classification. Journal of Ambient Intelligence and Humanized Computing 10, 10 (2019), 3889–3897.

[22] Fehmi Aziz, Faheem Tahir, Sadia Midhat, Shafaq Naz, and Naveeda Akhtar Qureshi. [n. d.]. Fuzzy soft set theory: Application of classification rules in decision making during medical diagnosis. Journal of Intelligent & Fuzzy Systems Preprint ([n. d.]), 1–9.

[23] AKM Rafid, Sami Azam, Sidratul Montaha, Asif Karim, Kayes Uddin Fahim, Md Hasan. 2022. "An Effective Ensemble Machine Learning Approach to Classify Breast Cancer Based on Feature Selection and Lesion Segmentation Using Preprocessed Mammograms." Biology 11.11 (2022): 1654.

[24] H Das, B Naik, and HS Behera. 2019. Medical disease analysis using Neuro-Fuzzy with Feature Extraction Model for classification. Inform. Med. Unlocked 18, 100288 (2020).

[25] Dheeru Dua and Casey Graff. 2017. UCI Machine Learning Repository. http://archive.ics.uci.edu/ml
[26] Sarah A Ebiaredoh-Mienye, Theo G Swart, Ebenezer Esenogho, and Ibomoiye Domor Mienye. 2022. A Machine Learning Method with Filter-Based Feature Selection for Improved Prediction of Chronic Kidney Disease. Bioengineering 9, 8 (2022), 350.
[27] Zarrin Tasnim, Sovon Chakraborty, F. M. Javed Mehedi Shamrat, Ali Newaz Chowdhury, Humaira Alam Nuha, Asif Karim, Sabrina Binte Zahir, Md. Masum Billah. 2021. "Deep learning predictive model for colon cancer patient using CNN-based classification." Int. J. Adv. Comput. Sci. Appl 12 (2021).
[28] SMM Hasan, MA Mamun, MP Uddin, and MA Hossain. 2018. Comparative analysis of classification approaches for heart disease prediction. In 2018 International Conference on Computer, Communication, Chemical, Material and Electronic Engineering (IC4ME2). IEEE, 1–4.
[29] LY Hu, MW Huang, SW Ke, and CF Tsai. [n. d.]. The distance function effect on k-nearest neighbor classification for medical datasets. Springerplus. 5, 1304 (2016).
[30] Ashir Javeed, Shijie Zhou, Liao Yongjian, Iqbal Qasim, Adeeb Noor, and Redhwan Nour. 2019. An intelligent learning system based on random search algorithm and optimized random forest model for improved heart disease detection. IEEE Access 7 (2019), 180235–180243.
[31] Sunil Kr Jha, Zhaoqing Pan, Ehsan Elahi, and Nilesh Patel. 2019. A comprehensive search for expert classification methods in disease diagnosis and prediction. Expert Systems 36, 1 (2019), e12343.
[32] Vinod J Kadam and Shivajirao M Jadhav. 2019. Feature ensemble learning based on sparse autoencoders for diagnosis of Parkinson's disease. In Computing, communication and signal processing. Springer, 567–581.
[33] Pushpendra Kumar and Ramjeevan Singh Thakur. 2021. Liver disorder detection using variable-neighbor weighted fuzzy K nearest neighbor approach. Multimedia Tools and Applications 80, 11 (2021), 16515–16535.
[34] D Malathi, R Logesh, V Subramaniyaswamy, V Vijayakumar, and Arun Kumar Sangaiah. 2019. Hybrid reasoning-based privacy-aware disease prediction support system. Computers & Electrical Engineering 73 (2019), 114–127.

[35] Bagyamathi Mathiyazhagan, Joseph Liyaskar, Ahmad Taher Azar, Hannah H Inbarani, Yasir Javed, Nashwa Ahmad Kamal, and Khaled M Fouad. 2022. Rough Set Based Classification and Feature Selection Using Improved Harmony Search for Peptide Analysis and Prediction of Anti-HIV-1 Activities. Applied Sciences 12, 4 (2022), 2020.

[36] Senthilkumar Mohan, Chandrasegar Thirumalai, and Gautam Srivastava. 2019. Effective heart disease prediction using hybrid machine learning techniques. IEEE access 7 (2019), 81542–81554.

[37] P Mohapatra, Sreejit Chakravarty, and Pradipta K Dash. 2015. An improved cuckoo search based extreme learning machine for medical data classification. Swarm and Evolutionary Computation 24 (2015), 25–49.

[38] Nicholas Pudjihartono, Tayaza Fadason, Andreas W Kempaliehr, and Justin M O'Sullivan. 2022. A Review of Feature Selection Methods for Machine Learning-Based Disease Risk Prediction. Frontiers in Bioinformatics 2 (2022), 927312.

[39] Omesaad Rado, Najat Ali, Habiba Muhammad Sani, Ahmad Idris, and Daniel Neagu. 2019. Performance analysis of feature selection methods for classification of healthcare datasets. In Intelligent Computing-Proceedings of the Computing Conference. Springer, 929–938.

[40] Bendi Venkata Ramana and Raja Sarath Kumar Boddu. 2019. Performance comparison of classification algorithms on medical datasets. In 2019 IEEE 9th annual computing and communication workshop and conference (CCWC). IEEE, 0140– 0145.

[41] Dharavath Ramesh and Yogendra Singh Katheria. 2019. Ensemble method based predictive model for analyzing disease datasets: a predictive analysis approach. Health and Technology 9, 4 (2019), 533–545.

[42] Alqahtani Saeed, Maryam Zaffar, Mohammed Ali Abbas, Khurrum Shehzad Quraishi, Abdullah Shahrose, Muhammad Irfan, Mohammed Ayed Huneif, Alqahtani Abdulwahab, Sharifa Khalid Alduraibi, Fahad Alshehri, et al. 2022. A Turf-Based Feature Selection Technique for Predicting Factors Affecting Human Health during Pandemic. Life 12, 9 (2022), 1367.

[43] Máximo Eduardo Sánchez-Gutiérrez and Pedro Pablo González-Pérez. 2022. Multi-Class Classification of Medical Data Based on Neural Network Pruning and Informationentropy Measures. Entropy 24, 2 (2022), 196.

[44] Alok Kumar Shukla, Sanjeev Kumar Pippal, Srishti Gupta, B Ramachandra Reddy, and Diwakar Tripathi. 2020. Knowledge discovery in medical and biological datasets by integration of Relief-F and correlation feature selection techniques. Journal of Intelligent & Fuzzy Systems 38, 5 (2020), 6637–6648.

[45] Girish Kumar Singh, Rahul K Jain, and Prabhati Dubey. 2019. Study of classification techniques on medical datasets. In Computing, Communication and Signal Processing. Springer, 557–565.

[46] Pronab Ghosh, Asif Karim, Syeda Tanjila Atik, Saima Afrin, Mohd Saifuzzaman. 2021. "Expert cancer model using supervised algorithms with a LASSO selection approach." International Journal of Electrical and Computer Engineering (IJECE) 11.3 (2021): 2631.

[47] Qubo Xie, Ke Zhou, Xiao Fu, and Xiaohu Fan. 2019. Feature attention-based detection model for medical text. Journal of Intelligent & Fuzzy Systems 37, 4 (2019), 4585–4594.

[48] Qing Zhou, Wei Peng, and Dai Tang. [n. d.]. Automatic recommendation of medical departments to outpatients based on text analyses and medical knowledge graph. Journal of Intelligent & Fuzzy Systems Preprint ([n. d.]), 1–11.

[49] Changsheng Zhu, Christian Uwa Idemudia, and Wenfang Feng. 2019. Improved logistic regression model for diabetes prediction by integrating PCA and K-means techniques. Informatics in Medicine Unlocked 17 (2019), 100179.

[50] J. Stirling, T. Chen, and M. Adamou, "Autism spectrum disorder classification using a self-organising fuzzy classifier," in Fuzzy Logic, pp. 83–94, Springer, 2021.

[51] M. M. Rahman, O. L. Usman, R. C. Muniyandi, S. Sahran, S. Mohamed, and R. A. Razak, "A review of machine learning methods of feature selection and classification for autism spectrum disorder," Brain sciences, vol. 10, no. 12, p. 949, 2020.

[52] M. Hasan, M. M. Ahamad, S. Aktar, and M. A. Moni, "Early stage autism spectrum disorder detection of adults and toddlers using machine learning models," in 2021 5th International Conference on Electrical Information and Communication Technology (EICT), pp. 1–6, IEEE, 2021.

6

Exploring the Promises and Perils of Implementing Generative AI into Mental Healthcare and Emotional Well-being Support of General Public: A Comprehensive Overview

Chintalapalli Arshita[1], Kishor Kumar Reddy C.[2], Nagari Apoorva[3], Srinath Doss[4], and Herat Joshi[5]

[1,2,3]Department of Computer Engineering, Stanley College of Engineering and Technology for Women, India
[4]Faculty of Engineering and Technology, Botho University, Botswana
[5]Great River Health Systems, USA
E-mail: carshithasharma@gmail.com; kishoar23@gmail.com; apoorvanagari7@gmail.com; srinath.doss@bothouniversity.ac.bw; heratjoshi@gmail.com

Abstract

In today's rapidly growing world, generative AI has found its use-cases in a multitude of domains. Its impact in the mental healthcare field is of special interest. With the rising need for mental and emotional health services, the traditional therapy industry can be effectively transformed and enhanced using generative AI in various ways. The proposed chapter is an overview of the opportunities and adversities faced on implementing generative AI into the mental healthcare industry. First, different technologies used in the industry like natural language processing (NLP), machine learning (ML) and deep learning are studied, then the various ways in which generative AI is leveraged into the industry for patient and clinician/mental health provider support are studied. Further, the chapter explores the current mental health app market for effective AI tools accessible by the general public. The chapter

DOI: 10.1201/9788743801764-6

also analyzes the potency of utilizing the popular LLM model, Chat-GPT for treatment of mental health issues and support. Moreover, the necessity of ensuring safety and responsible use of AI in the domain is highlighted considering the ethical challenges and the intricacies of human cognition.

Keywords: AI in Mental Health, Chat-GPT, Generative AI, Mental Health Apps, NLP, Virtual Therapy.

6.1 Introduction

In the modern era, mental health issues like anxiety, stress, and depression are growing in prevalence, due to various demographic, behavioral and educational factors [1]. The landscape of traditional healthcare is demanding as there is acute shortage of mental healthcare professionals, high costs of treatment and social stigma. In response to these needs, several effective breakthroughs have found innovative applications in the mental health sector. AI could be used in key areas of mental healthcare such as increasing awareness, assessment, diagnosis, treatment, therapy, self-care, tracking and monitoring, providing recommendations, feedback etc.

Artificial intelligence (Gen AI) has made great strides in the months and years since ChatGPT was launched in November 2022 [2]. Every month brings the introduction of a new technology, code, or technological innovation. While many people fear ChatGPT (and AI and machine learning), it is clear that machine learning has great potential. Since its widespread use, machine learning has made an impact in many industries, completing tasks such as medical image analysis and weather forecasting. A survey done by McKinsey and Company in 2022 [2] establishes that AI adoption has multiplied significantly in the past five years, and investment in AI is also hiking rapidly. It is true that AI creation tools like ChatGPT (GPT acronym for generative pre-training transformer) and DALL-E (image generator) have the capacity to change many ways of working. But the full extent of this impact and the dangers are still unknown. In simple terms, the word "build" means "to make," "to create," or "to construct" – generative artificial intelligence (Gen AI) that defines algorithms (like ChatGPT) that could be used to produce new content, including code, audio, images, simulations, text, and video [2, 3].

Mental illness is characterized by a significant impairment in a person's cognition, emotional control, or behavior, and is often associated with abnormalities in anxiety or work fear. Because many types of mental illness fall under the broad mental health umbrella, mental health services have always faced challenges such as low access, long wait times, and the scarcity of psychiatrists. In addition, the negative perceptions associated with mental illness can also prevent people from seeking help. In response to these issues, AI has been developed to provide the benefits of psychological support at increasingly affordable prices. AI-powered chatbots and virtual doctors can provide immediate help, reduce wait times, and potentially circumvent healthcare laws. Additionally, intelligent algorithms can analyze large amounts of data to customize interventions to individual needs, potentially improving treatment outcomes. While AI cannot replace humans, it can supplement traditional care by providing additional support and assistance.

The proposed chapter explains the technologies used to implement Gen AI into mental health support including natural language processing (NLP), machine learning (ML), and deep learning (DL). The chapter gives a review of the implementations of Gen AI into mental healthcare such as mental disorder diagnosis, Gen AI-driven therapy, treatment, clinical education, consultation, tracking and monitoring, etc. The chapter also explores some mental health support apps available to the general public. Further, it addresses some ethical challenges like data protection and information security, bias and fairness, dangers of human-AI interactions such as emotional dependence, etc.

6.2 Generative AI Technologies in Mental Health Support

The application of generative AI within the domain of mental health presents several opportunities and challenges. Many advanced algorithms are being leveraged in the industry to provide efficient delivery of care. Some technologies are discussed below.

6.2.1 Natural language processing (NLP)

Natural language processing (NLP) is defined as a process where computers are empowered to understand human language. In present times computers are capable of analyzing, understanding text-based information as well as voice-based information, including intentions and emotions of the speaker. This has been made possible due to improved technology in natural language processing (NLP). NLP is playing a significant role in delivering mental health support. The manner in which therapeutic care is provided has been dramatically altered by the utilization of natural language processing (NLP) and chatbots for mental health. Large-scale linguistic dataset analysis and mental health treatment research are discovering advantages from AI and

NLP technology. Chatbots use natural language processing (NLP) techniques like sentiment analysis, word embeddings, and models like the sequence-to-sequence model and attention mechanism [4]. A chatbot is a software application that uses natural language processing (NLP) to decode one or more human languages and interacts with the speaker through text or speech [4]. Patients undergoing therapy can make use of chatbots as a beneficial asset. When patients interact with chatbots befittingly, chatbots can help manage mental health issues of the patient. Chatbots offer a practical and effective way to get mental health support, which aids in overcoming the stigma connected to mental illness [4].

Sentiment analysis (one of the NLP methods) is a process in which the data provided by the user is classified based on the mentality expressed in the text, which can be positive, negative, and neutral [4, 5] technique has exhibited the potential for objective results and accuracy in treating neuropsychiatric disorders. It is becoming increasingly evident how valuable NLP is in improving mental health interventions. For nearly a decade, the Internet has enabled psychologists to integrate affordable psychotherapy techniques into their work. NLP is utilized in automated assessment tools in health to aid doctors and help people's understanding of a certain disease [6].

AI applications in mental health offer substantial ethical advantages such as heightened patient responsiveness by providing immediate support to the patient, novel treatment modalities such as personalized therapy plans, interactive exercising sessions to enhance the outcomes, opportunities to reach hard-to-target populations, and time savings for medical professionals [7]. Additional applications of chatbots in mental health include texting therapies, online support groups and interactive self-guided interventions [6].

6.2.2 Machine learning (ML) and deep learning (DL)

Articles primarily intended to assist in detecting mental diseases were sourced for a study that was done and is cited at [8]. After thorough examination of the approaches of ML and DL used by various scientists to conduct this study as well as the databases used. The study found that when applied to diagnose mental health issues, ML and DL technologies have both yielded outstanding results. To find the optimal method, the effectiveness and performance of several algorithms were also assessed. Many methods are being used to find patterns and therefore detect mental issues, like naïve Bayes, LSTM-RNN, logistic regression, support vector machines, random forests, neural networks, among others [8]. According to the study, combining DL approaches can aid in the diagnosis as well as the prediction of various mental health challenges, even though ML was previously effective in understanding and diagnosing mental health issues. When used with visual modalities, DL approaches may aid in the diagnosis of certain illnesses. Upon closer examination, other data modalities – like sensors – have proven to be useful in determining patients' mental states. The study does advise researchers to evaluate several ML and DL algorithms in order to select the most effective ones.

Another study, cited in [9], demonstrated that taking additional options into account, like transfer learning, can also produce excellent results.

Numerous further research demonstrates the potential benefits of machine learning in understanding psychiatric disorders. Furthermore, it might help identify and categorize patients' mental health conditions to provide them with additional care. Recent studies have shown that utilizing data from the combination of different sensor modalities found in IOT devices might be helpful in identifying patient responses and emotions, among other things.

It is evident that the substantial portion of groundwork and studies still face troubles validating their observations because of a lack of satisfactory, accepted, substantiated evidence, specifically from external origins. Only a subset of machine learning algorithms perform equally well in every problem, which makes implementing machine learning into the domain trickier. The properties of the data and the data samples that are obtained will determine how well the machine learning models function. Furthermore, preparatory functions like data cleaning and parameter tuning can have an effect on machine learning models so as to get the best results.

6.3 Applications of Gen AI into Mental Healthcare

The mental health services industry is ready to undergo a paradigm shift with the opportunities possible with innovation in generative AI. By leveraging the above-discussed technologies, inventive solutions are developed to confront the growing demand for mental health services/support. This section further explores some of the key applications of Gen AI in mental healthcare, discussing its possible merits and demerits.

6.3.1 For assessments and initial patient referral

Integration of generative AI into the backdrop of clinical challenges is another use-case which could hugely benefit mental support seekers. One hurdle patients face is the extended wait times between seeking appointment and beginning the actual treatment. These lengthy wait-times can even cause patients to drop-out of the waitlist before even receiving the cure. Furthermore, the scarcity of mental healthcare professionals also made seeking support difficult. Several studies earlier provide evidence that implementing digital tools and innovation into healthcare could possibly solve problems related to availability, ease of use, accessibility and service capacity. Therefore, testing and studying the potential and performance of Gen AI in supporting mental health support providers in clinical settings could allow us to unleash great potential solutions to the problems faced as stated above. Patients using chatbots/assistants are more likely to report accurate symptoms which help the mental health professionals easily assess the situation and establish an immediate strong connection with the patient as their details are already known to the mental health professional before-hand.

One application of Gen AI into actual-word clinical settings is studied by research cited at [10]. The research was conducted to judge the application of AI into clinical assessment and incoming patient consultation within the UK's National Health Service. A dataset of 64,862 patients was gathered from nine talking therapies facilities across England. It was observed that by integrating the AI tool (Limbic Access) into the assessment process of the nine healthcare centers, the overall time taken by the clinicians to assess their patients drastically reduced. This is critical in allowing mental health support providers to utilize their time well, with maximum efficiency. The report also indicated improved results in several aspects such as shorter delays, optimized care pathways, higher success rates, and lowered dropout rates. Thus, the study concluded that there is immense benefit of integrating AI (Gen AI) into clinical assessment of mental health issues. It further emphasizes on the efficiency of providing care, support to patients and achieving successful outcomes [10].

6.3.2 Chatbots for the rescue

Another use-case of implementing Gen AI into mental healthcare is by using chatbots or virtual assistants. Over the past years, chatbots and virtual assistants like Amazon Alexa, Google Assistant, Siri have all proved to be efficient to service customers for increasing productivity in their lives. However, doubts persist in usage of chatbots and virtual assistants to positively boost mental healthcare. This is because the chatbots seem to not understand the delicate nuances of the human mind. A study cited at [11] tested 10 apps meant for mental health support and treatment of mental health issues with in-built chatbot/assistant technology. Upon performing qualitative analysis of 3,621 customer ratings from Google Play Store and 2,624 reports from Apple App Store, it was learned that the users seemed to approve of the humanlike exchanges, and depended on these interactions as these chatbots/assistants are always available (24/7). A judgment-free environment fostered by these apps resulted in the customers feeling more at ease, which caused them to share even sensitive information. However, on the flip side, some users reported that they lost interest after the chatbot/assistant felt biased and gave improper answers.

Using chatbots or virtual assistants for mental support can seem dependable as they are available to the customer 24/7 unlike human mental healthcare providers, these tools seem to be especially effective when reaching out to friends/family/professional support is not possible or not preferred. Nevertheless, this situation poses the risk of isolation, over dependence and inefficient support at serious times. The study concluded that through further user-based refinements in chatbot-based apps, and balanced practice of use can allow us to tap into the endless potential of social and psychological support that these chatbots/assistants can provide.

6.3.3 Tracking and monitoring

With the substantial growth of modern AI and machine learning, there is huge potential of integrating prediction, detection and treatment solutions in the field. AI-based decision support systems can be used to predict the risks of developing mental health disorders along with detecting wild mood changes. On detection of harmful or extreme mood changes, alerts could be sent to either the patients themselves/family/friends or the patient's mental healthcare providers. This prediction and/or detection allows implementing proactive actions to avert or alleviate the onset of serious mental issues. This timely intervention can hugely benefit the patients and mental healthcare providers as well.

Chatbots or virtual assistants can be used to track patient conditions by actively engaging with them by inquiring various aspects of patient health – such as mood, stress levels, energy and sleep durations. Furthermore, the chatbots could also provide therapeutic measures and relief to help patients feel better – such as recommending to engage in physical activities (walking, playing), meditation methods, or even leading the patient to seek professional help in serious situations. In addition, chatbots could effectively alert the mental health providers in case their patient is in immediate danger due to their mental troubles. The continuous tracking of patient data could be used to generate insights on the patient's healing journey and help mental health providers view the aggregate data and suggest further treatment plans. The bots could also provide personalized feedback to the patients that could foster a positive environment allowing them to reflect on their mental growth and personal journeys [12].

6.3.4 Generative AI exposure therapy

Exposure therapy is another application of generative AI-based technology. According to the American Psychological Association [13], exposure therapy is a type of psychotherapy where people are slowly exposed to their fears. This is done to help people confront their fears and reduce their anxiety. Often, people tend to avoid the things/situations/activities they fear, this might make the fear worse, especially if the fear is deterring the person from living their personal lives comfortably and safely. In such situations, mental healthcare providers recommend exposure therapy so that the patient overcomes their fear and decreases their avoidance towards it [13].

One of the most widely used variations in exposure therapy is Virtual reality exposure. Oftentimes when a person is not willing to directly face their phobia, mental healthcare providers use VR technology to stimulate conditions matching the patient's fear to mimic the sights, sounds, and smells related to the patient's fear. This allows the patient to undergo graded exposure while being assured that they are (physically) in a safe and monitored environment. With time, the psychotherapists might recommend the patient to face their phobia directly, as the VR exposure can weaken the patient's fear associated with any object/activity/situation, etc.

Further, there is blooming research being done on virtual reality exposure therapy (VRET) approaches. One such research cited at [14] proposes a personalized VRET approach to enhance the patient experience, implementation and outcome of VRET. This approach is studied to be hugely beneficial for the patients and mental healthcare providers alike.

6.4 Exploring Mental Health App Markets

With the increasing awareness of mental health among the general public, and the easy access to digital tools, the app markets have tons of options which integrate AI into their apps to support users in their mental healthcare journeys. However, we observe a limited number of generative AI-based apps

Table 6.1 Review of generative AI-based apps in the mental health market space.

App	Type	Total downloads	Description
Wysa	Chatbot-based therapy	Over 1 million users	Offers relief to people with anxiety and depression [16]
Talkspace	Chatbot-based therapy	Over 500 thousand users	Offers online therapy along with an option to schedule therapist appointments [17]
BetterHelp	Chatbot-based therapy	Over 1 million users	Offers a platform to connect to therapists using AI [18]
Woebot	Chatbot-based therapy	Over 1 million users	Offers help through CBT-based online therapy [19]
Kintsugi	Smart mental health tool	10+ users	Offers help through providing support by analyzing facial and voice patterns of the users [20, 21]

being used indicating a need to investigate the effectiveness and outreach of Gen-AI-based apps in the practical world.

A study cited at [15], evaluated the biggest space-holder in the huge world of mental health apps in the market – Headspace. This study assessed everyday perceived stress and data interaction at two time points with moderate and perceived stress content for Headspace app members. Cognitive strain was considered with the stress scale (PSS-10), and collaboration was measured with headspace days and minutes and user time. Descriptive statistics were performed for all variables. Findings showed that members who used headspace experienced less stress in the real world. Data also showed that participants who used the application routinely were more probable to observe positive changes in tension/stress and anxiety levels. The study provided concrete proof that the DMH headspace platform effectively alleviates user stress. Their results have implications for treatment, including mediation and mental health in relation to mental illness or barriers to stress reduction.

Further, Table 6.1 takes a deeper dive in exploring some of the popularly used mobile apps/web applications in the current market space. It is to be noted that we only include apps that implement generative-AI technology directly into their apps or indirectly (e.g. Kintsugi).

6.5 Use of Chat-GPT for Mental Health Support

Ever since its launch on November 22, Chat-GPT has been a popular go-to LLM with over 200 million weekly active users as of September 2024

[21]. With the model being trained on a huge amount of data, Chat-GPT performs extremely well in producing human-like texts based on the user prompts [22]. This LLM developed by the company OpenAI is extensively studied by a great deal of researchers. Chat-GPT has found a multitude of use-cases in today's fast-paced world. Specifically, it is found to be tremendously impactful in allowing the general public to make impactful decisions about their health [23].

> "ChatGPT puts the power of AI in everyone's hand."
> - Fredrick Godin [21]

A qualitative study [24] conducted a two-week experiment followed by semi-structured interviews of 24 experimental subjects who used Chat-GPT for mental health support for various mental health issues. The study examined the performance of the LLM in 12 main categories (psychoeducation, emotional wellbeing, goal setting, motivation, guidance and resource information, self-awareness and monitoring, cognitive behavioral therapy, crisis intervention and psychotherapy exercises, ethical and legal issues, accuracy and reliability, limited evaluation competence and cultural issues) [24]. The results of the study are assessed in Table 6.2.

The study [24] further concluded that AI-powered tools like Chat-GPT possess immense capacity to provide essential support for people with mental health issues. However, this implementation poses certain challenges and

Table 6.2 Performance results (positive/negative) of study qualitative study conducted by research cited at [24].

S no	Factor considered	Performance
1.	Psychoeducation	Positive
2.	Emotional support	Positive
3.	Objective setting, inspiration	Positive
4.	Referral and resource information [24]	Positive
5.	Self-evaluation and monitoring [24]	Positive
6.	Cognitive behavioral therapy [24]	Positive
7.	Crisis mediations [24]	Positive
8.	Psychotherapeutic exercises [24]	Positive
9.	Ethical, legal considerations	Negative
10.	Accuracy and reliability	Negative
11.	Assessment capabilities	Negative (Limited)
12.	Cultural and linguistic considerations	Negative

risks which require us to explore the field further in depth and enact methods ensuring absolute safety of the users.

Another study cited at [25] explores the possibilities of implementing Chat-GPT into child mental healthcare. It concludes that although Chat-GPT has immense potential to positively alter approaches towards child and teen mental healthcare, it must be done so with great caution. It is essential to ensure responsible use of the LLM into a child's mental health journey, particularly because of the child's vulnerable age. Hence, it is concluded that Chat-GPT cannot replace human therapist treatment entirely, and it is important to utilize it with great accountability and care.

6.6 Opinions about Patients' Use of Generative AI (Source: Blease C, Worthen A, Torous J, 2024)

Apart from streamlining the processes involved in total patient care, Gen AI proves to be beneficial for mental health practitioners. Pulling through simple administrative duties such as clerical work, interpretation of data, and contacting patients, AI allows the clinicians to concentrate on more sophisticated and patient oriented aspects of their work. Improvement in operational effectiveness can result in enhanced patient outcomes and job satisfaction.

As well as addressing these issues, Gen AI provides insights for and support to mental health professionals. The use of AI technology in the treatment of patients allows professionals to gain insights from the data collected that helps formulate guidelines for future treatment. Furthermore, Gen AI is able to provide patients with individualized suggestions regarding the further modalities used and help with creating new paradigms.

Through the use of Gen AI, mental health practitioners would be able to improve their practice and that of the patient, and also help develop mental health as a practice.

A study cited at [30] surveyed 138 psychiatrists to rate their agreements and disagreements with several statements regarding the possible pros and cons of Gen-AI-driven therapy.

Table 6.3 provides insightful information on the outlooks of mental health professionals regarding the role of generative AI in healthcare. By analyzing these opinions, we can identify areas of consensus and potential areas of concern [30].

Table 6.3 Percentages of mental healthcare professionals agreeing/disagreeing on statements regarding role of generative AI in healthcare.

	Disagree	Somewhat disagree	Somewhat agree	Agree	Do not know
Better understand their health	8.0%	10.9%	39.1%	15.9%	26.1%
Worry more about privacy	4.3%	13.8%	29.0%	28.3%	24.6%
Consult Gen-AI before seeing a doctor	2.9%	5.1%	36.2%	39.1%	16.7%
Use these tools to better understand their health	8.0%	7.2%	33.3%	29.0%	22.5%

6.7 Ethical Challenges and Considerations

There has been a significant shift in the field of psychotherapy due to the invention and innovation in generative AI [26] there are multiple advantages of Gen AI in the medical field but it poses serious challenges on privacy of the user data. One of the major issues being the collection of large volumes of patients' personal data. This collected data is stored by a small number of powerful corporations which shifts the focus from patient-oriented care to profit motives, compromising service satisfaction [26]. It also alarms about the data use without the consent of the user, posing risks to user confidentiality and ethical standards. During users' interactions with Gen AI systems, unintentional collection of personal information such as names, identities, and contact information may occur, which hinders data privacy policy. The data being collected intentionally or unintentionally may cause potential revelation or misuse of personal data, particularly in mental healthcare [26, 27].

An example illustrating this issue is the application of emotion detection. Advanced Gen AI systems gather users' facial expression images to predict their mental health conditions. While this technique makes the job of recognizing the problem easier, there is potential risk for misuse of these images. This could violate individuals' privacy rights and disappoint patients and weaken their trust in mental health services [27].

Another significant problem is that people may undervalue the presence of traditional experts such as experienced psychologists, leading to less dialogue between therapist and patient, diminishing of human mastery, skill, conception, and perception in therapy. One of the key elements in therapy is showing empathy towards the patient and forming genuine human connections. Excessive reliance on Gen AI tools in therapy may lead to a reduction in the importance of genuine affinity and rapport in the therapy [26]. Instead of serving as a supportive element in the journey of therapy, Gen AI may become the central focus [26]. If biased data is used to train these models, the model may not be able to produce accurate results which may lead to discriminatory or life-threatening outcomes [27]. For example – if the model is only trained on white population data, it will be incapable of producing results for black population. The potential for algorithmic biases in training datasets could result in the discrimination of marginalized groups as well. Algorithms might fail to recognize or accurately present the specific requirements of diverse populations, resulting in healthcare disparity or misdiagnosis of marginalized communities [27].

6.8 Future Considerations

There has been substantial advancement in artificial intelligence, notably in generative AI. Gen AI has its extensive usage in the domain of mental health. However, there are aspects of Gen AI that are relatively underexplored [28].

There are numerous future trends of Gen AI in mental health, one being the employment of wearable gadgets such as smartwatches and fitness trackers [29]. These devices continuously track the user's heartbeat rate, sleep cycles, physical activity, and speech patterns. AI algorithms can analyze this data and can offer early insights into any behavioral disturbance. Healthcare providers can use this data and provide better treatments for their patients. For example – alterations in sleep patterns, physical activity or speech can be recognized by these devices and pose a red flag for the healthcare providers for timely interventions [29].

Images and visuals often enhance therapeutic interventions. Integrating generative AI to create photographs and images can increase the customization and efficiency of these mediations, sooner or later improving patient outcomes and the patient experience. [28]. In working with kids who may find it difficult to understand their thoughts, feelings, and behaviors, incorporating personalized images can help them comprehend more effectively. Visualizations can provide a new perspective, allowing children to see their behaviors in a different light and identify potential areas for growth [28]. Generative AI can make people feel calmer by showing them images that are relaxing and peaceful. It can also help people by generating fake scenarios, which can help patients deal and cope with their feelings in a safe environment. Utilization of Gen AI in art and music therapy can offer significant advantages [28].

6.9 Conclusion

In conclusion, this chapter has delved into the promising capacity of generative AI to revolutionize support and treatment of mental health issues. Easily accessible, personalized support is readily available to the general public through chat-bots, LLMs, etc. Advanced AI mechanisms like Natural language processing, Machine Learning and Deep Learning are already triumphing in detection, screening, counseling and clinical-decision making in the area of mental healthcare. It is certain that generative AI has great untapped potential. However, further research is required to unleash the full capacity of Gen AI into the industry.

Integrating Gen AI into mental healthcare comes with several ethical challenges. Data privacy, security, and algorithmic biases are some key areas that require strict rules and regulations to prevent any accidental harm to the user/patient. Guidelines must be extensively laid out to ensure AI is being used ethically and effectively. Nevertheless, it is essential to maintain human supervision to harness the maximum capacity of Gen AI in boosting mental health outcomes.

By cautiously navigating these difficulties and seizing the opportunities presented by Gen AI, we prepare for a future where people with mental health issues have access to effective support.

References

[1] Kishor Kumar Reddy C., Bhavya T., P. R. Anisha, and Hanafiah M. (2025) "Text-Based Prediction and Classification Model Of Stress, Anxiety and Depression Among Indians," in *Smart Sensors for Industry 4.0*, Wiley, pp. 131–147. Doi:10.1002/9781394214723.ch9.

[2] McKinsey and Company: "What is ChatGPT, DALL-E, and generative AI?". Available at: https://www.mckinsey.com/featured-insights/mckinsey-explainers/what-is-generative-ai [Accessed at: Sep. 16, 2024]

[3] Kalota F. (2024) "A Primer on Generative Artificial Intelligence," *Educ Sci (Basel)*, vol. 14, no. 2, p. 172, doi:10.3390/educsci14020172.

[4] Tewari A., Chhabria A., Khalsa A.S., Chaudhary S, and Kanal H. (2021) "A survey of mental health chatbots using NLP," *papers.ssrn.com*,

Available: https://papers.ssrn.com/sol3/papers.cfm?abstract_id=3833914 [Accessed:Sep. 16, 2024]

[5] Malgaroli M.,Hull T., Zech J.,Althoff T. (2023) "Natural language processing for mental health interventions- a systematic review and research framework," *nature.com*, doi:10.1038/s41398-023-02592-2.

[6] Calvo R., Milne D., Hussain M.S, Christensen H (2017) "Natural language processing in mental health applications using non-clinical texts," *cambridge.org*, vol. 23, no. 5, pp. 649–685, doi:10.1017/S1351324916000383.

[7] Fiske A., Henningsen P., Buyx A. (2019) "Your robot therapist will see you now: ethical implications of embodied artificial intelligence in psychiatry, psychology, and psychotherapy," *jmir.org*, Available at: https://www.jmir.org/2019/5/e13216 [Accessed at: Sep. 16,2024].

[8] Iyortsuun N. K., Kim S.H, M. Jhon, H.-J. Yang, and S. Pant, (2023) "A Review of Machine Learning and Deep Learning Approaches on Mental Health Diagnosis," *Healthcare*, vol. 11, no. 3, p. 285, doi:10.3390/healthcare11030285.

[9] López-Úbeda P., Plaza-del-Arco F. M, Díaz-Galiano M. C., and Martín-Valdivia M.-T. (2021) "How Successful Is Transfer Learning for Detecting Anorexia on Social Media?," *Applied Sciences*, vol. 11, no.4, p. 1838, doi:10.3390/app11041838.

[10] Rollwage M.*et al.* (2024) "Correction: Using Conversational AI to Facilitate Mental Health Assessments and Improve Clinical Efficiency Within Psychotherapy Services: Real-World Observational Study," *JMIR AI*, vol. 3, p. e57869, doi:10.2196/57869.

[11] Haque M.and Rubya S, (2023), "An Overview of Chatbot-Based Mobile Mental Health Apps: Insights From App Description and User Reviews," *JMIR Mhealth Uhealth*, vol. 11, pp. 11-e44838.

[12] Thakkar A.,Gupta A., and De Sousa A., (2024), "Artificial intelligence In positive mental health: a narrative review," *Front Digit Health*, vol. 6, doi:10.3389/FDGTH.2024.1280235.

[13] American Psychological Association: "What is Exposure Therapy?", Available at: www.div12.org , [Accessed: Sep. 20, 2024]

[14] Mahmoudi-Nejad A., (2021), "Automated Personalized Exposure Therapy Based on Physiological Measures Using Experience-Driven Procedural Content Generation," in *Proceedings of the AAAI Conference on Artificial Intelligence and Interactive Digital Entertainment*, vol. 17,no.1, pp. 232–235, doi:10.1609/aiide.v17i1.18914.

[15] Callahan C., Kimber J., Hu E. , Tanner L., and Kunkle S., (2024), "The Real-World Impact of App-Based Mindfulness on Headspace Members With Moderate and Severe Perceived Stress: Observational Study," *JMIR Mhealth Uhealth*, vol. 12, pp. e52968–e52968, doi: 10.2196/52968.
[16] Wysa: "Wysa - Everyday Mental Health." Available at: https://www.wysa.com/ [Accessed: Sep. 18, 2024]
[17] Talkspace: "Talkspace - #1 Rated Online Therapy, 1 Million Users.", Available at: https://www.talkspace.com/ [Accessed: Sep. 18, 2024]
[18] BetterHelp: "BetterHelp - Get Started & Sign-Up Today.", Available at:https://www.betterhelp.com/get-started/?go=true&transaction_id=102a2c8625bc5d7c8cdae804375629&utm_source=affiliate&utm_campaign=3612&utm_medium=Desktop&utm_content=&utm_term=babybubble&not_found=1&gor=start [Accessed: Sep. 18, 2024]
[19] Woebot Health: "About Us | Woebot Health.", Available at: https://woebothealth.com/about-us/ [Accessed: Sep. 18, 2024]
[20] Kintsugi: "About Us — Kintsugi.", Available at: https://www.kintsugihealth.com/about [Accessed: Sep. 18, 2024]
[21] DemandSage: "ChatGPT Statistics (SEP. 2024) – 200 Million Active Users." Available at: https://www.demandsage.com/chatgpt-statistics/[Accessed:Sep.18,2024].
[22] Khan I.U, Hajjami S.E, Ouaissa M., Belaqziz S., Bhatia T.K (2024) "Cognitive Machine Intelligence: Applications, Challenges, and Related Google Books."Available at: https://books.google.co.in/books?hl=en&lr=&id=aaAUEQAAQBAJ&oi=findpg=PA328&ots=XODpo8l49a&sig=uC154Uk7-BcGXizhHKLClCw-B4Y#v=onepage&q&f=false [Accessed: Sep. 18, 2024]
[23] Biswas S.S (2023) "Role of Chat GPT in Public Health," *Ann Biomed Eng*, vol. 51, no. 5, pp. 868–869, doi:10.1007/S10439-023-03172-7/METRICS.
[24] Alanezi F.(2024) "Assessing the Effectiveness of ChatGPT in Delivering Mental Health Support: A Qualitative Study," *J Multidiscip Healthc*, vol. Volume 17, pp. 461–471, doi:10.2147/JMDH.S447368.
[25] Imran N., Hashmi A., and Imran A. (2023) "Chat-GPT: Opportunities and Challenges in Child Mental Healthcare," *Pak J Med Sci*, vol. 39, no.4, doi:10.12669/pjms.39.4.8118.
[26] Haber Y., Levkovich I., Dorit H.-S., Elyoseph Z. (2024) "The artificial third: a broad view of the effects of introducing generative artificial

intelligence on psychotherapy," *mental.jmir.org*, Available at: https://mental.jmir.org/2024/1/e54781 [Accessed: Sep.15, 2024]

[27] Xian X., Chang A., Xiang Y., Liu M.T. (2024) J. of Medical, "Debate and Dilemmas Regarding Generative AI in Mental Health Care: Scoping Review," *i-jmr.org*, Available at: https://i-jmr.org/2024/1/e53672 [Accessed: Sep. 15, 2024]

[28] Sezgin E.,McKay I., (2024) "Behavioral health and generative AI: a perspective on future of therapies and patient care," *nature.com*, doi: 10.1038/s44184-024-00067-w.

[29] Olawade D., Wada O., Ojima Z., Wada B., Aderonke Odetayo C., Aanuoluwapo Clement David-Olawade D., Fiyinfoluwa Asaolu E., Judith Eberhardt F.(2024), "Enhancing mental health with Artificial Intelligence: Current trends And future prospects," *Elsevier*

[30] Blease C.,Worthen A., Torous J. (2024) Psychiatrists' experiences and opinions of generative artificial intelligence in mental healthcare: An online mixed methods survey, Psychiatry Research, Volume 333, 115724, ISSN 0165-1781, DOI:https://doi.org/10.1016/j.psychres.2024.115724.

[31] Kishor Kumar Reddy, C. (2023). An Efficient early Diagnosis and Healthcare Monitoring System for Mental Disorder using Machine Learning. In Sustainable Science and Intelligent Technologies for Societal Development, IGI Global.

[32] Thirupathi, L., SrihaReddy, E., & Deepika, J. V. (2024). Challenges and Innovations in the Creation of Digital Twins in Healthcare. In A. Dubey, C. Kumar Reddy, S. Doss, & M.Hanafiah (Eds.), Exploring the Advancements and Future Directions of Digital Twins in Healthcare 6.0 (pp 69-85). IGI Global. DOI: https://doi.org/10.4018/979-8-3693-5893-1.ch004

[33] G. H. Lee, K. J. Lee, B. Jeong and T. Kim. (2024). Developing Personalized Marketing Service Using Generative AI, in IEEE Access, vol. 12, pp. 22394-22402. Doi:10.1109/ACCESS.2024.3361946.

7

Navigating Autism Spectrum Disorder: A Fusion of Deep Learning and Explainable AI for Enhanced Detection and Classification

K. M. Danial Sadad[1], Anindya Nag[1], Nitesh Upadhyaya[2], Salman Islam[1], Kaysun Molla[1], and Dip Ranjan Dutta[3]

[1]Department of Computer Science and Engineering, Northern University of Business & Technology, Bangladesh
[2]GlobalLogic Inc, USA
[3] Department of Computer Science and Engineering, Guru Nanak Dev University, India
E-mail: danialsadad042@gmail.com; anindyanag@ieee.org; salmancse.i77@gmail.com; kaysun430@gmail.com; dipranjanduttad@gmail.com

Abstract

Autism spectrum disorder (ASD) is a neurodevelopmental disease that impairs communication, conduct, and social interactions. Early discovery is crucial for effective management. This study investigates the application of deep learning algorithms to predict ASD in children using a freshly constructed dataset. Several models were tested, including feed forward neural networks (FFNN), deep neural networks (DNN), convolutional neural networks (CNN), long short-term memory (LSTM), and gated recurrent units (GRU), with the DNN model outperforming the others with a 99.22% accuracy. Furthermore, this study employs explainable AI, namely local interpretable model-agnostic explanations (LIME), to give insights into model predictions. Explain ability integration guarantees that forecasts are interpretable, which improves model confidence and transparency. This study

DOI: 10.1201/9788743801764-7

contributes a valuable dataset and demonstrates the efficacy of deep learning approaches and explainable AI in early ASD detection.

Keywords: Deep Learning, Explainable AI, Autism Spectrum Disorder, FFNN, CNN, DNN, LSTM, GRU, Lime.

7.1 Introduction

The problem of ASD is becoming more and more common among people of all ages nowadays. The renovation of the patient's bodily and intellectual well-being can be notably aided by way of the early identity of this neurological condition. The increasing use of deep know-based total models to forecast a wide variety of human illnesses has made it seem viable to identify these ailments early on with the use of a variety of physiological and fitness parameters [1]. This something spurred us to turn out to be greater inquisitive about the identification and evaluation of ASD issues a good way to expand more effective therapeutic methods. the issue of autism spectrum disease has to do with how the human brain develops. it is commonly now not viable for a person with ASD to engage socially or communicate with others [2]. This often has an impact on a person's life at some point in their lifespan. The opportunity that this infection is a result of an aggregate of hereditary and environmental elements is exciting. The aforementioned difficulty may additionally take place with signs and symptoms as early as age 3 and can persist until old age. Although the patient's situation cannot be completely handled, if the symptoms are diagnosed early on, its consequences may be temporarily mitigated. because scientists accept as true that ASD is caused by human genes, they have not yet identified the best origins of the disorder. Human genes affect the environment, which in turn impacts development [3]. ASD is encouraged with the aid of some chance factors, including low birth weight, having an elderly dad and mom, and having a sibling with ASD. As opposed to this, there are a few issues with conversation and social interplay along with: the inability to make eye touch, incorrect response to sound, Social and verbal exchange challenges, loss of preference for cuddles, incapacity to talk gestures, loss of social interplay, beside the point attachment to objects, preference to stay by myself and so forth. The most critical movements that may be made to lessen the signs of autism spectrum sickness and decorate the lives of folks who are afflicted by ASD are early identity and remedy. But there is not a system for scientific examination to discover autism. ASD signs are often identified by remark. teachers and parents are normally those who recognize the signs of ASD in older and teen students. A faculty-affiliated unique schooling crew then assesses symptoms of ASD. The school group encouraged the students to see their medical doctor for essential exams [4]. For the reason that ASD symptoms can also overlap with the ones of other mental health conditions, it could be much more difficult to diagnose ASD signs in adults than in older youngsters and young people. Remark can detect behavioral issues in children as soon as six months old, whereas autism-specific brain imaging can only reveal changes after two years. Toddlers expand language through social interactions, which might be precise to humans and assist them in communicating and learning about their surroundings [5]. Adults direct newborns' attention to objects and activities via shared experiences such as imitation and collaborative attention. both receptive and expressive language development are concepts to arise at some stage in the first years of life through social conversation, which incorporates serial games, gestures, and mimics used to percentage shared interests and communicate wishes.

ASD is neurodevelopmental contamination that causes confined hobbies, repetitive behaviours, and problems with social communique and interaction. It commonly appears earlier than the age of three and lasts during existence. Signs encompass difficulties with social conversation, nonverbal behaviors, and building social relationships, as well as stereotypical behaviors, rigorous workouts, and obsessive interests [6]. Verbal exchange and language abilities are important to the phenotype and prognosis of autism. In keeping with the DSM-five, ASD is defined by main characteristics: continual deficits in social verbal exchange and interaction across more than one context, constrained, repetitive patterns of behavior, which appear early in development, and purpose sizeable impairment in each daily functioning. ASD is identified and controlled by measuring social responsiveness with devices such as the SRS [7]. To grow social interaction, behavioral therapy and social skill education are often used as interventions. Although speech and language impairments frequently accompany ASD, they are not clear markers of the diagnosis. Professional evaluations are required for effective interventions.

The goal of this chapter is to enhance ASD identification using a variety of deep learning methods. We will test and compare these algorithms on a dataset, analyze feature importance, and select essential traits to ensure accurate detection. Our objective is to create a high-performance model with superior accuracy, recall, F1 score, and precision. We will also use XAI to improve model interpretation. The dataset we used is quite fresh, with little prior study done on it. It contains a significant quantity of data and features.

To improve model interpretability and transparency, we want to use a variety of deep learning models and XAI techniques.

The remainder of the chapter is organized into the following sections. Section 7.2 provides an overview of the previous research related to ASD detection, highlighting the algorithms used in our study and their foundation. Section 7.3 discusses the dataset in detail, including its attributes, system architecture, and various aspects. Section 7.4 presents the results of our experiments using different models. We provide a comparative analysis of the model's performance. Section 7.5 Here, we conclude our findings and discuss potential future directions.

7.2 Literature Review

Maenner et al. [8] used deep learning models and eye-tracking technologies for early ASD screening investigated in this work. The following models obtained high accuracy: BiLSTM (96.44%), GRU (97.49%), CNN-LSTM (97.94%), and LSTM (98.33%). These findings show the promise of sophisticated computational approaches in ASD classification, with future studies focusing on bigger, more diverse datasets for greater application.

Thabtah et al. [9] investigated how ASD disrupts speech and interaction beginning in early childhood. This study compares deep learning and machine learning models (Naïve Bayes, SVM, Logistic Regression, KNN, Neural Networks, and CNN) across children, adults, and adolescents. CNN models excelled, with accuracies of 99.53% for adults, 98.30% for children, and 96.88% for adolescents. These findings indicate that CNNs are more successful than traditional machine learning methods for detecting ASD.

Kim et al. [10] presented a CNN model for early ASD identification based on fMRI data from 126 participants (56 ASD, 70 controls). The model, trained on 22,176 samples, obtained outstanding results, including 98.39% accuracy, 98.80% recall, 99.85% precision, and a 99.32% F1 score. The CNN proved its capacity to discern between ASD and generally developing youngsters using hierarchical feature extraction. While very accurate, this model requires more validation across varied populations, as well as the integration of multi-modal data, before it can be used in clinical settings for early ASD screening and personalized therapies.

Bolton et al. [11] found diagnosis of ASD has become more accurate and efficient with the use of machine learning (ML) approaches. Before and after addressing missing values, support vector machines (SVMs) obtained 97.95% and 98.30% accuracy, respectively. Similarly, artificial

Table 7.1 Summary of literature review.

Author	Model	Dataset	Accuracy
Maenner et al. [8]	LSTM	DEAP	98.33%
Thabtah et al. [9]	CNN	Self-Collected	98.30%
Kim et al. [10]	CNN	KAGGLE	98.39%
Bolton et al. [11]	ANN	Self-Collected	98.30%
Abraham et al. [12]	Xception	KAGGLE	91%
Elsabbagh et al. [13]	DNN	Online platform	88%
Bengio et al. [14]	CNN	DEAP	97.07%

neural networks (ANNs) achieved 97.60% accuracy before and 98.30% after addressing missing variables. CNNs, which were not assessed before handling missing values, achieved 98.30% accuracy thereafter.

Abraham et al. [12] investigated deep learning models for identifying ASD by analyzing face characteristics with two pre-trained CNNs, Xception and VGG16, using a dataset of 2,940 photos. Xception scored 91% accuracy, surpassing VGG16's 73%. The findings imply that deep learning may efficiently extract essential face traits, providing a scalable, non-invasive technique for early ASD identification that will help health professionals make faster, more objective diagnoses.

Elsabbagh et al. [13] created a deep learning model for identifying ASD based on multisite resting-state fMRI data and four brain atlases (CC200, AAL, BASC, and Power). The BASC atlas produced the greatest results, with 88% accuracy, 90% sensitivity, 87% F1 score, and 96% AUC. The deep neural network (DNN) classifier outperforms conventional approaches such as random forest and k-nearest neighbors in ASD identification.

Bengio et al. [14], used "ASD Classification Using Deep Learning" which uses CNNs to categorize ASD based on neuroimaging data from the NITRC. After optimizing hyperparameters, the CNN obtained 97.07% accuracy, beating the support vector machine (SVM), which had just 66.36% accuracy. This shows that deep learning approaches are more successful for ASD categorization. An overview of previous research is given in Table 7.1.

7.3 Methodology

The workflow diagram of the proposed system is as follows. They are data preprocessing, missing value handling, encoding, data splitting, Implementing models, model training, testing, and evaluation. Figure 7.1 represents the flow Diagram of our proposed work.

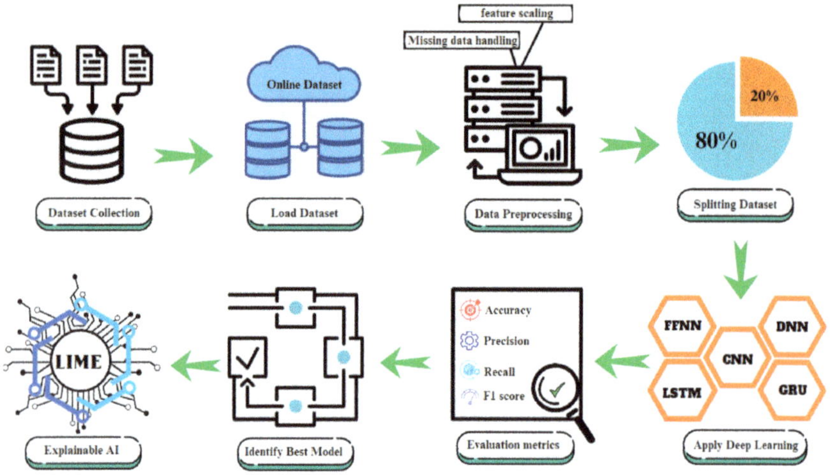

Figure 7.1 Flow diagram of our proposed work.

7.3.1 Dataset description

In this work, a Kaggle dataset centered on neurodevelopmental disorders with substantial healthcare costs – ASD – is employed. Early diagnosis is critical, but existing treatments are sluggish and expensive. With the global increase in ASD incidence, there is a need for efficient and accessible screening procedures. It consists of 18 features (categorical, continuous, and binary) and 1,054 examples targeted at enhancing ASD categorization.

7.3.2 Data preprocessing

Preprocessing is critical while preparing the ASD screening dataset in CSV format for deep learning tasks. To achieve optimal neural network performance, this includes managing missing values, encoding categorical variables, and normalizing/standardizing numerical features and feature scaling are critical for avoiding biases during training. Furthermore, feature engineering can improve the dataset's structure, allowing models to capture more complicated patterns.

7.3.2.1 Missing data handling

Missing values in datasets can lead to biased or inaccurate analyses if not addressed properly. In our study, to ensure the robustness and reliability of the data, we removed rows where missing values were present, thereby ensuring a complete and consistent dataset for our modeling efforts.

7.3.2.2 Data scaling

After cleansing the dataset via changing specific variables to binary and addressing lacking values, facts scaling is applied to make certain uniformity throughout functions. We applied StandardScaler to standardize the statistics, adjusting functions to have a median of zero and a popular deviation of one. This scaling method complements the reliability of the dataset by normalizing the variety of values, which is crucial for correct model performance and powerful diagnostic outcomes. Algorithm 7.1 depicts the data scaling algorithm.

Algorithm 7.1: Data Scaling Algorithm

Input: Original data matrix $X\ of\ size\ m \times n$

Output: Scaled data matrix X_{Scaled}

Steps:

Step 1: Compute the mean for each feature (column):

$$\mu_j = \frac{1}{m}\sum_{i=1}^{m} X_{ij} \text{ for each } j = 1, 2, \ldots, n$$

Step 2: Compute the standard deviation for each feature (column):

$$\sigma_j = \sqrt{\frac{1}{m}\sum_{i=1}^{m} (X_{ij} - \mu_j)^2} \text{ for each } j = 1,\ 2,\ \ldots, n$$

Step 3: Standardize each value by subtracting the mean and dividing by the standard deviation:

$$X_{\text{scaled}}[i, j] = \frac{X_{ij} - \mu_j}{\sigma_j} \text{ for each } i = 1,\ 2, \ldots, m \text{ and } j = 1, 2, \ldots, n$$

Step 4: Return the scaled data matrix X_{Scaled}

7.3.3 Dataset splitting

Dataset splitting is an important step in getting data ready for deep learning tasks. We used a stratified splitting strategy to divide the dataset into training and testing sets, ensuring that the distribution of target classes remained consistent across both. This strategy, which employs an 80:20 ratio, aids in assessing the model's capacity to generalize to new data and gives insights into its prediction performance for ASD-related traits.

7.3.4 Applied models

The goal of this effort is to develop a model that can minimize the number of instances. The goal of this work is to develop a trustworthy model for reliably screening ASD using deep learning approaches.

7.3.4.1 Feed forward neural network

A FFNN is a basic neural network in which data goes one way from input to output via hidden layers. It is used for tasks like classification, with learning accomplished by modifying weights to reduce mistakes [15]. The equation for FNN is given by eqn (7.1).

$$y = w_{\text{out}} \cdot a + b_{\text{out}}. \tag{7.1}$$

7.3.4.2 Convolutional neural network

A CNN is a specialized neural network that processes grid-like input, such as pictures. It is commonly used in image identification, object detection, and other applications that require the automated extraction of characteristics such as edges or textures via convolutional layers. CNNs excel in capturing spatial hierarchies in data because of their layered nature [16]. Eqn (7.2) shows convolutional calculation done in convolutional layer.

$$(f * g)(i, j) = \sum_{m} \sum_{n} f(m, n) \cdot g(i - m, j - n) \tag{7.2}$$

7.3.4.3 LSTM recurrent neural network

An LSTM recurrent neural network is a form of RNN that detects long-term relationships in sequential input. It employs memory cells to store information over time, making it useful for time series prediction, language modeling, and voice recognition. LSTMs overcome the vanishing gradient problem, allowing for more accurate pattern recognition in longer sequences [17]. Eqn (7.3) and (7.4) show the output equation for LSTM.

$$o_t = \sigma\left(W_o \cdot \left[h_{t-1}, x_t\right] + b_o)\right], \tag{7.3}$$

$$h_t = o_t \cdot \tan\text{h}\left(C_t\right). \tag{7.4}$$

7.3.4.4 GRU recurrent neural network

A GRU recurrent neural network is a form of RNN that captures sequence dependencies and addresses vanishing gradient concerns. GRUs govern the flow of input using gating mechanisms (reset and update gates), making

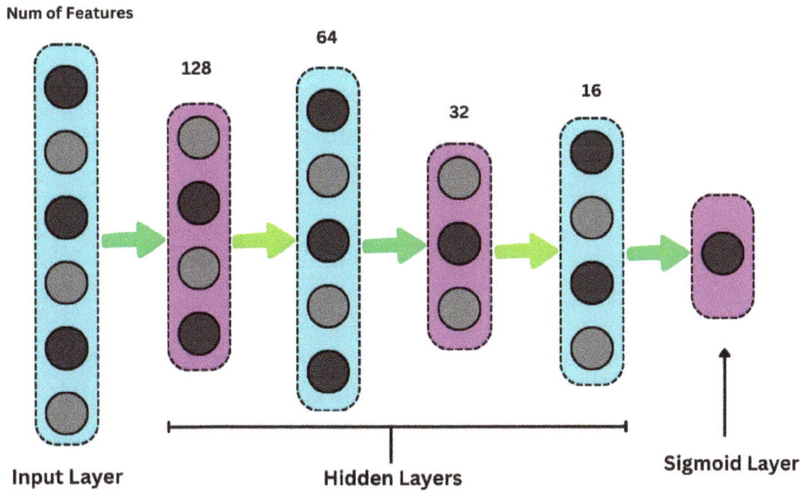

Figure 7.2 Proposed model architecture.

them more efficient than typical RNNs for applications such as time-series prediction and natural language processing [18]. Eqn (7.5) shows the output gate equation for GRU.

$$h_t = (1 - z_t) \cdot h_{t-1} + z_t \cdot \widetilde{h_t} \tag{7.5}$$

7.3.4.5 Deep neural network (proposed)

A DNN is a feed forward network with additional hidden layers between input and output. This deeper design allows the model to learn complicated patterns and representations, making it useful for applications [19]. The visual representation of DNN is given in Figure 7.2.

7.3.5 Evaluation metrics

Evaluation metrics are crucial tools for assessing the performance of deep learning models. They give quantitative assessments of a model's accuracy, precision, recall, and other essential performance characteristics [20].

7.3.5.1 Accuracy

Accuracy is the percentage of correctly classified cases out of all occurrences. It is best suited for balanced datasets and evenly distributed classes [21]. It is defined as:

$$\text{Accuracy}=\frac{\text{TP}+\text{TN}}{\text{TP}+\text{TN}+\text{FP}+\text{FN}}. \tag{7.6}$$

7.3.5.2 Precision

Precision measures the proportion of accurate positive predictions to all positive forecasts [22]. The equation for precision is:

$$\text{Precision}=\frac{\text{TP}}{\text{TP}+\text{FP}} \tag{7.7}$$

7.3.5.3 Recall

Recall, often called sensitivity or true positive rate, is the ratio of accurate positive forecasts to positive instances [22]. The equation for the recall is:

$$\text{Recall}=\frac{\text{TP}}{\text{TP}+\text{FN}}\ . \tag{7.8}$$

7.3.5.4 F1 score

We can reduce feature space and improve model training speed and accuracy by identifying the primary prediction factors [22]. The equation for the F1 score is:

$$\text{F1 score}= 2\times\frac{\text{Precision}\ \times \text{Recall}}{\text{Precision}\ + \ \text{Recall}}. \tag{7.9}$$

7.3.6 Explainable AI (LIME)

LIME is an XAI approach for interpreting deep learning models. It works by using smaller, interpretable models (such as linear models) to approximate the predictions of a more sophisticated model, such as a neural network, for individual data points. LIME enables consumers to understand why a deep learning model generated a certain prediction, increasing transparency and confidence in AI systems. Transparency is essential for verifying the dependability of the models and understanding the fundamental patterns in the data, which eventually enhances the credibility and comprehensibility of detecting responsible features for ASD [23].

This method detects (ASD) using deep learning models. It preprocesses the dataset, trains models such as FFNN, CNN, and LSTM, and assesses them using precision, recall, and F1 scores. LIME is used to explain predictions, and the top-performing model is chosen for deployment. It is shown in Algorithm 7.2.

Table 7.2 Comparison of model performance.

Models	Accuracy (%)	Precision (%)	Recall (%)	F1-Score(%)
FFNN	98.44	99.52	99.52	99.52
CNN	96.10	96.28	96.28	96.28
LSTM	78.18	99.24	99.24	99.24
GRU	96.62	95.89	95.89	95.89
DNN (Proposed)	**99.22**	**99.53**	**99.53**	**99.53**

7.4 Result and Discussion

In this chapter, we employed five distinct deep-learning models: FFNN, DNN, CNN, LSTM, and GRU. DNN achieves a higher accuracy of 99%, while FFNN achieves an accuracy of 98%, and LSTM has the lowest accuracy of 78%. A comparison of the performance of the models is provided in Table 7.2.

Algorithm 7.2. Algorithm for classification using deep learning models

Input:

- Data CSV file df
- Categorical columns cat_cols
- One-hot encoding columns two_col
- Models Mbase (e.g., FFNN, Dropout FFNN, CNN, LSTM, GRU)

Output:

- Best model Mbest
- Saved model file

Steps:

Step 1: Dataset Preparation

1. **Load and preprocess data:**
   - df = pd.read_csv('data_csv.csv')
   - Remove missing values and encode categorical columns
   - One-hot encode specified columns

2. **Split data and scale features:**
   - X_train, X_test, y_train, y_test = train_test_split(X, y, test_size=0.2, random_state=42)

- X_train = scaler.fit_transform(X_train)
- X_test = scaler.transform(X_test)

Step 2: Model Creation
Define and compile models using base models Mbase:

- Initialize with Adam optimizer and binary_crossentropy loss

Step 3: Model Training
Train each model:

- model.fit (X_train, y_train, epochs=10, batch_size=32, validation_split= 0.2)

Step 4: LIME Explanation
Use LIME to explain model predictions:

- explainer = lime.lime_tabular.LimeTabularExplainer (...)
- Explain a sample instance from X_test

Step 5: Model Evaluation
Evaluate models:

- Calculate precision, recall, f1_score, and plot performance metrics

Step 6: Identify Best Model
Select a model with the highest F1 score as Mbest

Step 7: Model Deployment

We used a confusion matrix to test the performance of several models, including FFNN, DNN, CNN, LSTM, and GRU. The DNN model outperformed the others, achieving 99.22% accuracy while maintaining good precision and recall. The confusion matrix revealed a few false positives and false negatives, demonstrating the DNN's ability to accurately categorize ASD patients. It is defined in Figure 7.3.

The accuracy and loss curves indicate how the model performed at each epoch. The DNN achieved 99.22% accuracy, and the accuracy curve climbed while the loss curve lowered, demonstrating efficient learning. Compared to FFNN, CNN, LSTM, and GRU, the DNN regularly outperforms them all in terms of accuracy and loss. It is defined in Figure 7.4.

An XAI framework, such as LIME, is essential for explaining black box models like DNN in ASD detection. It aids in determining how certain properties influence predictions, hence increasing confidence in the model.

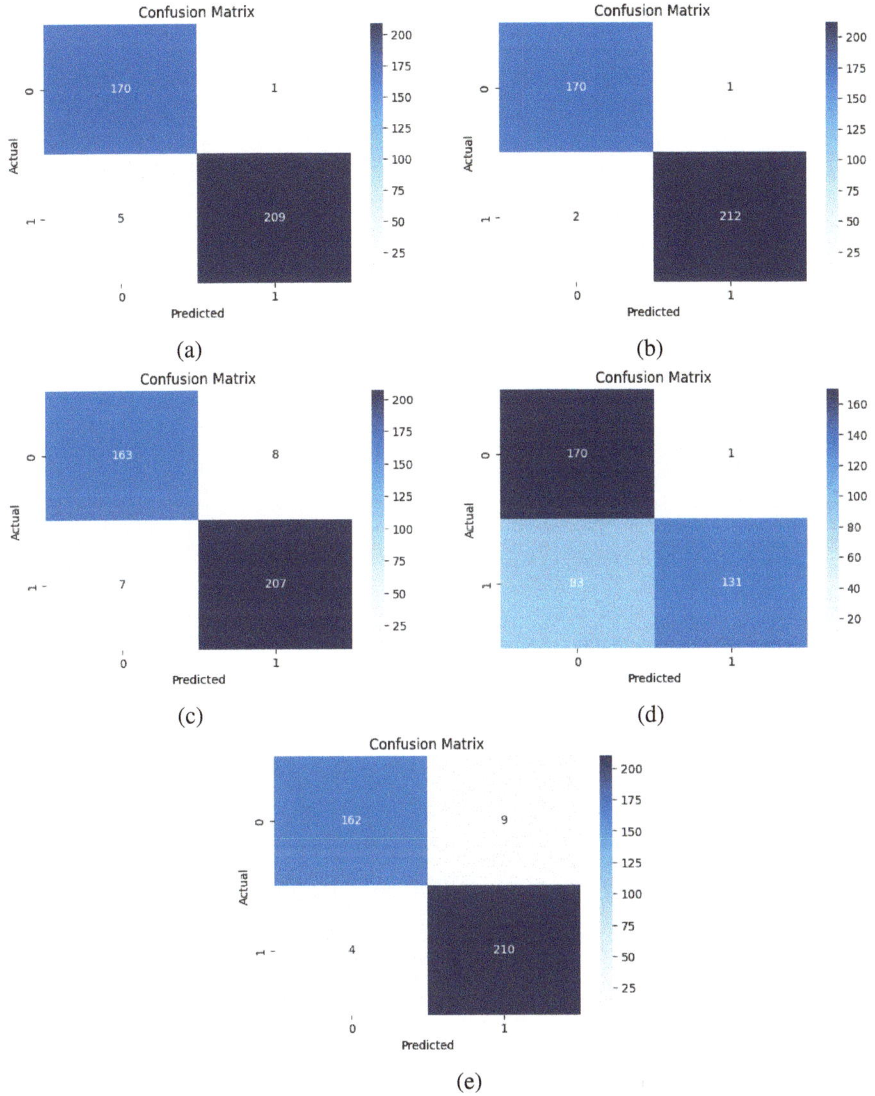

Figure 7.3 Confusion matrix of all models: (a) FFNN, (b) DNN, (c) CNN, (d) LSTM, (e) GRU.

By identifying critical characteristics, we can narrow the feature space and increase training efficiency. This chapter utilizes LIME and a DNN classifier to investigate how behavioral features contribute to ASD predictions. As a consequence, the model obtained 99.22% accuracy, with precision, recall, and

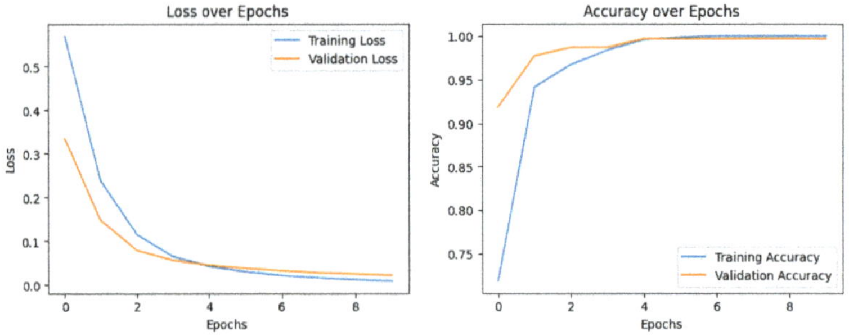
Loss over Epochs
Training Loss
Validation Loss
Loss
Epochs
Accuracy over Epochs
Training Accuracy
Validation Accuracy
Accuracy
Epochs

(a)

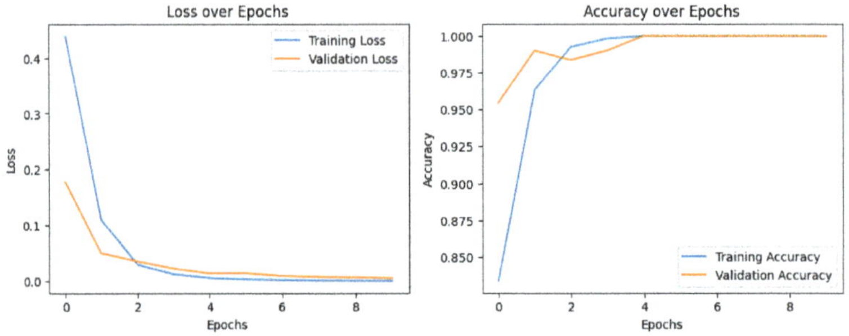
Loss over Epochs
Training Loss
Validation Loss
Loss
Epochs
Accuracy over Epochs
Training Accuracy
Validation Accuracy
Accuracy
Epochs

(b)

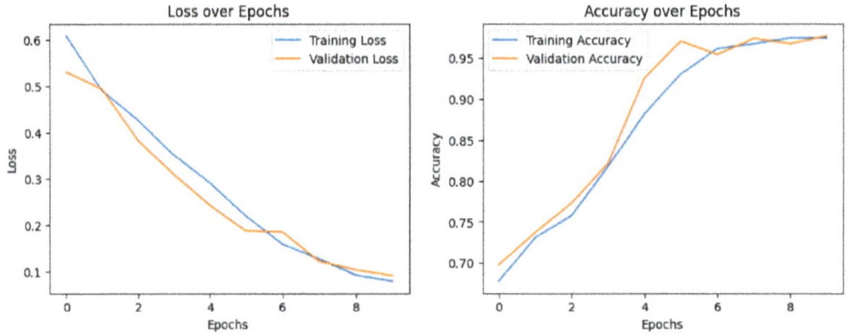
Loss over Epochs
Training Loss
Validation Loss
Loss
Epochs
Accuracy over Epochs
Training Accuracy
Validation Accuracy
Accuracy
Epochs

(c)

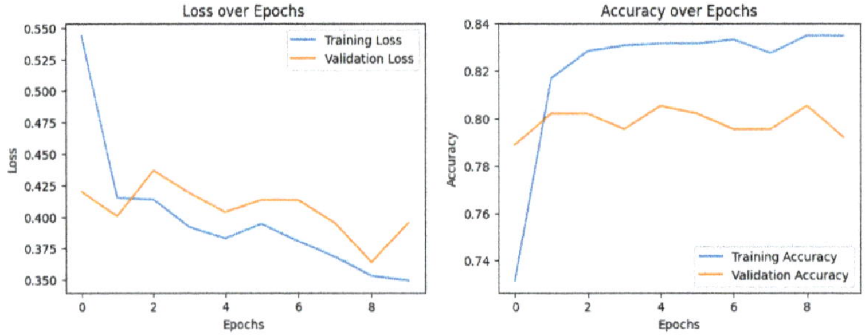
Loss over Epochs
Training Loss
Validation Loss
Loss
Epochs
Accuracy over Epochs
Training Accuracy
Validation Accuracy
Accuracy
Epochs

(d)

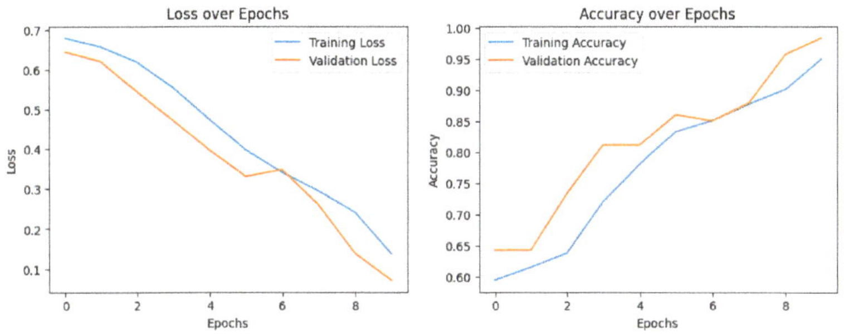

(e)

Figure 7.4 Accuracy and loss curve of all models: (a) FFNN, (b) DNN, (c) CNN, (d) LSTM, (e) GRU.

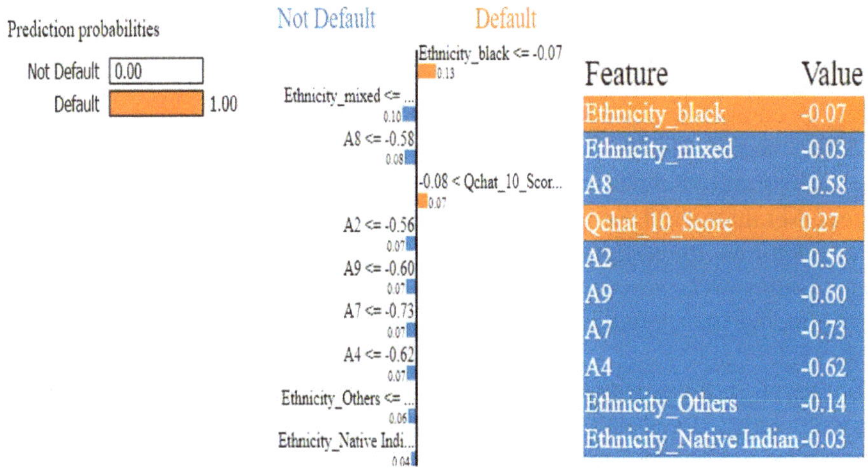

Figure 7.5 Explanation of DNN generated by LIME.

F1-scores of 0.9953, which improved the classifying process's representation as shown in Figure 7.5.

The dataset, while large, may not adequately capture the varied spectrum of ASD presentations across different populations, therefore limiting the model's generalizability. High-accuracy models like as DNN and FFNN need large processing resources, making them difficult to use in some clinical or therapeutic situations. Furthermore, the interpretability of these models remains an issue, making it difficult for healthcare practitioners to comprehend and trust their forecasts. Future research should concentrate on testing these models on bigger, more diverse datasets, improving interpretability,

Table 7.3 Comparison of the performance of the model to that of earlier research.

Author	**Model**	**Model exploitability**	**Accuracy**
Maenner et al. [8]	LSTM	NO	98.33%
Thabtah et al. [9]	CNN	NO	98.30%
Kim et al. [10]	CNN	NO	98.39%
Bolton et al. [11]	ANN	NO	98.30%
Abraham et al. [12]	Xception	NO	91%
Elsabbagh et al. [13]	DNN	NO	88%
Proposed	**DNN**	**Yes (LIME)**	**99.22%**

and increasing computing efficiency. Furthermore, approaches such as SHAP might be investigated to give more robust explainability in AI-powered diagnostics.

7.5 Comparison with State-of-the-Art Techniques

Table 7.3 compares multiple models used to classify ASD. Maenner et al LSTM model was 98.33% accurate, while [9] and [10] CNN models were 98.30% and 98.39%, respectively. Bolton et al ANN obtained 98.30%, whereas Abraham et al Xception scored 91%. Elsabbagh et al DNN scored 88%. In contrast, the suggested DNN model surpassed all others, achieving an astonishing 99.22% accuracy while using the LIME explainability tool to improve model interpretability. Comparisons with earlier research are given in Table 7.3.

Numerous critical aspects contribute to our model's exceptional performance. First, the DNN architecture was fine-tuned using appropriate hyperparameters, which increased learning efficiency. Second, the incorporation of LIME allowed for transparent inspection of the model's predictions, providing insights into which attributes contributed the most to categorization and solving the "black box" problem. This not only increased trust in the model but also allowed for a more in-depth knowledge of ASD-related patterns, resulting in a DNN model that is not only accurate but also interpretable and therapeutically useful.

7.6 Conclusion and Future Scope

This study explored the application of deep learning techniques for predicting ASD in toddlers using a newly developed dataset. Several preprocessing steps were taken, including handling missing values and scaling features, to ensure the data was suitable for training the models. Among the models tested, the DNN achieved the highest accuracy at 99.22%, highlighting its effectiveness in ASD detection. Additionally, explainable AI was incorporated through LIME, providing transparency into the model's decision-making process. The combination of preprocessing, model accuracy, and interpretability make this approach a valuable contribution to early ASD diagnosis. Future research could build on this study by expanding the dataset to include more diverse samples, potentially improving model generalization. Additionally, implementing real-time ASD detection in clinical settings could validate the practical applicability of these models. Further investigation into alternative preprocessing techniques, model architectures, and advanced explainability methods may offer additional improvements. Collaborations with healthcare professionals would also enhance the clinical relevance of the models, moving closer to real-world implementation for early ASD diagnosis and intervention.

Data Availability Statement

The used dataset of this study "ASD Dataset" is publicly available at https://www.kaggle.com/code/afarinbargrizan/autism-spectrum-disorder-detection-with-classifier. The code associated with this research is also found at this link with the special request of the corresponding authors [31].

References

[1] Rylaarsdam, Lauren, and Alicia Guemez-Gamboa. "Genetic causes and modifiers of autism spectrum disorder." *Frontiers in cellular neuroscience* 13 (2019): 385.

[2] Raj, Suman, and Sarfaraz Masood. "Analysis and detection of autism spectrum disorder using machine learning techniques." *Procedia Computer Science* 167 (2020): 994-1004.

[3] Abdelhamid, Neda, Fadi Thabtah, and Hussein Abdel-Jaber. "Phishing detection: A recent intelligent machine learning comparison based on models content and features." *2017 IEEE international conference on intelligence and security informatics (ISI)*. IEEE, 2017.

[4] Cantin-Garside, Kristine D., et al. "Detecting and classifying self-injurious behavior in autism spectrum disorder using machine learning techniques." *Journal of autism and developmental disorders* 50 (2020): 4039-4052.

[5] De la Marche, Wouter, et al. "Quantitative autism traits in first degree relatives: evidence for the broader autism phenotype in fathers, but not in mothers and siblings." *Autism* 16.3 (2012): 247-260.

[6] Kuhl, Patricia K. "Is speech learning 'gated' by the social brain?." *Developmental science* 10.1 (2007): 110-120.

[7] Al Otaiba, Stephanie, Amy Gillespie Rouse, and Kristi Baker. "Elementary grade intervention approaches to treat specific learning disabilities, including dyslexia." *Language, Speech, and Hearing Services in Schools* 49.4 (2018): 829-842.

[8] Maenner, Matthew J. "Prevalence and characteristics of autism spectrum disorder among children aged 8 years—autism and developmental disabilities monitoring network, 11 sites, United States, 2018." *MMWR. Surveillance Summaries* 70 (2021).

[9] Thabtah, Fadi. "Machine learning in autistic spectrum disorder behavioral research: A review and ways forward." *Informatics for Health and Social Care* 44.3 (2019): 278-297.

[10] Kim, Hyopil, Chae-Seok Lim, and Bong-Kiun Kaang. "Neuronal mechanisms and circuits underlying repetitive behaviors in mouse models of autism spectrum disorder." *Behavioral and Brain Functions* 12 (2016): 1-13.

[11] Bolton, Patrick, et al. "A case-control family history study of autism." *Journal of child Psychology and Psychiatry* 35.5 (1994): 877-900.

[12] Abraham, Alexandre, et al. "Deriving reproducible biomarkers from multi-site resting-state data: An Autism-based example." *NeuroImage* 147 (2017): 736-745.

[13] Elsabbagh, Mayada, et al. "Global prevalence of autism and other pervasive developmental disorders." *Autism research* 5.3 (2012): 160-179.

[14] Bengio, Y. "Learning Deep Architectures for AI." (2009).

[15] Mythili, M. S., and AR Mohamed Shanavas. "A study on Autism spectrum disorders using classification techniques." *International Journal of Soft Computing and Engineering* 4.5 (2014): 88-91.

[16] Nag, Anindya, et al. "Application of artificial intelligence in mental health." *International Conference on Intelligent Systems Design and Applications*. Cham: Springer Nature Switzerland, 2022.

[17] Rahman, Arafat, Anindya Nag, and Anupam Kumar Bairagi. "A Hybrid Model for Recognizing Human Activity Using Extreme Learning." *2023 26th International Conference on Computer and Information Technology (ICCIT)*. IEEE, 2023.

[18] Vaishali, R., and Rajamma Sasikala. "A machine learning based approach to classify autism with optimum behaviour sets." *International Journal of Engineering & Technology* 7.4 (2018): 18.
[19] Kim, Hyopil, Chae-Seok Lim, and Bong-Kiun Kaang. "Neuronal mechanisms and circuits underlying repetitive behaviors in mouse models of autism spectrum disorder." *Behavioral and Brain Functions* 12 (2016): 1-13.
[20] Jubayer, Fahad, et al. "Detection of mold on the food surface using YOLOv5." *Current Research in Food Science* 4 (2021): 724-728.
[21] Eslami, Taban, et al. "ASD-DiagNet: a hybrid learning approach for detection of autism spectrum disorder using fMRI data." *Frontiers in neuroinformatics* 13 (2019): 70.
[22] Allison, Carrie, Bonnie Auyeung, and Simon Baron-Cohen. "Toward brief "red flags" for autism screening: the short autism spectrum quotient and the short quantitative checklist in 1,000 cases and 3,000 controls." *Journal of the American Academy of Child & Adolescent Psychiatry* 51.2 (2012): 202-212.
[23] American Psychiatric Association. "Diagnostic and statistical manual of mental disorders." *Text revision* (2000).
[24] Wang, Jessica, et al. "Assessing autistic traits in a Taiwan preschool population: cross-cultural validation of the Social Responsiveness Scale (SRS)." *Journal of autism and developmental disorders* 42 (2012): 2450-2459.
[25] Aljero, Mona Khalifa A., and Nazife Dimililer. "A novel stacked ensemble for hate speech recognition." *Applied Sciences* 11.24 (2021): 11684.
[26] Alsaade, F. Waselallah, Theyazn HH Aldhyani, and M. Hmoud Al-Adhaileh. "Developing a recognition system for classifying covid-19 using a convolutional neural network algorithm." *Computers, Materials & Continua* 68.1 (2021): 805-819.
[27] Paula, Cristiane S., et al. "Brief report: prevalence of pervasive developmental disorder in Brazil: a pilot study." *Journal of autism and developmental disorders* 41 (2011): 1738-1742.
[28] Du, Yuhui, Zening Fu, and Vince D. Calhoun. "Classification and prediction of brain disorders using functional connectivity: promising but challenging." *Frontiers in neuroscience* 12 (2018): 525.
[29] Murray, Donna S., et al. "Transforming an autism pediatric research network into a learning health system: lessons learned." *Pediatric Quality & Safety* 4.2 (2019): e152.

[30] LeCun, Yann, Yoshua Bengio, and Geoffrey Hinton. "Deep learning." *nature* 521.7553 (2015): 436-444.

[31] UNIVERSITY OF ARKANSAS Computer Science Dept, https://www.kaggle.com/code/afarinbargrizan/autism-spectrum-disorder-detection-with-classifier

[32] Akter, Tania, et al. "Improved machine learning based classification model for early autism detection." *2021 2nd International Conference on Robotics, Electrical and Signal Processing Techniques (ICREST).* IEEE, 2021.

[33] Omar, Kazi Shahrukh, et al. "A machine learning approach to predict autism spectrum disorder." *2019 International conference on electrical, computer and communication engineering (ECCE)*. IEEE, 2019.

8

Generative AI-augmented Mental Health Support: The Impact of Generative Models on Therapeutic Practice

Monika Singh T.[1], Kishor Kumar Reddy C.[1], and Kari Lippert[2]

[1]Stanley College of Engineering and Technology for Women, India
[2]University of South Alabama, United States
E-mail: thakursingh.monika@gmail.com; drckkreddy@gmail.com; klippert@southalabama.edu

Abstract

The rapid development of generative artificial intelligence (AI) models, such as ChatGPT, has significantly impacted various fields, including mental healthcare. This chapter investigates the potential effects of generative AI on therapeutic practice, exploring both its opportunities and challenges. Through a comprehensive literature review, the study evaluates the social and practical implications of using generative AI in mental health support, drawing from key sources that assess the broader societal impact of these technologies. The findings indicate that while generative AI offers promise in enhancing personalized care, streamlining administrative processes, and expanding access to mental health resources, it also raises critical concerns. These include issues related to privacy, ethical considerations, and the risk of perpetuating or amplifying societal biases embedded in the training data or algorithms of AI models. It also examines AI models like GPT in the context of mental health, focusing on their role in transforming therapy, from conversational agents to personalized cognitive behavioral therapy (CBT) interventions. Generative AI improves accessibility, engagement, and scalability of care, particularly in underserved regions, by offering 24/7 support. However, ethical concerns such as data privacy and overreliance on AI require careful attention. This section presents case studies of AI-powered mental health chatbots, such as

DOI: 10.1201/9788743801764-8

Woebot and Wysa, and discusses the benefits and limitations of using artificial intelligence to support and enhance therapeutic practices. This chapter advocates for a hybrid approach that integrates AI automation with human-centered care. It also addresses ethical and regulatory challenges, offering strategic recommendations for researchers, mental health professionals, and policymakers to guide the responsible and equitable integration of generative AI into therapeutic practice.

Keywords: Generative Artificial Intelligence, Mental Health Support, Therapy Practices, AI-driven Solutions, ChatGPT, AI-assisted Therapy, Care, Cognitive Behavioral Interventions, Human–AI Integration.

8.1 Introduction

The rapid development of generative AI models has significantly impacted numerous sectors, including the realm of mental healthcare and support. These advanced AI systems, exemplified by groundbreaking tools like ChatGPT, have the potential to revolutionize the way mental health professionals approach therapeutic practices, offering novel opportunities and presenting unique challenges that warrant careful consideration. As the adoption of generative AI models continues to grow, it is crucial to explore the implications of this technological shift on the delivery, accessibility, and efficacy of mental health interventions [1]. The rapid development of generative AI models has significantly impacted numerous sectors, including the realm of mental healthcare and support. These advanced AI systems, exemplified by groundbreaking tools like ChatGPT, have the potential to revolutionize the way mental health professionals approach therapeutic practices, offering novel opportunities and presenting unique challenges that warrant careful consideration. As the adoption of generative AI models continues to grow, it is crucial to explore the implications of this technological shift on the delivery, accessibility, and efficacy of mental health interventions [1].

The global mental health crisis continues to intensify, leaving millions without sufficient access to care. Traditional mental health services, such as therapy and counseling, are struggling to keep pace with the growing demand due to several challenges. These include a shortage of mental health professionals, high treatment costs, lengthy waiting periods, and the persistent stigma surrounding mental healthcare. Geographic limitations, particularly in rural or underserved areas, further compound the problem, resulting in many individuals being deprived of timely and effective treatment. To address these gaps, innovative solutions are essential. Technology, especially generative AI and other digital tools, offers promising ways to expand mental health services, improve accessibility, and deliver personalized care. These emerging tools present a significant opportunity to create more inclusive, adaptable, and scalable mental health support systems to meet the growing needs of individuals seeking accessible and effective mental health care [19].

The integration of generative AI models into mental health [3] support systems can yield a multitude of benefits. These models can be leveraged to enhance the personalization and customization of therapeutic experiences, tailoring interventions to the unique needs and preferences of each individual client [2]. Moreover, the ability of generative AI to engage in natural language processing and generate human-like responses can facilitate more seamless and relatable interactions between clients and AI-powered therapeutic assistants, fostering a sense of rapport and trust [1]. This, in turn, can lead to improved client engagement, increased treatment adherence, and ultimately, better therapeutic outcomes. Furthermore, the scalability and accessibility of generative AI-powered mental health support can be particularly advantageous, especially in regions or communities with limited access to mental health professionals. By providing AI-driven therapeutic services, mental health support can be made more widely available, potentially reducing barriers to care and reaching individuals who may have previously been underserved.

AI is playing a transformative role in mental healthcare by improving early detection, diagnosis, and treatment. Through AI-powered tools, data from speech, text, and even social media can be analyzed to detect subtle signs of mental health conditions like anxiety and depression, often before healthcare providers notice them. Machine learning algorithms enable the creation of personalized treatment plans by evaluating individual patient data and adjusting therapeutic strategies in real time. Virtual therapists and chatbots also offer scalable, immediate support, providing cognitive behavioral therapy (CBT) and crisis intervention when needed. Moreover, AI helps expand access to care, especially in underserved areas, ensuring more people receive timely and effective treatment. This combination of early intervention, customized care, and greater accessibility is revolutionizing mental healthcare.

8.2 Generative AI in Mental Health: An Overview

Generative artificial intelligence [11] is a kind of AI that generates new data like text, pictures, or sound that are based on the training it has been exposed

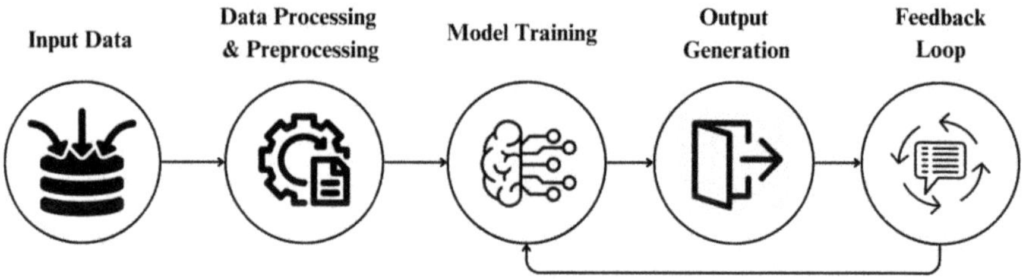

Figure 8.1 Working of generative AI.

to. These models do not only obey predetermined guidelines; rather, they learn patterns that make them produce content that appears similar to the one human beings create. This process uses neural networks, especially deep learning algorithms that have been trained over large data sets so as to grasp context and meaning. Among the many models of note in this trajectory is the Generative Pretrained Transformer (GPT), a voluminous language model that processes human speech and produces meaningful replies. This works by contrasting the anticipated word with the previous ones in the series, such that it can take in input and produce entire paragraphs or even conversations. These models are mostly dependent on an architecture known as transformers which help them to look at different sections of the input data at once thus making it super-efficient when it comes to contextually aware responses.

Because of its flexibility and adaptability, generative AI is especially useful in mental health applications. While conventional AIs mainly work on classification or diagnosis, generative AIs can imitate human interactions and help with mental health issues in a personalized way. At this point, AI-driven therapy tools, as well as chatbots that provide real-time assistance, adaptive interventions, and context-specific advice to patients, are powered by this mechanism.

As shown in Figure 8.1, a system of generative AI is established. This flowchart provides a detailed account of the procedures a machine learning model uses to take in data, process it, analyze it, and give an output from which it can learn and develop through feedback.

8.2.1 Evolution of AI applications in healthcare

AI utilization for medical attention has experienced a noteworthy transformation recently from its mere usage as basic diagnostic instruments to highly sophisticated systems presently aiding people with mental health issues. The primer function of artificial intelligence was mainly centered on improving diagnostic precision by the use of algorithms to recognize trends in medical photographs or patient information. But then, while strides were being taken in the development of technology, AI spread to different medicinal realms including predicting analytics, human-based care plans, and dealing with depression via its calculations.

The expansion of AI on mental well-being has been indeed tremendous. The treatment of mental illness used to be determined by subjective human emotions rather than concrete evidence. Despite that, breakthroughs in natural language processing (NLP) and machine learning techniques made it possible for some parts of this field to be automated while still retaining a sense of empathy. Specifically, artificial intelligence can now help us assess an individual's psychological state by analyzing their speech patterns or text messages and even anticipate their moods, as well as future psychiatric issues based on them. Modeling advanced generative AI such as the GPT [7] model has exhibited gigantic possibilities concerning support for mental healthcare in therapy and counseling. Information from these models can help mental healthcare workers through ideas, inputs, or even preliminary therapy for patients in less privileged regions. The process of integrating these technologies into mental healthcare [3] is in progress but initial outcomes imply that generative AI may greatly enhance both access and efficiency of therapeutic practices.

8.2.2 Types of generative models used in mental health (GPT, transformer models)

A variety of generative models have been utilized in the domain of mental health to provide more tailored and adaptive solutions. Specifically, the GPT family, particularly GPT-3 and GPT-4, are the most sophisticated. These models are trained on extensive text data so that they can produce responses that are coherent, context-aware, and human-like conversations. Due to their capacity to produce text, they appear suitable for applications such as chatbots which are capable of providing prompt support for mental health issues. Most of the contemporary generative AI [10] frameworks are backed by transformer models. These models process all data sequences (for instance sentences or paragraphs) at once, which is different from working them one after another as other designs do. As a result, they are very efficient in capturing long-distance relationships in texts that exist between different words in a line, thus facilitating an accurate contextual answer. The use of transformer models in mental health includes analyzing patient self-reports, predicting moods, and offering individual-based interventions.

Generative AI systems like variational autoencoders (VAEs) and generative adversarial networks (GANs) alongside transformer models and GPT have a lot to offer in regard to mental health interventions. For instance, VAEs can come up with fresh therapeutic activities that take into account patients' preferences; on the other hand, GANs can produce artificial patient data necessary for research studies. These models' versatility makes them most appropriate for mental healthcare which is a field that constantly evolves across time periods due to the different individual needs of different patients.

8.2.3 Distinguishing generative AI from other AI technologies in mental health support

In contrast to various AI technologies utilized for mental health purposes by other developers, generative AI generates completely new material using given inputs, rather than merely searching similar patterns from continuously changing reams of documents without making any further transformations or synthesis, which were usual methods employed in conventional artificial intelligence applications dealing with such unique issues as depression detection based on voice tonality, so if someone talks about his depression, it will always identify it due to its similarity with archived voices showing sadness; though these models work exceptionally well concerning differential diagnosis, they offer no tailored therapeutic interventions nor offer inventive treatments. Conversely, generative artificial intelligence models like GPT can have instantaneous dialogues and offer specific advice or therapy sessions relying on the previous words of the user. They are therefore more interactive and dynamic than diagnostic AI [16] systems. For example, a chatbot that utilizes GPT may be able to hold a chat with a patient by giving advice, suggesting coping strategies, as well as therapeutic exercises that relate to his or her emotional state and still make necessary adjustments during the course of a conversation.

An important distinction lies in the adaptability of generative AI [4] in mental health interventions, as opposed to conventional AI models that adopt a generalized approach. In contrast to conventional AI models that adopt a generalized approach, the use of generative AI enables customized interventions for each client. Such an individual-centered strategy is important in mental healthcare because patients' experiences are different for every individual, and thus, addressing them generically may not always work. Generating novel therapeutic suggestions, exercises, or even conversation starters is how generative AI improves upon conventional manuals thereby making it more effective and tailored to the needs of various individuals suffering from mental illness.

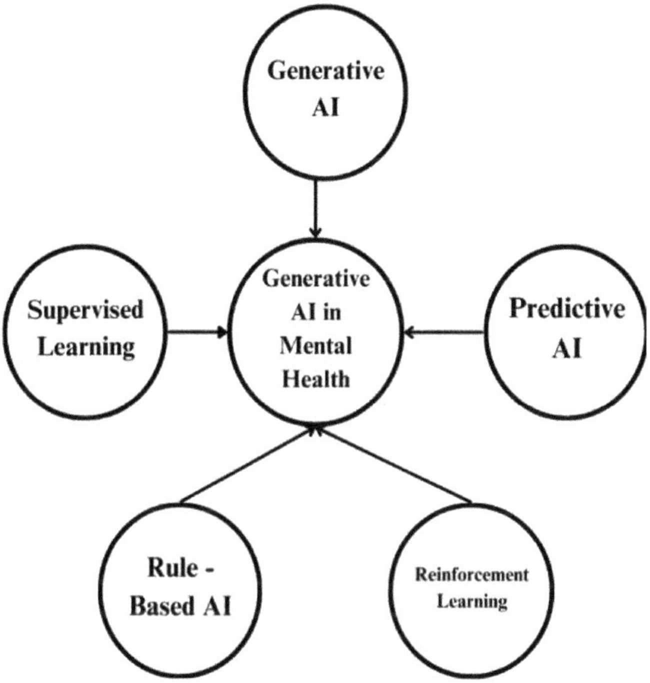

Figure 8.2 Generative AI in mental health.

As shown in Figure 8.2, the relationship between generative AI [9] and other prominent AI technologies used in mental health support can be seen. In the diagram, we have a central circle labeled "Generative AI in Mental Health" which is surrounded by smaller circles that represent various types of AI technologies. Each of the surrounding circles illustrates a unique approach to AI and its application to the mental health field.

8.3 Current Applications of Generative AI in Mental Health Support

Generative AI has found numerous applications, including in mental health support, where it offers innovative solutions to enhance care. They are as follows.

Conversational agents: AI-driven mental health chatbots

Among the most regular uses of generative AI in psychological wellness is conversational agents also known as AI-driven emotional wellness chatbots.

These chatbots use natural language processing (NLP) that enables them to mimic conversations with customers and provide suggestions, assistance, or therapeutic measures. Chronically depressed people can talk to such counseling assistants as Woebot and Wysa rather than waiting until office hours.

A notable benefit of using generative AI [4] chatbots is their accessibility. They can be reached 24 hours a day, 7 days a week, and they can offer quick help to persons in trouble, unlike human therapists. This proves helpful, especially to those who cannot access mental health practitioners or are afraid of asking for assistance because of stigma. Additionally, because these chatbots can handle multiple users simultaneously, they offer a scalable solution to the growing demand for mental health services. Nevertheless, chatbot systems do have their limitations as well. For instance, although they can help people by providing basic assistance and guidance in terms of handling emergency acute psychological crises, they are not equipped with emotions or compassion like human therapists. In addition, the chatbot [17] software that uses the language models is also subject to the quality of training data available to them hence at times it may give unhelpful suggestions. Nevertheless, even though these systems have certain constraints, AI-powered chatbots are still quite useful for initial support in mental health and for referring users to specialists if necessary.

Figure 8.3 shows the flow of how an AI chatbot processes user input using natural language processing, generates responses, and at last, passes user feedback.

Generative AI in cognitive behavioral therapy (CBT)

AI's generative capabilities are transforming cognitive behavioral therapy (CBT) by enabling the personalization of therapeutic interventions based on each patient's unique psychological and behavioral data. CBT, which is systematic psychotherapy, assists people in detecting and altering their troublesome negative thinking habits, as well as conduct. In the past, therapists usually facilitated exercises that would help patients see things differently, but now with AI, such can happen automatically and individualized during its performance.

In generative [2] AI models, they could assess similar patterns of fake thoughts or behaviors that require changing among patient engagements. Take for instance, when one case will always think in a manner that is negative about capabilities; there are some exercises that can be generated by the AI that use such techniques such as cognitive restructuring to address these negative feelings through CBT interventions. This capacity to adapt therapy while

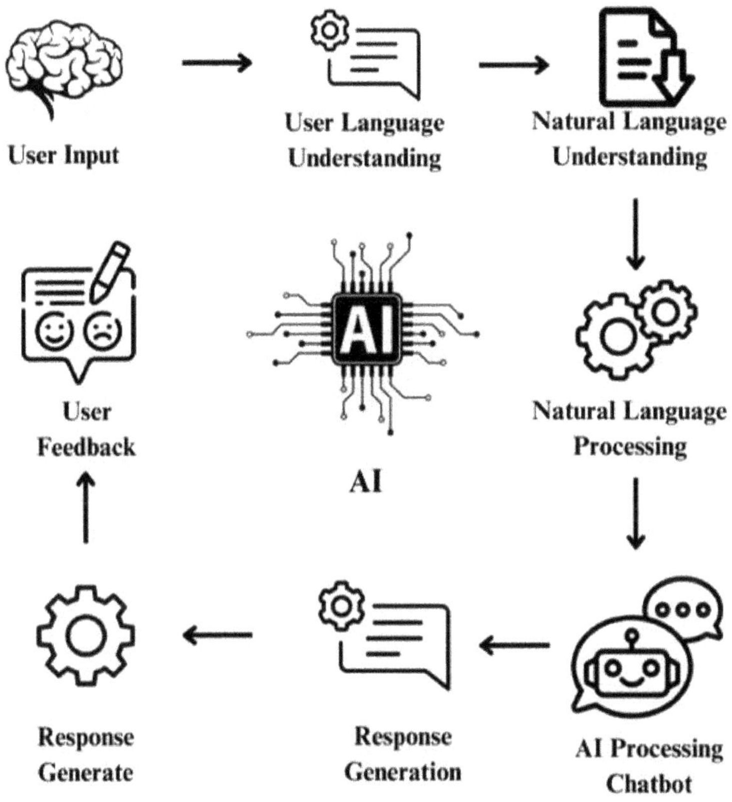

Figure 8.3 AI-driven mental health chatbots.

still within these conversations increases their potency in so far as making them cognizant and immersive to the recipient. In addition to that, patients can use AI to practice CBT methods between their therapy sessions hence enabling support that is continuous. Through AI-based platforms, patients get continuous reminders to perform exercises and track their progress, as well as feedback on their thought processes. In this way, consistent interactions are facilitated; thus, promoting good alterations and guaranteeing the continuation of psychotherapy beyond conventional environments so that it improves patient results who are receiving the treatment.

Personalized mental health interventions

A personalized treatment plan is one of the major contributions of generative AI [6] to mental health services. For example, mental health is more of an individual thing and what helps one patient may not help another. By accessing various data sets ranging from patient history, behavior patterns, and sometimes genetic makeup, generative AI [17] can provide personalized therapeutic solutions that take care of their individual needs.

If someone has depression and anxiety, for example, CBT and mindfulness might be a good match. An AI system will not only look at the symptoms but could also recommend some form of exercise or diet changes to enhance mental well-being. It is important to note that the continuous collection of patient data enables real-time adjustments in therapeutic strategies by learning how individuals respond to care over time. However, there is concern about mood fluctuations during the first week-when patients often experience lower energy levels-which may affect early engagement and outcomes. Through the improvement of personalized mental health treatments, not only is it made more effective but also we empower the patient who feels they have some control over their own treatment. In addition, if patients receive tailored suggestions from professionals, they become more involved in their treatment plans and fulfill their therapeutic exercises. This unique type of personalization constitutes a radical change in the mode of delivering mental healthcare services and makes such services more patient-centered, as well as flexible.

AI for early diagnosis and predictive analytics in mental health

Moreover, predictive analytics is being done by generative AI for early diagnosis of mental illness. AI models identify patterns that inform of the beginning phases of mental illness even before one experiences serious symptoms, through big data analysis. For instance, depression, anxiety, or even schizophrenia may have warning signs that include slight variations in spoken language, speech patterns, or even social media behavior.

In contrast, employing AI predictive analytics allows healthcare providers to take early action before mental illness worsens. This is essential in cases of anxiety disorders and bipolar depression where the fate of the patient significantly depends on prompt reaction. Both patients and health professionals would be warned by AI concerning possible problems for them to intervene immediately. No doubt that predictive analytics has its challenges when it comes to mental health. The most worrying issue is whether the predictions are accurate because wrong predictions may cause wrongful fears and unwanted treatments. Furthermore, there are issues of privacy regarding how this information is collected and analyzed. All these considered, the early identification of mental problems through artificial intelligence could help clinicians achieve better patient outcomes while decreasing the load on health services associated with psychosocial diseases.

Virtual mental health assistants: benefits and limitations

Virtual mental health assistants are AI-powered platforms that provide round-the-clock support for people with mental illness. With these virtual assistants available as mobile applications or desktop platforms, they can initiate conversations with users, monitor their mental well-being over time, and offer tailored recommendations or coping methods. In addition, they utilize a generative AI [4] algorithm which makes it possible for them to adjust their responses based on the emotional state and requirements of the user thus making it more individualized compared to conventional mental health applications. Handling with care, 24 hours every day, and 7 days a week are the greatest advantages of using virtual assistants. These tools come in handy for those living in remote areas or who cannot afford psychological counseling because they are not able to arrange therapy sessions. Users can keep track of how they are faring emotionally using your service and this leads to over time noting down progresses such as patterns development. With such unending connections between a user and the system, it would be easier for the individual to stick to their own path toward healing by taking all preventive measures required.

Nevertheless, the capability of virtual assistants in mental health may really not give you support, and cannot comprehend complex emotional issues. Support may be provided by AI for difficulties that are mild to moderate but cannot serve as a substitute for the cases where there are severe instances with human therapists. In addition, while it may recognize people's feelings, AI-based assistants might not detect the more delicate ones that would be understood by a therapist taking care of them. Despite these deficits, virtual aides form part of valuable tool in an ecosystem that deals with mental illness providing affordable help to the needy on a large scale.

As shown in Table 8.1, an elaborate contrast is shown between the benefits and drawbacks of using virtual mental health assistants. These automated

Table 8.1 Virtual mental health assistants: benefits and limitations.

Aspect	Benefits	Limitations
Cost	Lower cost compared to human therapists	May require subscriptions for advanced features
Accessibility	Available 24/7, no need for scheduled appointments	Lack of internet access can hinder usage
User experience	Easy-to-use interfaces and instant responses	Lack of empathy and understanding compared to human therapists
Effectiveness	Helpful for providing immediate coping strategies	Limited ability to handle complex mental health issues
Personalization	Can be tailored to user needs based on data analysis	Less personalized than human-led therapy sessions

chatbots and online therapists-supported mental health services are being provided with the help of these AI-powered tools. The table contains advantages such as 24/7 availability, scalability, and cost efficiency in dealing with mentally ill patients and some limitations which include the absence of profound empathy and possible data protection issues in the future.

8.4 The Impact of Generative AI on Therapeutic Practices

Generative AI is transforming therapeutic practices by providing on-demand, scalable mental health support through chatbots and virtual therapists. It enables personalized interventions like cognitive behavioral therapy (CBT) and creates customized self-care resources. AI-driven tools also enhance accessibility, offering immediate support, particularly in underserved areas. This integration is making therapy more efficient, responsive, and widely available.

Enhancing access and engagement through AI-augmented therapy

A vast storehouse of options lies in the view that generative AI may alter the functioning of psychologists and their interface with patients, especially in regard to mental health treatment. Regular therapy may not be available to many people but the use of AI tools can help greatly because they are accessed online. Psychotherapy given via the internet is one way through which generative AI can solve the problem posed by inadequate services for mental health treatment through counselors using chatbots owing to cognitive behavioral therapy (CBT).

Not only does generative AI enhance accessibility but it also improves patient involvement. Usually, traditional therapy needs regular face-to-face consultations; however, this is made possible by AI through persistent and immediate interaction. In a case where an AI-driven application might prompt someone to carry out therapeutic activities, provide them with feedback about their performance, or recommend ways of dealing with emotions depending on their situation. By doing so, patients remain committed to therapy and actively participate in it.

In addition, the use of AI-supported therapy can lessen the belief that people looking for mental health treatment are weak. People who might feel bad talking about their mental disabilities can receive assistance through AI without facing any judgment, hence allowing them to mask their identities. The inclusion of AI into therapeutic care will probably increase accessibility to mental health services and enhance the results for patients.

AI-driven customization of therapy approaches

Generative AI provides a high level of customization in therapeutic approaches, allowing treatments that are well-tailored to the individual needs and circumstances of the patients. While therapists base their approach on patient feedback and progress in traditional therapy, AI serves to improve this process by perpetually analyzing patients' data in order to render real-time recommendations. For instance, it is possible for AI to regulate the intensity of CBT exercises depending on how a particular patient responds so as to keep the treatment effective and exciting.

Therapists are assisted in understanding their patients using AI through the analysis of big data that is impossible for a human to process. Aside from having the responses provided by patients who are undergoing therapy, AI is capable of studying other sources of data, for instance, wearable gadgets that are used in tracking physical health and social media activities. Therefore, the combination of all this information will help in forming a better perspective on the emotional wellbeing of an individual hence generating more accurate and speedy interventions. Moreover, generative AI helps psychotherapists obtain new tools to tailor treatment. From a different perspective, an AI tool could mention specific ways of coping based on the person's unique stresses or indicate when he/she may want to pause in order to be mindful. This level of individualization ensures treatment effectiveness and personal relevance, thus contributing to improved recovery outcomes.

Virtual counseling and real-time mental health monitoring

With generative AI, virtual counseling opens new doors for patients to receive mental health support that does not require a face-to-face meeting. Chatbots or mobile applications that act as online therapists provide immediate assistance for monitoring and keeping track of emotional states through conversation, thus resulting in therapy-related recommendations. This form of counseling has proven useful, especially to people who cannot afford common therapy methods, as well as those who just want comfort when seeking help.

Virtual advice givers have been made possible through generative AI which provides tailored assistance by evaluating what the users say and altering its answers simultaneously. For instance, if a user's messages indicate signs of anxiety, the platform (e.g., Tui) can recommend interventions such as deep-breathing exercises or cognitive behavioral therapy (CBT) sessions to help manage their emotional state. Additionally, artificial intelligence can analyze mood patterns over time and alert users to emerging mental health concerns, enabling timely and appropriate support. AI-based real-time emotional health tracking has a lot of advantages, but it also has its challenges. Although AI gives uninterrupted assistance, it might find it hard to handle emotional challenges that call for compassion and understanding of humans. Furthermore, there are worries regarding confidentiality and security of data as the effective functioning of AI mechanisms involves the use of confidential personal data (PPD). Regardless of these limitations, remote counseling and real-time mental health monitoring present serious improve in making mental treatment more open and quick to respond.

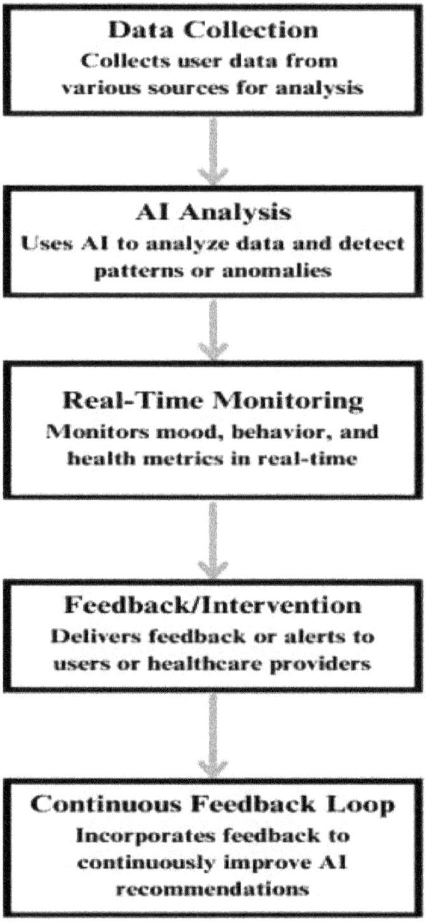

Figure 8.4 Real-time mental health monitoring workflow with AI.

As shown in Figure 8.4, the diagram for virtual counseling and real-time mental health monitoring would depict the key processes and components involved in using AI and technology to support mental healthcare.

Complementing human therapists: enhancing effectiveness or replacing human connection?

One of the largest arguments in favor of the integration of generative AI into mental health systems is whether it would augment or substitute human therapists. On the plus side, therapy may become more effective with AI since therapists would take well-informed decisions as a result of personalized and data-driven insights provided by this technology. For instance, AI can be used to analyze a single patient's behavior patterns and recommend specific interventions or coping strategies allowing psychologists enough time to concentrate on other areas of the treatment process. AI methods are being improved to provide additional support between therapists' sessions. They provide real-time advice that can help in tracking progress, as well as reminding patients to carry out prescribed therapeutic exercises. This can help patients adhere to their treatment regime ensuring better results. The inclusion of AI in mental healthcare means that such services will reach more people and be more efficient. But, it really worries that AI might eventually take over the jobs of human therapists, particularly in places where mental health services are scarce. Though AI-powered [13] tools can be of great assistance, they do not possess the emotional profundity and empathetic qualities that characterize a good therapist. In most cases, mental health issues are deeply rooted and need a human healing touch, otherwise, if not careful, may result in decreased quality of care when previously mentioned overdependence on AI gets established. It is important to have an equilibrium between the improvement of mental health support by means of artificial intelligence and retaining human connection which plays a very significant role during therapy sessions, hence as these technologies continue changing every day, we should become more cautious especially with the use of them in the psychiatric field because if not done right, this may lead us back to where we began from.

Shifting the therapeutic landscape: integrating AI into routine practice

Generative AI [5] not only makes for technological advancement in mental healthcare but also shifts its therapeutic terrain. The use of artificial intelligence (AI) in psychiatry is revolutionizing the method of administering therapy making it more accessible personalized and scalable. As artificial intelligence (AI) amasses to become an integral component of routine practice, therapists and mental health practitioners must adjust to new ways of carrying out their tasks. This entails acquiring skills on how to efficiently employ AI tools while at the same time comprehending what they can or cannot do. One of the most essential alterations AI to therapy may have is the possibility for real time, data-supported insights into a patient's psychological well-being. Rather than depending on patient self-reports alone, therapists can utilize AI-generated data in order to comprehend better their patients' emotional states and behavioral patterns. This once again leads them to make better decisions, as well as customize treatment plans according to individual requirements; which will ultimately result in healthier servicing. The advance of artificial intelligence is such that it is bound to take a central position in mental healthcare. Nevertheless, the incorporation of this technology in everyday activities warrants careful consideration of some ethical aspects like data privacy and the possible displacement of psychologists by computers. If we want to preserve and improve human connection in order to have effective therapies, there must be a balance between taking advantage of AIs' potential and keeping them out as much as possible from human relationships.

8.5 Benefits of AI-augmented Mental Health Support

The various benefits of AI-augmented mental health support are as follows.

8.5.1 Scalability: expanding mental health services in underserved areas

A primary benefit of AI-augmented [8] mental health support is its scalability. For instance, there are geographic and resource constraints in traditional mental health services that make it impossible for communities to access such services, especially those that are heavily populated with many at-risk people. Generative AI [2] answers this question by making it possible for the provision of mental health support online and hence does not require physical infrastructure or face-to-face meetings. Chatbots and virtual mental health assistants driven by AI may be used, especially for people living in remote areas or places with few doctors. They can provide simple forms of mental healthcare like cognitive behavior therapy (CBT) practices, coping mechanisms, and emotional listening, thus making them more widely available to those who require such services. Furthermore, the provision of mental health [14] assistance augmented by artificial intelligence can be done at a lesser price that is unlike the typical therapy providing an avenue for its accessibility to those who cannot be in a position of regularly utilizing human therapists. When it comes to mental healthcare, the ability of artificial intelligence to make it more available to everyone has been argued as one way in which this problem can be addressed internationally by reducing the burden of psychiatric disorders and improving outcomes for persons who may otherwise remain untreated.

8.5.2 Personalization: tailoring support to individual needs

An extra considerable benefit of AI-enabled mental wellness assistance is its capacity to deliver individualized attention. Conventional mental health [3] service delivery normally adopts a generic approach; however, AI provides a specific treatment experience. By interpreting information from many places like self-reports given by patients, the use of portable gadgets, and online dealings, artificial intelligence will generate an elaborate representation of whether one's psychiatric needs should be addressed in some particular way. For instance, AI-based mental health applications can modify suggestions for cognitive-behavioral therapy tasks based on an individual's reactions to prior tasks. For instance, in the case of an anxious user, the AI might suggest techniques aimed at relaxation or mindfulness exercises which are known to reduce stress levels. This way, mental healthcare becomes more efficient and interesting because it is personalized through AI. As well as customizing treatment strategies, artificial intelligence can assist patients in monitoring their development through time. AI [15] can track changes in emotional states, circumstances, or habits across periods of time used for therapeutic purposes and provide information on whether the patient is improving or not by comparing various indicators that are relevant to treatment progress. Moreover, it may recommend some adjustments if necessary for an effective cure. The practice of this degree of individualization incorporates a flexible and accommodating approach that takes into account the fluctuation nature of an individual's mental health assistance.

8.5.3 Cost-effectiveness: reducing the economic burden of mental healthcare

If you seek for an efficient and effective solution to your mental health issues, seek in the direction of artificial intelligence-augmented care. Traditional mental healthcare is expensive, especially for patients that require on-going therapy or treatment. On the contrary, virtual mental health assistants and chatbots offer AI-based assistance at reduced prices as compared to human therapists. For healthcare systems, support for mental health augmented with artificial intelligence can help reduce the economic burden of mental health disorders through intervention that comes in early hence preventing conditions from getting worse. Through the identification of mental health, which are psychological problems in their incipient states, and the provision of timely support, AI reduces future intensive and costly treatments. Apart from helping achieve good patient outcomes, this contributes to easing the strain on healthcare resources. Moreover, AI [13] can help healthcare providers improve their resources by automating repetitive tasks such as patient intake and follow-up. This results in mental health employees not wasting much time on easy cases, and thus, delivery of mental healthcare services can be done with a more optimal layout. For this reason, AI-assisted mental health support is aimed at increasing efficiency and sustainability in basic primary care for all patients in the near future.

8.5.4 Personalization and adaptability in mental health interventions

With greatness, generative AI [2] is great at professionalizing and personalizing mental illness interventions that are fit for use, thereby boosting therapeutic efficacy. Thus, when put among many platforms, the AI notes the differences and makes the adjustments necessary. For instance, suppose someone suffers from anxiety attacks press-ups or breath control methods crafted for this reason will be given by means of such systems. One more important benefit of AI is its real-time adaptability. The system continues to learn from user feedback and modifies its recommendations as the user engages with AI-powered instruments. Thus, this enables AI to make interventions that become increasingly relevant and successful over time, increasing the overall quality of mental healthcare. Moreover, various factors like wearable gadgets such as fitness monitors or smart watches can also be merged into artificial intelligence systems to better understand the totality of the human being's physical and mental wellness. By incorporating self-reporting with these other forms of knowledge, machine learning machines may assist individuals in promptly handling their emotional disorders through individual feedback which are true to them.

8.5.5 Patient empowerment and self-management through AI tools

When these AI tools are used in the field of mental healthcare, they empower patients by providing them with resources and support for self-management.

Table 8.2 Patient empowerment and self-management through AI tools.

AI tool	Features	Device compatibility
Mood tracking apps	Track daily moods, offer visual charts of mood trends	Smartphones, tablets
Virtual mental health assistants	Provide coping strategies, goal-setting, reminders	Smartphones, computers
Meditation and mindfulness apps	Guided meditations, breathing exercises, stress relief tips	Smartphones, wearables
AI-based CBT platforms	Cognitive-behavioral therapy exercises, self-assessments	Smartphones, tablets, computers
Wearable health devices	Track heart rate, sleep patterns, physical activity	Smartwatches, fitness trackers

These tools can come in various forms such as mental health apps or even virtual assistants that allow individuals to have an active part in the management of their own minds. For instance, AI-driven applications are being used by patients in order to keep track of their moods, set therapeutic targets, and also access coping mechanisms at any time when necessary. AI is empowering because it gives patients information on their mental health patterns. By examining the information being collected from different contacts, AI can provide users with valuable feedback on how far they have come and pinpoint what should be focused on. As a result of this heightened consciousness, individuals become more cognizant of their own mental illnesses thus prompting them to commit themselves to seeking remedy for the same. Moreover, constant round-the-clock assistance is provided to support self-management by AI tools. Patients may obtain help anytime they need it since this constant presence eliminates the waiting duration of planned therapy sessions. The empowerment of patients and improved mental health results are brought about by AI applications which are these days making such resources available and individualized.

As shown in Table 8.2, how AI tools can enhance people's capacity to manage their mental health is discussed. The chapter will focus on self-monitoring tools driven by AI, personalized feedback, data-driven insights, and improved accessibility as such methods of empowering patients.

8.6 Challenges and Ethical Considerations

The use of generative AI in mental healthcare [3] raises challenges like ensuring data privacy, managing the risk of misdiagnosis, and addressing the lack of human empathy in AI-driven support. Ethical concerns include potential bias in algorithms, informed consent, and ensuring accountability for AI's decisions. Striking a balance between innovation and patient safety is crucial. Some of them are as follows.

Data confidentiality and safety: protecting information of patients

In the field of mental healthcare, certain patient data that are sensitive and confidential are prior medical records, psychiatric diagnoses, therapy notes, and direct communication between therapist and patient. Consequently, organizations that build AI healthcare systems in the United States are bound to comply with rigorous privacy laws including the Health Insurance Portability and Accountability Act (HIPAA) or the General Data Protection Regulation (GDPR) in Europe. These statutes seek to protect patient data against illicit access and abuse. In order to protect data, AI creators need to integrate some important security features. One way is to encrypt information in transit and storage to prevent unauthorized ones from accessing it. Moreover, PII can be eliminated through methods such as deidentification and anonymization that make it difficult or impossible for an outsider to relate data to individuals. Also, there should be access control mechanisms in place so that only those who are authorized by virtue of their positions are able to view or change any information. In addition, audits and monitoring are essential for fast detection and response in case of breaches. The loss of patient trust and legal issues may follow if privacy is not preserved.

Figure 8.5 shows the importance of having a robust data security system in healthcare because it helps protect patient information, increases the organization's reputation, and lowers litigation costs. This diagram also stresses the necessity of obeying data security requirements and how this can contribute to maintaining continuous business operations.

Honest utilization of artificial intelligence: openness, responsibility, and faith

AI must show transparency, accountability, and reliability for it to be used ethically in mental healthcare. This is particularly important during diagnosis or treatment, as both patients and clinicians need to know why AI makes certain decisions. Transparency means that users should be able to comprehend why certain recommendations or outcomes are made by AI algorithms. This is really hard when we have "black-box" models like deep learning which are inherently obscure and unexplainable in their internal workings. Accountability needs well-defined rules that outline who is responsible for instances when AI systems go wrong or generate results that were not intended. By putting the blame on developers, clinicians, or healthcare institutions, trust develops, prompting adherence to ethical values. Over time it builds up trust in AI through its uniformity and dependability. Working machines

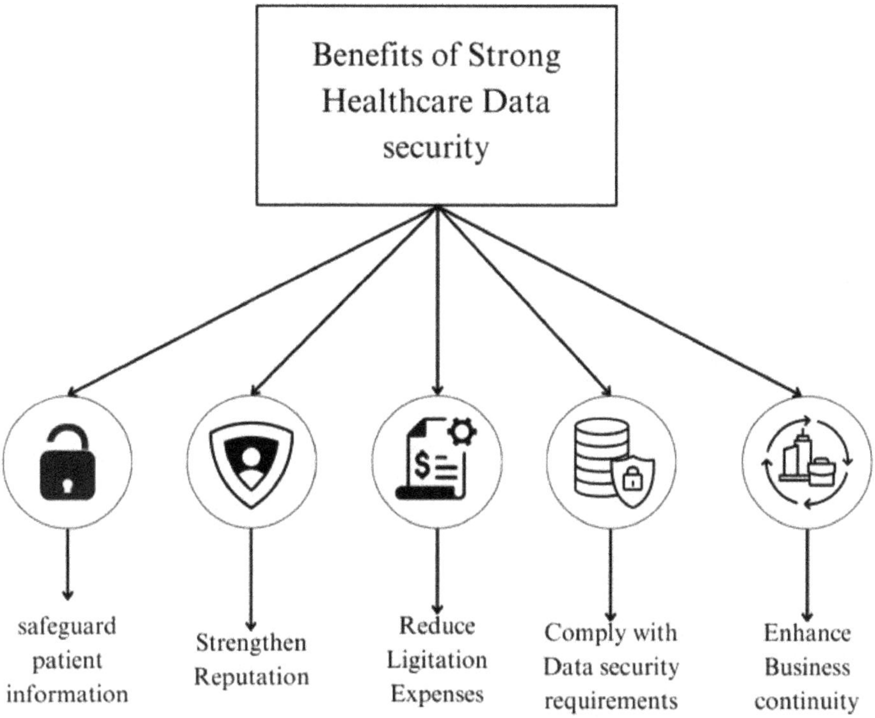

Figure 8.5 Benefits of strong healthcare data security.

encouragingly gives weight to human values, and therefore, tenants of safety and privacy while still observing due process strengthen users' confidence. Further, enhancing the relationship between patients, doctors, and AIs is to involve human oversight like clinicians in decision-making using AI systems.

Unfairness and bias in AI-made mental health solutions

Human beings have biases that arise out of their conditioning and upbringing. Similarly, AI systems have the potential to adopt or sustain such biases depending on the training data utilized. Consequently, this leads to varying levels of service delivery among various demographic groups characterized by factors like race, sex, or income levels. For example, an artificial intelligence model trained mainly using input from one community may prove ineffective when it comes to serving less frequent respondents' communities. Diverse training data sets should be used, and monitoring mechanisms need to be put in place in order to remove predisposition and promote equality. AI must be trained using input data that captures different communities including those from minority groups, hence heterogeneous training sets are essential in avoiding biased results. This would allow for fairer results during mental healthcare [3] by ensuring that there are no preferences for any particular group when creating such systems.

The subsequent phase that is as crucial as any other is bias detection, as well as mitigation during the model development. In these systems, developers can implement algorithms that are meant to detect potential biases and then take corrective measures to minimize them. Moreover, AI systems must be continually monitored for signs of bias after deployment in real-world applications. Ethical guidelines should guide regular audits and evaluations to ensure sustained fairness and accuracy in AI systems. Inadequate measures taken toward bias might impel AI systems to yield unequal diagnoses or recommendations for treatment, especially in mental healthcare. For instance, Kubernetes when poorly handled might unintentionally deploy biased AI; thereby, causing some sections of society not to have access to and receive medical attention unfairly.

Table 8.3 summarizes some important bias issues happening in the field of AI within mental health and proposes approaches for overcoming these problems.

Therapeutic practices are highly dependent and overreliant on AI system

AI can help in the realm of mental healthcare through faster diagnoses, individualized therapeutic courses, and broader reach. However, there exists a danger of professionals relying too much on AI systems to the detriment of key components that demand human compassion, judgment, and intuition.

Concerns regarding the overdependence are:

Loss of humane touch: mental healthcare encompasses emotional intelligence, empathy, and understanding which are not possible to imitate by present AI systems. If doctors overly depend on AI, the human touch will dissipate and this will negatively impact patient outcomes.

Diminished clinical judgment: no AI system is fail-proof and excessive reliance on it may cause physicians to rely on advices from it rather than applying their own clinical judgment. This may bring about wrong diagnoses or ineffective treatment.

Ethical limits: it is important to set ethical boundaries on how AI ought to be deployed in therapeutic practices. AI is supposed to act as a tool that enhances instead of replacing human decision-making capabilities. Thus, it is essential that specific guidelines be put in place so that human clinicians still dominate in making critical decisions.

Table 8.3 Various biases in AI-generated mental health solutions.

Aspect	Description	Mitigation strategy
Bias in training data	AI may inherit biases from data sets, especially if under-represented groups are not adequately included.	Use diverse, representative training data sets that include data from various demographic and socioeconomic groups.
Demographic disparities	AI may perform better for certain demographics (e.g., racial, gender, or age groups) than others.	Conduct performance evaluations across demographic groups to ensure equal accuracy and fairness.
Algorithmic fairness	AI systems may favor certain populations due to imbalanced data or biased.	Implement fairness-aware algorithms that account for and correct any demographic imbalances in the predictions.
Unconscious bias	Biases may unintentionally be introduced by developers or data curators.	Train developers and curators on bias detection and conduct ethical reviews of the AI models.
Bias detection	Identifying and quantifying bias can be challenging, especially when bias is not obvious.	Use statistical and machine learning techniques to detect, measure, and mitigate bias during model development. Implement ongoing monitoring of AI systems to detect bias in real-world applications and update models as needed.
Continuous monitoring	Bias may arise after deployment as AI systems interact with new data.	Ensure clinicians have final oversight and are involved in decision-making to prevent reliance on biased AI outputs.
Fairness in decision-making	AI may unfairly prioritize treatment options or access to resources based on biased predictions.	This table summarizes key bias issues in AI for mental health and suggests strategies for mitigating these challenges.

Legislation and rules regulating AI in psychological healthcare

The AI usage for mental healthcare is under a complex legal and regulatory environment that is still evolving. Current laws governing AI in healthcare include data protection regulations (GDPR, HIPAA, etc.), but there are also other challenges affecting mental health AI systems, especially concerning liability, safety, and efficacy issues.

The key considerations encompass:

Regulation of AI algorithms: several governmental organizations, for example, the Food and Drug Administration (FDA) of America and the European Medicines Agency (EMA), have initiated the management of artificial intelligence-driven decision support systems. However, there exist unique concerns about mental health disorders due to the fact that psychiatric tests tend to be subjective. Hence, it is essential for artificial intelligence systems to be aligned with the laws on effectiveness and security.

Liability: who should be held responsible when there is harm caused by AI systems or when they fail to give accurate diagnoses? Clinicians, developers, and institutions must deal with issues of liability, as well as malpractice in AI-assisted care.

Informed consent: the patients need to know what role AI plays in their care process so as to give informed consent. It involves; understanding how their data are being utilized; and knowing about the limitations of the involved AI systems.

Global disparities: there are significant differences among countries regarding regulations which could lead to disparities in how different regions use an AI system for healthcare purposes. While some countries possess comprehensive legal frameworks governing its use in healthcare others may not have the necessary infrastructure for regulation or monitoring of these systems successfully.

8.7 Emerging Trends and Future Directions

Emerging trends in AI for mental health include the integration of wearable devices for real-time monitoring, advancements in personalized therapy through predictive analytics, and the rise of virtual reality (VR)-based mental health interventions. Future directions point to more seamless AI–human collaboration in therapy, expanding access to care globally, and improving AI's emotional intelligence for more empathetic interactions.

8.7.1 Teletherapy with AI enhancement: blending human assistance and AI

Teletherapy, which is enhanced by AI, is a promising advancement in the field of mental healthcare as it combines human expertise with the efficiency and availability of AI systems. This approach allows for constant monitoring and support 24/7 especially in between sessions when there is no therapist around. AI can be helpful in understanding mood variations, giving real-time feedback, and even suggesting methods to cope with distress according to patients' data. Utilizing machine learning besides analyzing progress, AI can also adjust to the individual requirements of the patient and reveal things that could not be caught during regular therapy sessions. Human therapist skills are not supplanted but improved by way of the use of artificial intelligence. For example, artificial intelligence is able to analyze large amounts of data at supersonic speed, giving mental health professionals an overall picture of a client's condition throughout the years. Such a combination results in a more thorough and successful therapeutic process. Furthermore, with the increasing availability of teletherapy practice, AI-supported platforms help ensure that every patient receives individual, steady treatment from any place.

8.7.2 Mental health self-improvement using AI models for digital therapeutics

The development of digital therapy has transformed the way people receive treatment for their mental health problems through the use of artificial intelligent self-directed devices that help manage one's well-being. These platforms integrate artificial intelligence in order to facilitate interventions such as cognitive behavioral therapy (CBT), meditation, and mood-tracking interventions thereby enabling individuals to gain access to solutions they can use on their own within the domain of their psychological issues. Adaptive feedback usually comes from analyzing user input and progress over time which informs AI models on new activities and strategies which one should undertake based on emotional and mental clues provided by different users. For anyone desiring to be independent in terms of their mental health or who cannot access conventional therapy, this self-help approach will be particularly useful. It also provides the opportunity for confidentiality and convenience that may not be available with face-to-face consultations. Moreover, as these AI systems continue developing, digital therapeutics are getting smarter at understanding user habits and customizing their interventions for optimal results.

Table 8.4 conveys a synopsis of prominent aspects of digital therapies powered by artificial intelligence which emphasizes their ability to offer individualized interventions for mental health problems based on scientific proof, as well as monitor user's progress.

8.7.3 Generative AI in predictive models of mental health crisis

As time goes by, generative AI [4] holds a vital position in preventing impactful mental health crises by creating predictive models to recognize signs of trouble before they escalate. AI can mark slight behavioral changes which could mean a mental health crisis is approaching through examining wide

Table 8.4 Features of AI-driven digital therapeutics for self-guided mental health improvement.

Feature	Description
Personalized recommendations	AI models tailor mental health exercises and interventions based on individual user data and preferences.
Behavioral tracking	Continuous monitoring of user interactions, mood reports, and progress to adjust therapeutic strategies.
Evidence-based interventions	Uses techniques that work with CBT and mindfulness, as well as other confirmed therapeutic methods adjusted by AI algorithms according to the needs of the users.
Engagement techniques	AI incorporates gamification, reminders, and motivational messages to encourage consistent use and engagement.
Real-time adjustments	Immediate updates to therapeutic content and recommendations based on user feedback and behavior.
Accessibility	Provides self-guided mental health support that is accessible anytime and anywhere, enhancing availability.
Data privacy	AI systems implement measures to protect user data and maintain confidentiality while providing personalized care.
Limitations	Challenges include a potential lack of human empathy, user adherence, and effectiveness compared to traditional therapy.

ranges of information such as posts on social media, outputs from wearable sensors, and ways used in therapy apps. With these models, caregivers or therapists get alerts that warrant a prompt response. Apart from risk identification, generative AI can simulate many intervention techniques to know which one works best. For instance, it can help identify therapeutic techniques or coping techniques that would work well for a person who is undergoing a crisis. This preventive approach not only saves lives but also helps patients understand their triggers better and manage their mental health with more precision and assistance.

8.7.4 Multimodal therapy using AI: speech, text, and emotion identification

Developments in mental diagnoses and treatments are being realized as AI integrates with as many modalities as possible including text, speech, and emotional cues. Multiple forms of input contribute to better insights into patients' minds. For instance, NLP allows computers to notice variations in language that indicate possible episodes of depression or anxiety among the afflicted. The tone or pace variations can also suggest intense feelings of tension according to voice analysis tools (specially designed software). Finally,

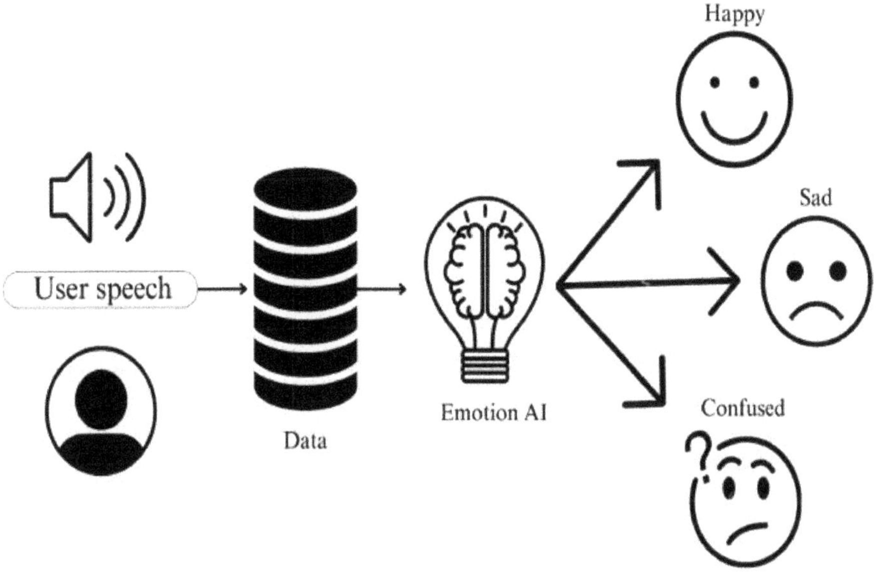

Figure 8.6 AI-based speech analysis for emotion detection.

facial recognition technologies check individuals' unspoken emotions by evaluating their facial expressions.

Figure 8.6 shows an emotion-analyzing system diagram using AI to analyze user speech. Speech data is captured and then processed by "Emotion AI" which can tell if the speaker or listener is happy, sad, or confused, thus, demonstrating the ability of AI to understand human emotions based on sound. This kind of treatment requires every aspect of a multimodal approach to better understand and care for patients in real time. Hence, therapists use it to observe the emotional trends of their patients over time, as well as some hidden patterns that cannot be easily perceived through traditional means. More so, with better AI technologies coming up all the time, this kind of emotional analysis will definitely become more accurate and precise; therefore, therapists will be able to offer really tailored and effective help.

8.7.5 A hybrid method for the future of mental health human–AI collaboration

A modified version of hybrid mental healthcare, using both AI and human psychotherapists together, can improve the results for patients. While doing errands such as data collection or progress tracking, and even assessing patients' problems, AI systems may assist therapists in their work so they can address complex patient issues within them. Automated therapy processes leave more time for human therapists to develop meaningful relationships with their clients – this is the main element in effective psychotherapy. Additionally, in this partnership model, the delivery of mental healthcare can be made more reachable and scalable so that it is accessible to underprivileged populations within reach of anybody who cannot have regular exposure to human therapists. The therapist's capacity for empathy, critical reasoning, and tailored assistance complements AI's ability to offer continuous observation and early intervention. They are supposed to work alongside one another hence making therapy more effective; precise and broadly used but not to replace them instead.

8.8 Case Studies

The various case studies are as follows:

Woebot and Wysa as mental health aides: application of AI chatbots

AI chatbots such as Wysa and Woebot are other pioneering examples in healthcare advocacy for mental well-being, for example. This is what Woebot, a product of clinical experts, is all about: it uses conversational artificial intelligence (AI) to create an environment similar to that of a therapist using CBT techniques that help users identify and challenge negative thought patterns, providing mood tracking, journaling prompts along with daily check-ins. On the other hand, Wysa combines CBT with mindful exercises that offer users the support of a trustworthy friend during conversations. Interaction between these bots remains anonymous as they help eliminate mental illness-related stigmas and make counseling services more approachable. In dealing with mild to moderate anxiety, stress, and depression, both chatbots are quite powerful. They provide round-the-clock support that the users can turn to in their times of trouble, offering timely interventions that would otherwise need a scheduled appointment with a therapist. Even if Woebot and Wysa cannot be used as substitutes for therapeutic professions, they help us in our daily lives with mental health issues, making us emotionally resilient and enabling us to develop coping strategies.

Cognitive behavioral therapy (CBT) applications utilizing generative artificial intelligence

Generative artificial intelligence has changed the business of delivering cognitive behavior therapy significantly, as it makes use of applications that can analyze user input and provide feedback tailored to their needs. It is in contrast to static self-help programs since generative AI can modify its communication style and therapeutic content in real time. For example, an AI can identify specific cognitive distortions such as catastrophizing or overgeneralization by studying user dialogue patterns and offer CBT techniques like reframing or thought balancing right away. This capacity to adjust makes for a more individualized experience that allows mental health support to seem more individualized and pertinent in relation to unique case scenarios of users. Generative AI can also provide structured interventions, leading users through exercises specifically aimed at their distinct mental health challenges. Similar to the kind of individualized therapy sessions, AI-based CBT apps can closely follow-up user's progression and suggest relevant recommendations during the process. As a result, this increases mental healthcare accessibility by allowing many more individuals to access it while at the same time, fostering a sense of control among patients in undertaking self-management with a therapist who monitors progress changes.

Patients' and therapists' impressions on AI-enhanced therapeutic approaches

Therapy that uses AI therapy solutions for patients is well-liked because it is quick to access, cost-effective, and available when the need arises. Many people feel safe talking to chatbots because there is no judgment involved unlike when you are talking to a human therapist. These interventions help with managing stress on a daily basis, reducing anxiety [12] levels, as well as facilitating emotional comprehension among other benefits according to users' reports. Additionally, the structured evidence-based format of AI interventions fosters reliance since they are based on scientifically proven methods similar to conventional ones in psychotherapy. Nonetheless, several patients admit that emotional depth and empathy present in human interaction are what makes these AI-designed tools inadequate. Yet, therapists are careful about its limits even though they tend to favor AI's ability to help mental health providers solve their problems. Seen in this way, an AI can manage trivial tension and nervousness but not intricate concerns within mental wellness such as trauma or major depression requiring profound knowledge of additional emotional involvement beyond AI. Thus, certain specialists believe that it is important for the use of artificial intelligence in psychology so that there will always be a human who is personally leading the patient during the process of treatment from beginning to end where such moments happen and they can get specialized treatment that is based on total understanding and compassion.

Contrastive study: artificial intelligence against normal psychotherapy programs

In various key differences, conventional therapy methods and AI [18] driven psychological health measures differ from each other. Some of these are like such solutions as CBT apps and chatbots that provide on-demand support available irrespective of where one is at any time creating an element of convenience and low cost specifically for users. For instance, this serves as a missing link for those who may be time-constrained, under-resourced, or do not feel comfortable enough going for conventional treatment procedures. Nonetheless, the development of authentic emotional connections between therapist and patient through AI remains gravelly limited since its responses are based on preset algorithms instead of emotional intelligence or human real-time feedback. Therapists [20] are skilled in analyzing nonverbal signals, providing emotional support, and adjusting their techniques based on the intricacy of feelings involved making them traditional models for addressing mental health. The dominant mode of psychotherapy is more suited for people suffering from serious or chronic forms of mental illness; however, it is less accessible as it requires payment which may not be affordable by many individuals, consumes time plus imposes societal stigma. It comes as a relief that the integration of artificial intelligence in a compassionate way is emerging as an effective model for scalable mental health services satisfying both the accessibility and the accuracy of care provided. Below is a summary of the main benefits and drawbacks of each approach based on the table, which says AI-driven interventions are generally better at being accessible and scalable while conventional therapy provides a greater depth to the individual care given.

Table 8.5 displays the major strengths, as well as limitations, of each method, showing that AI-based interventions have advantages when it comes to accessibility and scalability whereas traditional therapy provides more in-depth and tailor-made treatment options.

Table 8.5 Comparison between mental health interventions driven by AI and traditional therapy.

Aspect	AI-driven interventions	Traditional therapy	Notes
Accessibility	Available 24/7, accessible via smartphone or computer	Requires appointments, limited by therapist availability	AI tools are more accessible, especially in underserved areas accessibility
Cost	Low-cost or free for most platforms	Can be expensive, varies based on location and specialization	AI is more affordable, making mental healthcare more inclusive
Personalization	Provides real-time feedback and automated support based on user input	Highly personalized with therapist adapting based on sessions	AI can tailor responses but lacks deep emotional personalization
Scalability	Can support millions of users simultaneously	Limited to therapist's capacity (usually 1:1 sessions)	AI scales well and can alleviate the burden on the mental health system
Emotional depth	Lacks empathy and nuanced emotional understanding	Deep empathy, human connection, and tailored emotional support	Traditional therapy excels in emotional support, especially for complex cases
Effectiveness for mild issues	Effective for managing stress, anxiety, and mild depression	Effective across a wider range of issues from mild to severe	AI is suitable for low-risk conditions; traditional therapy covers the full spectrum
Complex issues	Limited capacity for addressing trauma, personality disorders, or deep-rooted emotional issues	Can handle complex mental health issues with depth and understanding	Traditional therapy is more suited for complex, multifaceted mental health problems
Therapist involvement	No human interaction, fully automated	Involves direct interaction with a trained professional	AI lacks the human element; therapist guidance is crucial in many cases
Hybrid potential	Can complement traditional therapy by handling routine tasks	Can provide depth and context to AI-driven support	A hybrid model can enhance mental healthcare delivery by combining both approaches

8.9 Conclusion

In conclusion, the integration of generative AI into mental healthcare marks a transformative shift in how support is delivered, addressing gaps in traditional systems. AI models like GPT are revolutionizing early detection and therapy by analyzing data patterns and offering personalized care through tools such as mental health chatbots and virtual assistants. These scalable solutions provide 24/7 support, especially for underserved communities, empowering individuals to manage their mental well-being. While AI enhances efficiency and customization, it cannot replace the human empathy central to therapy. The challenge lies in integrating AI to complement human therapists, maintaining a balance between automation and human connection. Despite the benefits, challenges like data privacy, security, and algorithmic bias must be addressed to ensure ethical AI deployment in mental healthcare. Strong legal and regulatory frameworks will be essential for building trust and safeguarding users. Looking ahead, AI's role will likely expand in areas like teletherapy and predictive mental health interventions, blending human expertise with AI-enhanced tools. This hybrid approach promises to revolutionize mental healthcare, combining AI's scalability and efficiency with the empathy and understanding of human caregivers.

References

[1] Michel-Villarreal, R.; Vilalta-Perdomo, E.; Salinas-Navarro, D.E.; Thierry-Aguilera, R.; Gerardou, F.S. Challenges and Opportunities of Generative AI for Higher Education as Explained by ChatGPT. Educ. Sci. 2023, 13, 856. https://doi.org/10.3390/educsci13090856.

[2] Maria Teresa Baldassarre, Danilo Caivano, Berenice Fernandez Nieto, Domenico Gigante, and Azzurra Ragone. 2023. The Social Impact of Generative AI: An Analysis on ChatGPT. In Proceedings of the 2023 ACM Conference on Information Technology for Social Good (GoodIT '23). Association for Computing Machinery, New York, NY, USA, 363–373. https://doi.org/10.1145/3582515.3609555.

[3] Koutsouleris, N., Hauser, T. U., Skvortsova, V., & De Choudhury, M. (2022). From promise to practice: towards the realisation of AI-informed mental health care. The Lancet Digital Health, 4(11), e829-e840.

[4] Mannuru, N. R., Shahriar, S., Teel, Z. A., Wang, T., Lund, B. D., Tijani, S., ... & Vaidya, P. (2023). Artificial intelligence in developing countries:

The impact of generative artificial intelligence (AI) technologies for development. Information Development, 02666669231200628.

[5] Gupta, P., Ding, B., Guan, C., & Ding, D. (2024). Generative AI: A systematic review using topic modelling techniques. Data and Information Management, 100066.

[6] Sedkaoui, S., & Benaichouba, R. (2024). Generative AI as a transformative force for innovation: a review of opportunities, applications and challenges. European Journal of Innovation Management.

[7] Budhwar, P., Chowdhury, S., Wood, G., Aguinis, H., Bamber, G. J., Beltran, J. R., ... & Varma, A. (2023). Human resource management in the age of generative artificial intelligence: Perspectives and research directions on ChatGPT. Human Resource Management Journal, 33(3), 606-659.

[8] Hitch, D. (2023). Artificial Intelligence (AI) Augmented Qualitative Analysis: The Way of the Future?. Hitch, D.(2023). Artificial Intelligence Augmented Qualitative Analysis: The Way of the Future.

[9] Mariani, M., & Dwivedi, Y. K. (2024). Generative artificial intelligence in innovation management: A preview of future research developments. Journal of Business Research, 175, 114542.

[10] Callison-Burch, C., Zhu, A., Dugan, L., Hwang, A., Callison-Burch, C., Lyu, Q., ... & Wong, E. (2023). Understanding generative artificial intelligence and its relationship to copyright. In Proceedings of the 13th International Joint Conference on Natural Language Processing and the 3rd Conference of the Asia-Pacific Chapter of the Association for Computational Linguistics (IJCNLP-AACL 2023) (pp. 370-387).

[11] Sandelin, F. (2024). A multi-case study on generative AI use in work and decision-making: exploring applications and potential departmental effects.

[12] Habicht, J., Viswanathan, S., Carrington, B., Hauser, T. U., Harper, R., & Rollwage, M. (2024). Closing the accessibility gap to mental health treatment with a personalized self-referral Chatbot. Nature medicine, 30(2), 595-602.

[13] Kishor Kumar Reddy, Advaitha Daduvy, R Madana Mohana, Basem Assiri, Mohammed Shauib, Sadaf Alam and Abdullah Sheneamer, “Enhancing Precision Agriculture and Land Cover Classification: A Self –Attention 3D Convolutional Neural Network Approach for Hyperspectral Image Analysis, IEEE Access, 2024, DOI:10.1109/ACCESS.2024.3420089

[14] Kishor Kumar Reddy, Palakurthi Anaghaa Reddy, Himaja Janapati, Basem Assiri, Mohammed Shauib, Sadaf Alam and Abdullah Sheneamer, "A Fine Tuned Vision Transformer (FTVT)based Enhanced Multi-Class Brain Tumor Classification using MRI Scan Imagery", Frontiers in Oncology Cancer Imaging and Image-directed Interventions, August 2024, DOI: 10.3389/fonc.2024.1400341

[15] Kishor Kumar Reddy C, Aarti Rangarajan, Deepti Rangarajan, Mohammed Shuaib, Fathe Jeribi and Shadab Alam, "A Transfer Learning Approach: Early Prediction of Alzheimer's Disease on US Healthy Aging Dataset", MDPI Mathematics, July 2024, 2204. https://doi.org/10.3390/math12142204

[16] Kishor Kumar Reddy C, Ritika Badam, Shauib Ahmed, "IoT Driven Accessibility:A Refreshable OCR-Braille Solution for Visually Impaired and Deaf-Blind Users through WSN",JETECH Elsevier, April 2024, DOI:10.1016/j.ject.2024.04.007

[17] Kishor Kumar Reddy, Vijaya Sindhoori Kaza, P R Anisha, Mousa Mohammed Khurbani, Mohammed Shauib and Sadaf Alam, "Optimizing Barrier Placement for Intrusion Detection and Prevention in WSNs" PLOS ONE, February 2024. https://doi.org/10.1371/journal.pone.0299334

[18] Malviya, R., Chilamkurti, N., Sundram, S., Dhanaraj, R. K., & Balusamy, B. (Eds.). (2023). Artificial Intelligence for Health 4.0: Challenges and Applications.

[19] Monika Singh T., Kishor Kumar Reddy C., Kari Lippert (2024) Advancing Human-Centric Solutions: The Future Trajectory of Soft Computing in Modern Society. IGI Global. DOI: 10.4018/979-8-3693-6806-0.ch001

[20] Narayanan, R. R., Durga, N., & Nagalakshmi, S. (2022). Impact of artificial intelligence (AI) on drug discovery and product development. Indian Journal of Pharmaceutical Education and Research, 56(3), S387-S397.

9

AI and Neurodegenerative Disorders: From Early Diagnosis to Advanced Care

Sridhar Arumugam[1], Gloriya Raju[2], K. S. Vimala[3], and Avneet Aneja[4]

[1]Lovely Professional University, Professor & Principal, TLM Institute of Health Sciences and Research Centre- Physio, India
[2]Galgotias University, HIMS College of Physiotherapy, India
[3]Sri A.R.M Physio Rehab and Research Centre, India
[4]Om Sai Physiotherapy Clinic, Canada
E-mail: gloriya.heritage@gmail.com;
aveneet.physio@gmail.com; vimala.pth@gmail.com

Abstract

Incorporating artificial intelligence (AI) into treating neurodegenerative disorders represents a profound transformation in care delivery. Across allied health professionals, AI is driving a more personalized and dynamic approach. Machine learning, wearable sensors, and robotic technologies enable precise diagnostics and treatment, particularly for conditions like Parkinson's, ALS, and MS. In physiotherapy, AI systems analyze motor functions to create tailored rehabilitation plans, often supported by virtual reality and wearable tech, allowing continuous care from home. Occupational therapy benefits from real-time data analysis, making treatment more adaptive and personalized. Speech therapy has been revolutionized by AI-driven tools that diagnose and treat language impairments with high accuracy, promoting consistent progress. Robotics, like exoskeletons, assist in physical recovery, offering personalized support. AI enhances multidisciplinary collaboration, integrating data across fields to ensure cohesive, patient-centered care. Despite challenges like infrastructure costs and data privacy concerns, AI promises to transform rehabilitation by improving outcomes and health

DOI: 10.1201/9788743801764-9

status of life. Overcoming these hurdles is essential to fully unlocking AI's potential in neurodegenerative care.

Keywords: Artificial Intelligence, Wearable Technology, Data Privacy, Robotics, Neurodegenerative Disorders, Machine Learning.

9.1 Introduction

Healthcare has been transformed in various ways starting from diagnosing a disease, monitoring, and treating. In addition, the arrival of artificial intelligence (AI) helped in real time assessment, diagnosis, and treatment of neurodegenerative (ND) conditions like Parkinson's disease (PD) and Alzheimer's disease (AD), and AI has become essential. Advancements in technological field and incorporation of machine learning (ML), neural language processing (NLP), computer vision, robotics, and wearable sensors are assisting and improving the overall outcome of the patient care [1]. When humans assess a neurodegerative disorder patient, there is a chance of missing important details while processing large data, identifying patterns and prediction models of treatment. ML, which is an influential aspect of AI, will help overcome the above deficits. The effective treatment and prognostic plan can be made available to the patient in real time by applying AI in our regular treatment [3]. NLP assists physicans and specialists to extract various data and provide the best option of treatment [2]. Adding robotics and computer vision are improving physical rehabilitation and cognitive assessments, while wearable sensors provide real-time health information [4]. Together, these technologies make healthcare more personalized, dynamic, and proactive [5].

9.2 Importance of AI in Managing Neurodegenerative Diseases

When dealing with neurodegenerative diseases, early treatment and personalized care are critical. AI provides insights that traditional methods might miss, like small changes in speech or movement that could be early signs of Parkinson's or Alzheimer's [7].

In rehabilitation, AI-driven technologies such as robotic exoskeletons and smart prosthetics adjust to a patient's progress [8]. AI's ability to predict and track patient progress allows for real-time therapy adjustments that lead to better outcomes. Wearable devices that monitor real-time health data also allow for more proactive care [7]. AI also benefits cognitive rehabilitation by offering personalized training programs to improve memory, problem-solving, and daily activities [9].

9.2.1 Scope and objectives of this chapter

This chapter looks at how AI is changing rehabilitation and patient care for neurodegenerative diseases. The main objectives include:

- **AI's role in early diagnosis:** Early diagnosis is crucial in neurodegenerative diseases, and AI assist in identifying minimal changes in health data to predict the start of these conditions.
- **AI in physical and cognitive rehabilitation:** AI aids in providing customized physical and cognitive rehabilitation programs to each patient's specific needs, using tools like robotic aids and virtual reality.
- **Wearable tech and real-time monitoring:** Wearable items with sensors collect real-time health data, and AI processes this information to predict changes and adjust treatments accordingly.
- **Ethical challenges in AI-driven patient care:** As AI grows in healthcare, there are important ethical issues to consider, such as data privacy and ensuring patient autonomy [13].
- **Case studies on AI in neurodegenerative care:** Real-life examples show how AI is making a big difference in how patients with neurodegenerative conditions are cared for.

9.3 Machine Learning Algorithms in Rehabilitation for Neurodegenerative Disorders

Machine learning has the potential to revolutionize physiotherapy treatment for patients suffering from Alzheimer's disease by providing personalized care that improves the patient's outcomes. This progressive neurodegenerative disorder affects memory, cognition, and movement in the individual; hence it is a real challenge to maintain physical function over time [15]. Physiotherapy can help in maintaining mobility, balance, and strength of patients, improving their quality of life. In physiotherapy, therefore, the integration of ML lets treatment become more personalized and responsive, increasing the efficacy of the treatment [16]. Machine learning thrives on data such as patient histories, physical assessments, and movement data. Applied to physiotherapy, ML can analyze this data to create customized rehabilitation plans that adapt to each patient's specific needs [15].

A dynamic system that continuously learns from a patient's progress allows therapy to evolve alongside the patient's physical condition, ensuring a more responsive and flexible treatment [17]. ML can also forecast the progression of Alzheimer's disease, predicting when motor skills will begin to decline and allowing physiotherapists to adjust treatments proactively [16]. Wearable technology and motion sensors, combined with ML algorithms, can analyze patient movements to provide real-time feedback, reducing injury risks and optimizing therapy outcomes [17]. In rural areas, ML facilitates tele physiotherapy, where patients receive remote monitoring and support. This ensures consistent care even when in-person visits are challenging [15]. Overall, ML transforms physiotherapy by personalizing and adapting treatments for Alzheimer's patients, enhancing their care [16].

9.3.1 Personalized rehabilitation plans

Machine learning is transforming the rehabilitation process for individuals with Alzheimer's disease by facilitating a more individualized treatment strategy. Conventional physiotherapeutic practices frequently utilize a uniform approach, potentially disregarding specific variances in disease development and symptomatology. The symptoms associated with Alzheimer's disease manifest across a wide spectrum and progress at differing velocities. Consequently, customizing therapy to accommodate each patient's distinct circumstances is essential, and machine learning can provide substantial advantages in this regard [15]. By analyzing diverse datasets, including medical histories, cognitive assessments, and motor function tests, machine learning algorithms can detect patterns in how individual patients respond to different therapies [16]. This advanced data analysis allows for the creation of highly customized rehabilitation plans. For instance, if one patient experiences balance issues while another faces coordination difficulties, the system can modify each therapy plan accordingly [18].

This approach individualizes therapy, targeting areas most in need and providing better results more effectively. Furthermore, machine learning is constantly adaptable to the improvement of patients through real-time adjustments in treatment plans. If an exercise is too challenging or not yielding a desired outcome, the system can suggest another approach. Dynamic changes of this nature are far more effective than any stagnant therapeutic program that often fails to consider the fluctuating needs of Alzheimer's disease patients [15]. Furthermore, machine learning possesses the capacity to anticipate possible future difficulties, thereby facilitating proactive modifications to therapeutic approaches. For example, should the system identify preliminary indicators of deterioration in motor abilities, it is able to suggest balance exercises aimed at averting future falls, thereby guaranteeing that the patient obtains prompt interventions [16]. This predictive functionality significantly augments the individualization and flexibility of treatment regimens.Essentially, the integration of machine learning into physiotherapy brings a more personalized, adaptive, and progressive approach toward the rehabilitation process in individuals with Alzheimer's disease. The emergence of this technology ensures patients receive specific treatments, thus improving physical skills and quality of life [18].

9.3.2 Predicting disease progression

Probably the most important use of machine learning is that it enables the functionality of forecasting future trends from historical data. This functionality becomes very important when dealing with degenerative disorders of neurological system. Throughout the progression of illness, affected patients show progressive impairment in both cognitive and motor abilities, hence rendering the importance of early intervention vital to maintain mobility and independence. Machine learning algorithms are capable of examining data gathered during routine physiotherapy appointments, including factors such as movement patterns, muscle strength, and coordination, in order to predict potential alterations in a patient's motor skills over time [16]. Such forecasts allow therapists to predict a disease process. Instead of waiting until the patient has suffered major losses in mobility, for example, machine learning can tease out subtle early signals of decline. For instance, when the system foresees that over the coming couple of months, the patient will show a decline in gait speed or deterioration in stability, then adjustments can be made in advance to their treatment program. Targeted exercises can be started that focus on the strengthening of specific muscle groups or the improvement of coordination; these can be used to slow down the physical decline and maintain the patient's independence as long as possible [15].

What really makes this effective, though, is that it can evolve with the patient: machine learning models learn from every session to make their predictions and recommendations more fine-tuned as more data becomes available. A very personalized treatment plan follows, changing in real time to the evolving needs of the patient. Such early intervention not only improves physical outcomes but also enhances the way patient's activities of daily living of life by extending the time they can remain active and independent [18]. In summary, machine learning presents an innovative strategy for the management of Alzheimer's disease by forecasting motor deterioration prior to its exacerbation. By equipping therapists with the means to initiate early interventions, it enhances their ability to deliver more efficient and individualized care, thereby enhancing both patient outcomes and overall quality of life.

9.3.3 Motion analysis and feedback systems

9.3.3.1 Machine learning transforming physiotherapy for Alzheimer's patients

The integration of ML and motion-sensing technology is a whole new ball game in physiotherapy, especially concerning Alzheimer's patients. This neurodegenerative condition does not just slowly eat away at memory; it also affects physical coordination, making once-simple tasks feel insurmountable over time. Physiotherapy, hitherto the first line of defence against the loss of motor function, has recently found a strong ally in technology. Thanks to ML, we are no longer limited to generic, one-size-fits-all approaches to treatment. Instead, therapy becomes tailored and an ever-changing process that can be adapted to every patient's needs, even in real time.

9.3.3.2 How machine learning and motion sensors work together

Picture an Alzheimer's patient going through the daily routine course of physiotherapy exercises. While going through each motion, they are under intense surveillance not by a human therapist, but by sensors of motion with high technological advancement. These sensors do not passively just sit but actively monitor down to minute details: muscle activation, joint dynamics, and over-all body posture alignment.

Here's how it works.

9.3.4 Data acquisition

Instantaneous information on the movements of the patient's body is collected by the motion sensors. Machine learning algorithm: Further, this data feeds into a potent machine learning framework. Thus, the algorithm checks the patterns of movement to find any anomaly or inefficiency.

As the patient goes through his exercises, the system provides feedback on each one, giving recommendations for further improvement or warnings where there are problems. Therapist involvement: If a critical problem in the system, such as wrong postures or injury threats, is detected, the system immediately sends an alert to the physiotherapist to take proper action. This mechanism is in place to ensure patient safety with respect to most effective therapeutic benefits to the patient.

Thus, the patient is provided with immediate guidance, while the therapy adjusts to their changing requirements, thereby guaranteeing they remain on a constructive path [19]. This situation can be likened to having a virtual coach who continuously observes, learns, and assists – alleviating the patient's burden and offering reassurance to both the individual and their healthcare team.

9.3.5 The role of ML in remote physiotherapy

As healthcare continues to evolve into more virtual models, ML plays a vital role in increasing access to care. For those suffering from Alzheimer's disease who reside in countryside, regular physiotherapy sessions may not be accessible at all times. Using telephysiotherapy, patients are now able to perform home exercises as ML systems observe their movements in real time. The system tracks everything from movement accuracy and long-term motor function trends to keep the patient going even when they are not at a clinic [20]. In places where travelling for medical services could pose problems like rural areas, this artificial intelligence provides an essential link for continuing healthcare provision. Physiotherapists can access patient information from remote locations and alter exercise programs accordingly ensuring that patients remain stable and progressive throughout recovery phases [39].

9.3.5.1 Proposed steps in rehabilitation

Patient performs exercise

- Patient begins daily physiotherapy movements.

Motion sensors capture data

- Real-time monitoring of muscle, joints, and posture.

Data fed into ML algorithm

- Information processed by machine learning to identify patterns and irregularities.

Instant feedback provided

- o System provides real-time guidance (e.g., “Correct your posture” or “Slow down”).

Alert physiotherapist (if needed)

- o If a serious issue is detected (e.g., risk of injury), the physiotherapist is notified immediately.

Improved and safe therapy

- o Patient receives personalized care, with the system continuously adapting to their needs.

Over time, that technology becomes more than just a passive bystander. It learns from the unique movement patterns of the patient, improving its feedback. The longer it learns, the more the system can adapt an exercise program to the patient’s aptitudes and changing condition throughout his or her disease progression [11]. If a patient begins to struggle with their balance, for example, it can recommend additional stability exercises before a catastrophic fall occurs. The key to personalized therapy goes beyond error detection. It evolves with the patient. In the past, a patient would complete a set of physiotherapy exercises and get feedback later often days or even weeks after doing them. ML allows for instant feedback. When the system spots a patient moving incorrectly – maybe they are not rotating enough during a stretch – it suggests a change right away. The patient has a digital personal trainer working with them around the clock [21]. The learning process never ends. Machine learning does not just help improve performance now; it keeps evolving to anticipate future challenges. If the data points to an upcoming decline in strength or mobility, the system can suggest new exercises to address the problem before it happens. This ability to look ahead lets therapists step in before the patient’s condition gets worse offering care that prevents issues rather than just reacting to them [12].

Boosting safety and stopping injuries injury risk always worries people Alzheimer’s patients. Their mental decline can make it tough to follow workout instructions. This is where ML-powered systems help out. They can watch movements as they happen warning patients if they might hurt themselves. Picture a patient about to lose their footing during a standing workout – the system can spot the wobble and right away suggest ways to fix it maybe stopping a risky fall [37]. These systems also change how hard the workouts are based on how the patient is doing. If a workout is too tough, the system can make it easier or suggest changes. This on-the-fly tweaking makes sure the therapy stays within what the patient can do cutting down on frustration and keeping them interested. The patient is led along a therapy path that grows with them instead of being pushed through a stiff, one-size-fits-all plan [14].

9.4 Long-term Advantages for Alzheimer's Victims

Applying machine learning in physical therapy for people with Alzheimer's disease has potential implications that go beyond what we can imagine today. It could greatly improve patient care if it were able to make adjustments according to individual progress and to keep on learning. By predicting possible changes of gait or movements, it would permit early interventions that are able to slow down physical deterioration. This entails longer periods of autonomy, reduced number of accidents, and overall better life standard [26]. So far this year, we have seen how machine learning and physiotherapy contribute to better management of Alzheimer's disease cases. Doctors can deliver changing treatments along with their patients who receive highly personalized care that is impossible in conventional therapies. Such circumstances do not only lead to more effective treatment options but empower patients and relatives always believing they can improve not only the quantity but also quality of life even when battling against difficult conditions like Alzheimer's disease.

9.4.1 AI in physiotherapy for neurodegenerative disorders

Diagnostic and therapeutic approaches for neurodegenerative disorders are exceedingly complex. AI significantly contributes to this feature. AI has a potential impact in the clinical management of NDs. AI encompasses a diverse array of technologies, including computer vision, natural language processing, neural networks, and machine learning. These innovations permit machines for picking up knowledge from data, identify trends, and make judgments that frequently exceed human capacities in terms of precision and speed [23].

9.4.2 Artificial intelligence in AD

AD is a progressive neurological disorder characterized by the progressive deterioration of memory and cognitive abilities [24]. An inherent challenge of AD is that timely identification allows for appropriate therapeutic approaches and preventive measures to restrict the advancement of the disease. Artificial

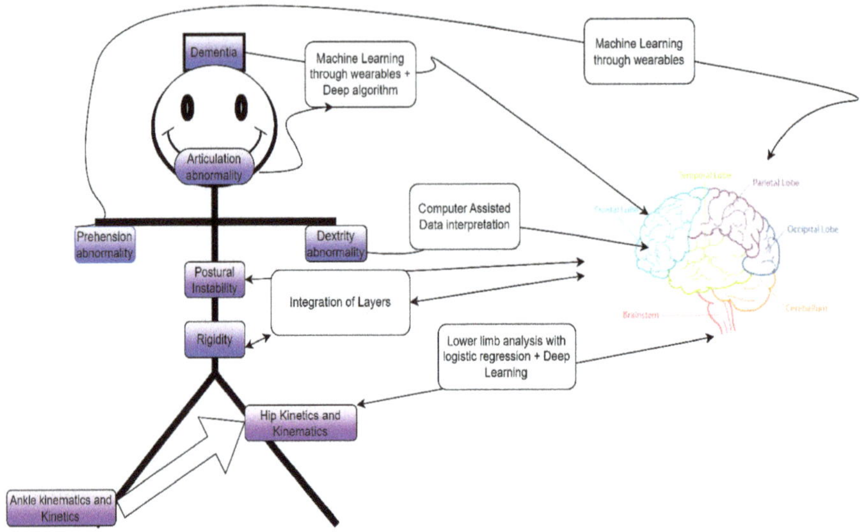

Figure 9.1 Diagrammatic illustration of a clinical decision-making system powered by AI for next-generation medications.

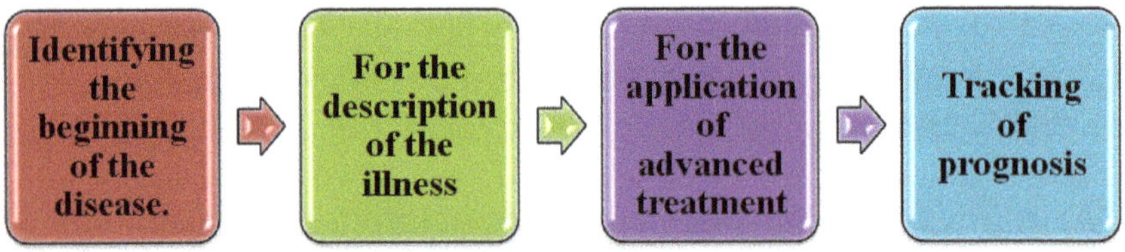

Figure 9.2 Prognosis pathway.

intelligence (AI) is beginning to demonstrate potential methodology to enhancing the accuracy and timeliness of AD diagnosis [25]. The application of AI in AD covers:

a. Early diagnosis of AI.
b. To analyze the medical data.
c. Analyzing the data of tests and assessments which includes, cognitive tests and neuropsychological assessment, retinal evaluation.
d. Yet another fascinating utilization of the AI in AD is the personal devices such as watches and mobile phones for verbal fluency (patients with AI suffered with reduced verbal fluency in AD-related dementia).
e. The patients with AD suffered with frequent falls. To prevent this, comfortable and easy-to-use devices can be given to the patients.

Figure 9.1 presents a diagrammatic representation of an AI-driven clinical decision-making system for next-generation pharmaceuticals, while Figure 9.2 delineates the prognosis pipeline.

9.5 Artificial Intelligence in PD

PD is the one of the most prevalent neurological condition globally, affecting both males and females at an increasing frequency, and regrettably, at present, there is no proven remedy. The disease originates with the degeneration of dopaminergic neurons, essential for dopamine synthesis. Dopamine is a predominant neurotransmitter that facilitates intercellular communication in the brain and throughout the body. The sensory, motor and autonomic symptoms that define PD are caused by the depletion of this function. The integration of AI in the diagnostic domain has enabled the development of systems capable of providing highly individualized and thorough evaluations. These artificial intelligence systems integrate many data sources such as clinical symptoms, genetic variations, and biomarker profiles to generate a customized diagnosis for every individual patient. In recent years, remote monitoring has gained significant popularity as it enables patients to effectively control their symptoms from the comfort of their own homes. Innovations in present technological era such as wearable and implantable gadgets and sensors, enable the routine visualization of patients in real time from the comfort of their own homes [36]. Existing research provides robust evidence for the capacity of AI-driven technologies to automate the administration of sophisticated professional development. In addition to reducing expenses for patients, these technologies greatly enhance the quality of care and provide substantial advantages to healthcare [27].

9.5.1 Wearable devices and remote monitoring for neurodegenerative disorders

The benefits of wearables for the surveillance of neurodegenerative disorders are vast. The integration of continuous tracking, reliable measurements, and telemetry capabilities results in accelerated diagnoses, tailored therapy interventions, and enhanced overall results. Wearable devices can monitor several factors like blood pressure, cardiac rate, mobility, sleep cycles, and neuronal activity, providing valuable information on both known and unknown neurological diseases. Moreover, machine learning algorithms has the capacity to examine the data generated by these devices, identifying patterns, and developing forecast models that can aid clinicians in making educated and timely decisions about patient care and therapy [28].

9.5.2 Robotics in rehabilitation for neurodegenerative disorders

Neurodegenerative disorders are primarily due to the loss of neurons within the brain and spinal cord system. Millions of individuals are affected by neurological disorders. Much appreciated to the advancement of the innovation presently there are a lot of treatments accessible to come across this issue. Artificial intelligence is one of the ways to treat patients which gives time successful productive results [29].

9.5.3 Role of robotics in assisting patient care

1. With the advancement of technology, the integration of robots in movement therapy and recovery is getting increasingly crucial. Robotic systems have demonstrated their use in assisting patients in their recuperation from sickness or injury. Furthermore, they assist physical therapists in enhancing the efficacy of patient treatment.
2. Robotic rehabilitation can help therapists by taking care of hard and time-consuming tasks.
3. It can also change to meet the needs of the people being treated.
4. The combination of this technology with virtual and augmented reality can provide a therapeutic experience that stimulates a range of senses. This could offer extra sensory cues that facilitate brain adjustments, enhancing understanding for people with cognitive difficulties.
5. Robotic technology holds significant potential to assist individuals in their recovery and with daily activities [30].

Examples of robotic devices used in therapy for neurodegenerative conditions as follows:

Sports rehabilitation robot: As individuals age, they may experience declines in physical skills such as strength, flexibility, balance, stamina, coordination, and speed due to health conditions associated with aging. This may cause problems with limbs and make it hard to do basic body actions. There is a wide range of rehabilitation robots for sports that are presently accessible to help improve poorly functioning body parts. For example, older people often have trouble with balance and walking, especially those with Parkinson's disease. This can be difficult for both the patients and their physical therapists. Sports rehabilitation robots make it easier for patients to walk. Straps are attached to their feet and legs, and the robot helps them move. It also alters the speed and duration. By implementing diverse methods, these robotic systems aid patients in restoring their physical capabilities and leading their usual lives once again [16].

1. Walking and talking with robots: The Ludwig project was developed by a research team at the University of Toronto in collaboration with Mitacs, a national nonprofit organization. At One Kenton Place, a senior living facility in North York that provides care for those with Alzheimer's and dementia, Ludwig was introduced. Some organizations are utilizing robots as a means of communication with children diagnosed with autism. According to him, engaging in dialogue with strangers may cause some anxiety, but having conversations with robots is both easy and pleasurable. The group is examining how the robot can recognize shifts in someone's feelings or mindset by analyzing their way of speaking. Rudzicz mentioned that a long-term initiative is underway to develop the capability to recognize when a person is confused or disinterested in engaging in conversation [32].

9.5.4 Impact on patient outcomes and quality of life

Using robots in physical therapy has greatly improved how well patients recover, making the treatment faster and more effective. One important benefit of robots is that they help with practice that involves repeating movements, which is essential for the brain's ability to change and adapt. Studies have shown that doing repetitive tasks helps patients with nerve problems improve their movement skills. Also, robotic devices can offer steady help and attention that human therapists may find hard to match. Many older people often feel isolated and lonely. Social robots can help both older adults and children. They can make people feel less lonely, reduce anxiety, boost mood, and ease pain by interacting with them [33]. Robots can help patients recover in good ways, but they cannot provide the comforting touch and hugs from people that help reduce stress. Children and older people need a little encouragement and support when they reach their goals. This makes them feel proud and happy. This negative effect can make recovery take longer [34].

9.6 AI in Speech Therapy for Neurodegenerative Disorders

The integration of artificial intelligence (AI) in speech therapy is revolutionizing how we approach neurodegenerative disorders like Parkinson's,

Table 9.1 The different types of wearable sensors.

SL. no	Wearable sensors	Types	Applications	Disadvantage
1	Pressure and strain sensor	Piezoelectric effect	For the fingers, Joints and Limbs	The sensor is not able to sense the static force and it is influenced by the temperature.
		Capacitance Change	For the joint movement and tactile pressure	The sensor is not able to sense the static force and it is influenced by the temperature.
		Accelerometer	For the assessment of tremor	The sensor is not able to sense the static force and it is influenced by the temperature.
2	Inertial Sensors	Gyroscope	For the detection of tremor and bradykinesia	Sensitivity to the gravity
		Magnetometer	For the detection of tremor and bradykinesia	Contain the disturbances due to magnet
3	EMG	Surface EMG	Detect the muscle activity	Changes will occur due to noise
		Needle EMG	To detect exact muscle activity	It is invasive in nature
4	EEG	Surface EMG	To find out the cognitive activity	Outside noise can impact the result
5	GPS	Radio waves	For assessing the daily living activities	Depends on the device battery life

Alzheimer's, and ALS. What used to be an incredibly challenging aspect of care – addressing the gradual loss of speech – has now become a dynamic process aided by technology that seems to understand, adapt, and improve with every interaction. AI is not just here to help therapists do their jobs more efficiently; it is providing capabilities we could only dream about a decade ago. Imagine an advanced system that can detect even the most subtle shifts in someone's speech – changes that are so slight, a human ear might miss them. But these systems catch everything. They dissect words, pitch, and cadence with such precision that early signs of speech decline are detected before anyone even knows there's an issue. This early intervention can make a world of difference in the progression of diseases like Parkinson's [16]. It's like having a silent partner in the room with you, continuously analyzing, learning, and providing feedback in real time. In one study, AI-driven tools were able to predict the development of speech disorders with an accuracy that has never been seen before in clinical settings [8].

9.6.1 Virtual speech therapy

Breaking down barriers for patients living with progressive conditions like ALS, the need for constant therapy can be a burden. Traveling to appointments becomes harder, and the sessions themselves may feel too few and far between. This is where AI steps in as a game changer. Virtual speech therapy offers a solution that is accessible from the comfort of one's home. Gone are the days where therapy is confined to a clinic. Now, with a device in hand, patients can engage in customized exercises without leaving their living room [35]. In many ways, AI bridges the gap between patient and therapist. It acts almost like a personal trainer, always there, giving feedback instantly. If a patient mispronounces a word, AI will catch it. If they are struggling with an exercise, AI adjusts the difficulty right there and then. Patients, especially those living with degenerative diseases, report feeling more engaged and in control of their therapy [6].

9.6.2 Real-time feedback: The new normal in therapy

The idea of real-time feedback is not new, but AI elevates it. It is not just about catching mistakes – it is about learning from every session. AI does not need time to process data the way a human might. Instead, it listens, learns, and adapts almost instantly. Let us say a patient's speech is starting to slur or they are having difficulty enunciating certain words. AI provides targeted corrections and adjustments, which can prevent further decline in speech [10]. Patients no longer have to wait for a follow-up session to get their progress evaluated. This instant adjustment is not just a luxury – it is a necessity for conditions that change rapidly, like ALS and Parkinson's. The real-time nature of these tools ensures that therapy is always relevant and effective. AI in occupational therapy for neurodegenerative disorders is making huge strides in occupational therapy, particularly for people dealing with neurodegenerative conditions. By using advanced data analysis, therapists can now assess daily activities with unmatched accuracy, develop highly tailored treatment plans, and seamlessly integrate AI into a patient's daily life. This combination of technology and therapy is paving the way for a more individualized, patient-focused future for those living with Parkinson's, Alzheimer's, ALS, and MS.

9.6.3 AI-powered tools for assessing daily activities

Picture a future where therapists no longer have to rely on occasional check-ins or subjective assessments to understand how well a patient manages daily tasks. Instead, AI-driven tools, such as sensors and data streams, provide continuous, real-time insights into how patients handle basic activities like getting dressed, eating, or moving around their homes. Far from being a distant dream, this technology is already starting to reshape occupational therapy. Using data from smart devices and wearables, AI provides a detailed understanding of a patient's capabilities far beyond what human observation could offer [19].

One of the greatest strengths of AI is its ability to detect small changes in motor skills or cognitive functions – things that might go unnoticed during a regular clinic visit but could signal the beginning of a decline. For instance, AI systems monitoring fine motor skills in Parkinson's patients have proven to be more accurate in identifying early issues than traditional methods, enabling timely intervention [42]. By capturing real-world data, AI allows therapists to make better, more informed decisions and adapt care as the patient's condition evolves [22].

9.6.4 Personalized treatment plans for neurodegenerative disorders

AI brings healthcare closer to achieving true personalization, especially when treating neurodegenerative disorders. Since these conditions vary significantly from one patient to another, a one-size-fits-all approach does not work. AI, however, can analyze a wide range of factors – such as medical history, current symptoms, genetics, and lifestyle choices – to create treatment plans that are uniquely tailored to each patient [41].

What makes AI stand out is its ability to update these plans in real time. Instead of sticking to a static treatment plan, AI allows therapy to change based on how a patient is doing. If a patient is struggling with a particular exercise or showing signs of fatigue, AI can adjust the exercises or treatment intensity to better suit the patient's current needs [38]. This makes therapy more engaging and effective, increasing the chances that patients will stick with their treatments and, in turn, achieve better results. The days of rigid, one-size-fits-all treatment plans are over – AI makes therapy flexible and highly responsive.

9.7 Integrating AI into Daily Life and Patient Care

Perhaps the most exciting development in AI's role in occupational therapy is how smoothly it integrates into a patient's daily life. Imagine a smart home environment where AI assists with everything from meal preparation to medication reminders, all while ensuring that patients can maintain their independence [24]. These smart technologies not only promote autonomy but also act as safety measures, reducing the likelihood of accidents or health issues. At the same time, AI is revolutionizing how healthcare providers and caregivers interact with patients. Rather than relying solely on scheduled appointments, AI can continuously monitor a patient's condition and send alerts to caregivers if something seems off. This kind of real-time monitoring allows for quicker adjustments in care, ensuring that a patient's needs are met as soon as they arise [40]. By embedding AI into everyday life, occupational therapy moves beyond the clinic and becomes a continuous part of rehabilitation and self-management. The integration of AI into occupational therapy for neurodegenerative disorders is nothing short of ground-breaking. With its ability to offer real-time assessments, highly personalized treatment plans, and seamless integration into daily life, AI is fundamentally changing the way Parkinson's, Alzheimer's, ALS, and MS are treated. As this technology continues to develop, it promises to enhance patient independence, improve therapy outcomes, and lead to innovative treatment approaches. The future of occupational therapy is not just promising – it is already here, powered by AI [9].

9.8 Future Directions and Innovations in AI-Powered Rehabilitation for Neurodegenerative Disorders

Wearable AI technologies hold immense potential, not only in the nuanced analysis of symptom progression but also in streamlining the delivery of rehabilitation regimens. However, as promising as these advancements are, rigorous prospective research remains essential. It is imperative to establish the reliability, accuracy, precision, and unbiased support these technologies offer to both patients and healthcare systems in order to gain broader acceptance and validation. In the grand scheme, we must acknowledge that AI is no longer an emerging presence but a deeply integrated component of modern healthcare, poised for continued expansion in addressing complex medical challenges. From developing individualized treatment plans to injury prevention and facilitating remote rehabilitation, AI is redefining the rehabilitation landscape. Its use in patient monitoring, automating repetitive rehabilitation tasks, and optimizing the efficiency of healthcare professionals highlights the transformative capabilities of these technologies. Not only do they increase healthcare accessibility, but they also enhance the productivity of practitioners while improving patient outcomes in rehabilitation. Yet, this progression is not without its caveats [31].

Legal and ethical considerations, particularly around privacy and data protection, loom large as AI continues to be interwoven with patient care. Another critical concern is the erosion of the human connection in healthcare, with AI potentially replacing essential interpersonal interactions. To ensure AI's successful integration into the rehabilitation field – while minimizing unforeseen negative consequences – education, research, and thoughtful legal deliberations must advance in parallel. Only through comprehensive exploration and strategic implementation can we maximize AI's benefits while safeguarding the human elements that remain central to effective healthcare delivery.

9.9 Conclusion

AI has brought a profound shift in the care of neurodegenerative diseases, far beyond just enhancing existing methods. By integrating AI into physiotherapy, occupational therapy, and speech therapy, patients now experience more tailored, dynamic rehabilitation that adapts in real time to their needs. Whether through advanced motion analysis, virtual reality environments, or wearable devices, AI is making rehabilitation more accessible and continuous, allowing patients to recover in the comfort of their homes. It transforms how diseases like Parkinson's, ALS, and MS are treated, empowering patients to regain mobility, independence, and quality of life. However, as promising as AI-driven care is, challenges remain, especially concerning data privacy, accessibility, and ethical concerns. AI's potential to revolutionize healthcare depends on ensuring it is equitable and inclusive, reaching all patients regardless of their circumstance. Moving forward, advancements in AI, such as biometrics and neuroprosthetics, hold the promise of further enhancing recovery. Ultimately, AI is not just improving care – it is opening new frontiers of possibility, offering hope to patients where there once was none.

References

[1] E. J. Topol, *Deep Medicine : How Artificial Intelligence Can Make Healthcare Human Again*. New York: Basic Books, 2019.

[2] A. Esteva *et al.*, "A Guide to Deep Learning in Healthcare," *Nature Medicine*, vol. 25, no. 1, pp. 24–29, Jan. 2019, doi: https://doi.org/10.1038/s41591-018-0316-z.

[3] A. Rajkomar, J. Dean, and I. Kohane, "Machine Learning in Medicine," *New England Journal of Medicine*, vol. 380, no. 14, pp. 1347–1358, Apr. 2019, doi: https://doi.org/10.1056/nejmra1814259.

[4] T. Davenport and R. Kalakota, "The Potential for Artificial Intelligence in Healthcare," *Future Healthcare Journal*, vol. 6, no. 2, pp. 94–98, 2019, doi: https://doi.org/10.7861/futurehosp.6-2-94.

[5] A. Ramesh, C. Kambhampati, J. Monson, and P. Drew, "Artificial intelligence in medicine," *Annals of The Royal College of Surgeons of England*, vol. 86, no. 5, pp. 334–338, Sep. 2004, doi: https://doi.org/10.1308/147870804290.

[6] R. Gassert and V. Dietz, "Rehabilitation Robots for the Treatment of Sensorimotor deficits: a Neurophysiological Perspective," *Journal of NeuroEngineering and Rehabilitation*, vol. 15, no. 1, Jun. 2018, doi: https://doi.org/10.1186/s12984-018-0383-x.

[7] N. Jalloul, "Wearable Sensors for the Monitoring of Movement Disorders," *Biomedical Journal*, vol. 41, no. 4, pp. 249–253, Aug. 2018, doi: https://doi.org/10.1016/j.bj.2018.06.003.

[8] C.-W. Park *et al.*, "Artificial Intelligence in Health Care: Current Applications and Issues," *Journal of Korean Medical Science*, vol. 35, no. 42, Oct. 2020, doi: https://doi.org/10.3346/jkms.2020.35.e379.

[9] R. Das, S. Paul, G. K. Mourya, N. Kumar, and M. Hussain, "Recent Trends and Practices Toward Assessment and Rehabilitation of Neurodegenerative Disorders: Insights From Human Gait," *Frontiers in Neuroscience*, vol. 16, Apr. 2022, doi: https://doi.org/10.3389/fnins.2022.859298.

[10] T. Feng, "Applications of Artificial Intelligence to Diagnosis of Neurodegenerative Diseases," *Studies in Health Technology and Informatics*, pp. 648–655, Nov. 2023, doi:https://doi.org/10.3233/shti230896.

[11] D. Putrino and J. W. Krakauer, "Neurotechnology's Prospects for Bringing About Meaningful Reductions in Neurological Impairment,"

Neurorehabilitation and Neural Repair, vol. 37, no. 6, pp. 356–366, Nov. 2022, doi: https://doi.org/10.1177/15459683221137341.

[12] A. Pantelopoulos and N. G. Bourbakis, "A Survey on Wearable Sensor-Based Systems for Health Monitoring and Prognosis," *IEEE Transactions on Systems, Man, and Cybernetics, Part C (Applications and Reviews)*, vol. 40, no. 1, pp. 1–12, Jan. 2010, doi: https://doi.org/10.1109/tsmcc.2009.2032660.

[13] D. D. Farhud and S. Zokaei, "Ethical issues of artificial intelligence in medicine and healthcare," *Iranian Journal of Public Health*, vol. 50, no. 11, Nov. 2021, doi: https://doi.org/10.18502/ijph.v50i11.7600.

[14] F. Lanotte, M. K. O'Brien, and A. Jayaraman, "AI in rehabilitation medicine: Opportunities and challenges," *Annals of Rehabilitation Medicine*, vol. 47, no. 6, pp. 444–458, Dec. 2023, doi: https://doi.org/10.5535/arm.23131.

[15] F. Angelucci, A. R. Ai, L. Piendel, J. Cerman, and J. Hort, "Integrating AI in fighting advancing Alzheimer: diagnosis, prevention, treatment, monitoring, mechanisms, and clinical trials," *Current Opinion in Structural Biology*, vol. 87, p. 102857, Aug. 2024, doi: https://doi.org/10.1016/j.sbi.2024.102857.

[16] H. Fröhlich *et al.*, "Leveraging the Potential of Digital Technology for Better Individualized Treatment of Parkinson's Disease," *Frontiers in Neurology*, vol. 13, p. 788427, Feb. 2022, doi: https://doi.org/10.3389/fneur.2022.788427.

[17] Y. Xing, K. Yang, A. Lu, K. Mackie, and F. Guo, "Sensors and devices guided by artificial intelligence for personalized pain medicine," *Cyborg and Bionic Systems*, vol. 5, Jan. 2024, doi: https://doi.org/10.34133/cbsystems.0160.

[18] C. Neiertz, E. J. M. Wouters, and I. Mannheim, "The association of technology-based ageism with using digital technology in physical therapy for older persons," *Healthcare*, vol. 11, no. 19, p. 2672, Oct. 2023, doi: https://doi.org/10.3390/healthcare11192672.

[19] S. Wongvibulsin, T. M. Frech, M.-M. Chren, and E. R. Tkaczyk, "Expanding personalized, data-driven dermatology: Leveraging digital health technology and machine learning to improve patient outcomes," *JID Innovations*, vol. 2, no. 3, p. 100105, May 2022, doi: https://doi.org/10.1016/j.xjidi.2022.100105.

[20] S. Setya, S. Talegaonkar, N. Manchanda, and A. Aggarwal, "Digital intervention for the management of alzheimer's disease," *Current*

Alzheimer Research, vol. 19, no. 14, pp. 909–932, Dec. 2022, doi: https://doi.org/10.2174/1567205020666230206124155.

[21] P. K. Moore, A. P. Thomas, G. Tadros, Fatos Xhafa, and L. Barolli, "Detection of the onset of agitation in patients with dementia: real-time monitoring and the application of big-data solutions," *International journal of space-based and situated computing*, vol. 3, no. 3, pp. 136–136, Sep. 2013, doi: https://doi.org/10.1504/ijssc.2013.056405.

[22] C. Fabrizio, A. Termine, C. Caltagirone, and G. Sancesario, "Artificial intelligence for alzheimer's disease: Promise or challenge?," *Diagnostics*, vol. 11, no. 8, p. 1473, Aug. 2021, doi: https://doi.org/10.3390/diagnostics11081473.

[23] E. H. Shortliffe and M. J. Sepúlveda, "Clinical decision support in the era of artificial intelligence," *JAMA*, vol. 320, no. 21, pp. 2199–2200, 2018, doi: https://doi.org/10.1001/jama.2018.17163.

[24] A. P. Porsteinsson, R. S. Isaacson, S. Knox, M. N. Sabbagh, and I. Rubino, "Diagnosis of early alzheimer's disease: Clinical practice in 2021," *The Journal of Prevention of Alzheimer's Disease*, vol. 8, no. 3, pp. 1–16, 2021, doi: https://doi.org/10.14283/jpad.2021.23.

[25] S. Mirkin and B. C. Albensi, "Should artificial intelligence be used in conjunction with Neuroimaging in the diagnosis of Alzheimer's disease?," *Front. Aging Neurosci*, vol. 15, pp. 1–18, Apr. 2023, doi: https://doi.org/10.3389/fnagi.2023.1094233.

[26] Katie Louise Bounsall, M. Milne-Ives, A. J. Hall, C. Carroll, and E. Meinert, "Artificial Intelligence Applications for Assessment, Monitoring and Management of Parkinson's Disease Symptoms: A Systematic Review Protocol (Preprint)," *JMIR Research Protocols*, vol. 12, pp. e46581–e46581, Jun. 2023, doi: https://doi.org/10.2196/46581.

[27] L. Perju-Dumbrava *et al.*, "Artificial intelligence applications and robotic systems in Parkinson's disease (Review)," *Experimental and Therapeutic Medicine*, vol. 23, no. 2, p. 153, Feb. 2022, doi: https://doi.org/10.3892/etm.2021.11076.

[28] F. Demrozi, L. Borzì, and G. Olmo, "Wearable sensors for supporting diagnosis, prognosis, and monitoring of neurodegenerative diseases," *Electronics*, vol. 12, no. 6, p. 1269, Mar. 2023, doi: https://doi.org/10.3390/electronics12061269.

[29] R. Lamptey, B. Chaulagain, R. Trivedi, A. Gothwal, B. Layek, and J. Singh, "A Review of the Common Neurodegenerative Disorders: Current Therapeutic Approaches and the Potential Role of

Nanotherapeutics," *ProQuest*, vol. 23, no. 3, p. 1851, 2022, doi: https://doi.org/10.3390/ijms23031851.

[30] Rehab Modalities, "Neuro robotics: Integrating technology into rehabilitation," *Rehab Modalities*, Mar. 06, 2024. https://rehabmodalities.com/neuro-robotics-technology-into-rehabilitation-programs-2/ (accessed Sep. 15, 2024).

[31] F. Ju, Y. Wang, B. Xie, Y. Mi, M. Zhao, and J. Cao, "The Use of Sports Rehabilitation Robotics to Assist in the Recovery of Physical Abilities in Elderly Patients with Degenerative Diseases: A Literature Review," *Healthcare*, vol. 11, no. 3, p. 326, Jan. 2023, doi: https://doi.org/10.3390/healthcare11030326.

[32] Dr. F. Rudzicz, "Robot designed to help alzheimer's patients," *Utoronto.ca*, 2016. https://rsi.utoronto.ca/news/dr-frank-rudzicz-robot-designed-help-alzheimers-patients (accessed Sep. 15, 2024).

[33] J. Zuijderwijk, A. Gomez Martos, M. Asensi Hérnandez, and C. Plate, "The effect on the quality of life using a social robot with elderly in sheltered housing," Jun. 2021.

[34] M. Eckstein, I. Mamaev, B. Ditzen, and U. Sailer, "Calming effects of touch in human, animal, and robotic interaction – scientific state-of-the-art and technical advances," *Frontiers in Psychiatry*, vol. 11, Nov. 2020, doi: https://doi.org/10.3389/fpsyt.2020.555058.

[35] L. Beijer and T. Rietvel, "Potentials of telehealth devices for speech therapy in parkinson's disease," *Diagnostics and Rehabilitation of Parkinson's Disease*, Dec. 2011, doi: https://doi.org/10.5772/17865.

[36] Ishita Guglani, Sanskriti Sanskriti, S. H. Joshi, and Ashish Anjankar, "Speech-Language Therapy Through Telepractice During COVID-19 and Its Way Forward: A Scoping Review," *Cureus*, vol. 15, no. 9, Sep. 2023, doi: https://doi.org/10.7759/cureus.44808.

[37] E. K. Oikonomou and R. Khera, "Artificial intelligence-enhanced patient evaluation: bridging art and science," *European Heart Journal*, Jul. 2024, doi: https://doi.org/10.1093/eurheartj/ehae415.

[38] R. Seccia, S. Romano, M. Salvetti, A. Crisanti, L. Palagi, and F. Grassi, "Machine Learning Use for Prognostic Purposes in Multiple Sclerosis," *Life*, vol. 11, no. 2, p. 122, Feb. 2021, doi: https://doi.org/10.3390/life11020122.

[39] U. Khalid, M. Naeem, Fabrizio Stasolla, M. Syed, M. Abbas, and A. Coronato, "Impact of AI-Powered Solutions in Rehabilitation Process: Recent Improvements and Future Trends," *International Journal*

of General Medicine, vol. Volume 17, pp. 943–969, Mar. 2024, doi: https://doi.org/10.2147/ijgm.s453903.

[40] R. R. Ileşan *et al.*, "Proof of Concept in Artificial-Intelligence-Based Wearable Gait Monitoring for Parkinson's Disease Management Optimization," *Biosensors*, vol. 12, no. 4, p. 189, Apr. 2022, doi: https://doi.org/10.3390/bios12040189.

[41] Ismail Dergaa *et al.*, "Using artificial intelligence for exercise prescription in personalised health promotion: A critical evaluation of OpenAI's GPT-4 model," *Biology of Sport*, vol. 41, no. 2, Jan. 2024, doi: https://doi.org/10.5114/biolsport.2024.133661.

[42] H. Liu, R. K. Tripathy, and P. Bhattacharya, *Clinical Practice and Unmet Challenges in AI-Enhanced Healthcare Systems*. IGI Global, 2024.

10

Prediction of Alzheimer's and Parkinson's Diseases: AI Perspectives

Monalisha Pattnaik[1], Deepti Rani Pattanaik[1], Sudev Kumar Padhi[2,3], Ashirbad Mishra[3], and Sadhu Charan Panda[4]

[1]Department of Statistics, Sambalpur University, India
[2]Department of CSE, Indian Institute of Technology Bhilai, India
[3]Department of CSE, Pennsylvania State University, United States
[4]Department of Community Medicine, VSS Institute of Medical Sciences and Research, India
E-mail: monalisha_1977@yahoo.com; 97deeptirani@gmail.com; sudevpadhi2011@gmail.com; ashirbadm@gmail.com; sadhu.p7@gmail.com

Abstract

Neurodegenerative disorders are a category of irreversible conditions, gradually progressing and marked by the death of neurons and the atrophy of brain tissue. Common disorders namely "Alzheimer's disease" (AD), "Parkinson's disease" (PD), "Huntington's disease," "Pick's disease," "ALS," and "Lewy body dementia" "cause cognitive decline," "motor impairment," and "challenges in daily tasks." This chapter proposes a deep learning-based neural network model for diagnosing the two neurodegenerative disorder diseases namely Alzheimer's and Parkinson's aimed at early prediction of the patients. This approach enhances prediction accuracy, potentially reducing the adverse effects of neurodegenerative disorders. We use more than 2000 patients' worth of data with 32 predictors using a random split of 70/30 for train/test using "root mean squared error" (RMSE) for performance in "decision tree" (DT). Furthermore, using the decision tree, we found that the functional assessment, memory complaints, behavioral problems, ADL, and MMSE were sufficient to diagnose AD without depending on the rest

DOI: 10.1201/9788743801764-10

27 attributes of patients with RMSE of 0.2055216. Similarly, we found that the UPDRS, postural instability, tremor, functional assessment, bradykinesia, rigidity, and MoCA were sufficient to determine PD without depending on the rest 25 attributes of patients with RMSE of 0.2895523. The efficiency of the diagnosis of these two neurodegenerative diseases is tested by "decision tree" (DT), "artificial neural network" (ANN) having a hidden layer of one, ANN having two hidden layers, hybrid ANN, different "deep neural network" (DNN), hybrid DNN, boosting algorithm-based machine learning, and "TabNet" models. TabNet model has shown the finest results for diagnosing Alzheimer's disease with an accuracy of 0.997 and 0.996, and Parkinson's disease with an accuracy of 0.997 and 0.996 with train and test data sets, respectively, which outperforms other models.

Keywords: TabNet Model, DNN, ANN, Decision Tree, Machine Learning Techniques, Boosting Algorithm.

10.1 Introduction

Neurodegenerative disorders are a category of steadily continuing, irreparable conditions marked by the death of neurons and the atrophy of brain tissue. Common disorders namely AD, PD, Pick's disease, Huntington's disease, ALS, and Lewy body dementia cause cognitive decline, motor injury, and challenges in daily tasks. More than 55 million people worldwide are exaggerated by dementia, with 60% residing in low- and middle-income countries. Approximately, 10 million new cases emerge each year from various brain-related diseases and injuries, with AD being the most prevalent cause. Dementia is the seventh leading cause of death, costing the global economy 1.3 trillion USD in 2019. Women are disproportionately affected by dementia, experiencing higher disability-adjusted life years and mortality. Additionally, Parkinson's disease cases have doubled in the past 25 years, with over 8.5 million individuals affected in 2019. Similarly, AD impairs memory and daily functioning. Millions of Americans, mainly aged 65 or older, may be affected. Early diagnosis and intervention are essential for managing these conditions.

10.2 Literature Survey

PD has been a prevalent disorder with motor symptoms like trembles and rigidity, as well as nonmotor issues. It is estimated that 6.3 million people suffer from PD worldwide. The incidence of PD in India is 70 out of 100,000. The Parsi community in Mumbai has the world's highest incidences of PD where it affects about 328 out of every 100,000 people. More than 55 million people worldwide are exaggerated by dementia, with 60% residing in low- and middle-income countries. Approximately, 10 million new cases come into sight each year from various injuries and brain-related diseases, with AD being the most prevalent cause. Dementia is the seventh leading cause of death, costing the global economy 1.3 trillion USD in 2019. Additionally, PD cases have increased twofold in the past 25 years, with over 8.5 million individuals affected in 2019. A spectrum of debilitating symptoms ranging from loss of motor reflexes to cognitive decline is seen in PD. Whether the cognitive decline is due to the aging process or due to PD is a difficult task. Similarly, in the case of AD, the initial asymptomatic stage remains around 20 years after which there may be a mild cognitive decline (MCD) [4]. Like PD, diagnosis of AD based on evidence of MCD is a challenge for physicians because MCD is also a part of the natural aging process. Both conditions are irreversible, not curable, and debilitating for which early and accurate diagnosis is necessary to develop new and effective interventions. This early detection concept helps to identify, analyze, and prevent its progression before the manifestation of clinical features. On one hand, substantial clinical, genetic/genomic, and demographic, data sets are available to diagnose these two disorders [18]. On the other hand, advancement in machine learning has prompted researchers to focus on this approach to come out with easy and accurate diagnostic algorithms of these neurodegenerative disorders [6].

Supervised ML techniques have been extensively used for detecting AD. Among the earliest and most widely used techniques are SVMs. For example, [30] showed that SVMs were able to classify MRI scans of patients having AD with approximately 89% accuracy by analyzing brain atrophy patterns. Likewise, RFs have demonstrated great effectiveness in detecting AD. The Alzheimer's Disease Neuroimaging Initiative (ADNI) data set is one of the larger which have been used by [10] with a deep learning method termed CNN. They carry out multiclass classification across the four stages of AD. They first use a simple CNN model to reduce the 2D and 3D scans of the structural part of the brain. Next, they apply pretrained models for classification such as VGG19. They achieve an accuracy of 93.61% for 2D and 95.17% for 3D image classifications. [28] also use the ADNI image data set for disease classification. Their proposed DNN uses three different types of activations, Leaky ReLU, ELU, and PReLU, for its hidden layers. They perform three different types of comparison, AD and CN, AD and MCI, and CN versus MCI, obtaining accuracy scores of 85.19%, 72.73%, and 76.93%, respectively.

Previously researchers such as [7] also used deep learning techniques on MRI images. They create a deep CAE architecture designed to work on very large size data sets achieving an accuracy of over 84%. They identify strong correlations with clinical variables such as age, tau protein deposits, and neuropsychological assessments.

Researchers [5] have looked at a variety of classifiers using machine learning, such as DT, RF, voting classifiers, Gradient Boosting, and SVM, which were applied to the OASIS data set, and this resulted in the highest accuracy of 83%. Another study utilized [34] ML algorithms significantly enhancing the forecasting accuracy of Alzheimer's disease with related dementia (ADRD). They used the One Florida+ Research data set with more than a million patients comparing using AUC scores for 0, 1, 3, or 5 years prior to diagnosis. They used models like GBT, RF, and LR, on the Employee Health Record (EHR) data. The highest AUC score (0.939) was for the 0th-year model and the worst was for the 5-year model with an AUC score of 0.856.

The data sets that we use in this work have been generated synthetically for educational and statistical research. The data set has been used to perform machine learning analysis [6]. They have used a variety of methods such as NB, DT, k-NN, and their Ensemble. Their Ensemble model's accuracy is 94.07% obtaining only 13 features. The 13 features were selected using the Spearman feature selection algorithm.

[8] compared different DNNs and regularized Cox proportional hazard models for predicting new events in the older general population. They trained three DNN algorithms and two Cox models. Tab transformer showed superior time-dependent balanced accuracy and specificity, promising for heterogeneous tabular data sets and handling censored data. [23] highlighted promising areas of machine learning research for preventing and correcting neurodegenerative and depressive disorders, exploring these areas by various scientific groups worldwide. [9] conducted an innovative framework using PCA, FDR, and SVM for feature extraction, selection, and classification of diseases, achieving 100% accuracy. An NDD classification algorithm was done by Nguyen et al. (2020) by using gait force and ML models. They validated the algorithm using used Synthetic minority oversampling technique and the Physionet NDD gait database. The algorithm achieved high classification accuracies for healthy controls and NDD, with satisfactory results.

[12] used five feature selection algorithms on 18F-fluorodeoxyglucose PET images to identify key features in PPA. The classification and clustering results were compared based on before and after selection, finding PCA to perform similarly by using all features. This study talks about the importance of ML in neuroimaging for better disease classification and reducing the gap between clinical diagnosis tools and image processing. [13] discussed a comprehensive analysis of ML techniques and data modalities utilized in diagnosing PD by applying PubMed and IEEE Xplore databases. Various metrics evaluated the efficiency of machine learning models, with voice recordings, movement, and MRI data commonly used in methodology studies. Clinical applications mainly focused on MRI, movement, and SPECT imaging data. Various machine learning models such as SVM, Several Neural Networks, KNN, Decision Tree, and Naïve-Bayes algorithms were implemented in diagnosing PD. The chapter offers a high-level summary of studies, showcasing the use of machine learning methods in PD diagnosis, potential biomarkers for precise diagnosis, and databases to enhance smaller data sets. [17] developed a model using genomic machine learning to enhance multi-omic predictions of PD by combining machine learning with multimodal data from PPMI. The model, validated in the PDBP data set, improved diagnosis accuracy by optimizing classification thresholds. Networks identified PD-specific gene communities. UPSIT and PRS were key predictors. The used model is ideal for selecting individuals for further testing in health registries or biobanks. [2] used ML methods on PD data to identify the type of patients and predict the progression of the disease. Three distinct subtypes were found with varying progression rates, and serum neuro filament light was identified as a key biomarker. [32] applied DL and ML techniques to discern between individuals with PD and healthy individuals on the basis of voice signals. They utilized k-NN and FNN models, implemented SMOTE for class imbalance, conducted feature selection, and tuned hyperparameters. FNN and KSVM models showed the best results on an 80-20 data set split. [14] studied using machine learning to predict PD by grouping factors connected with cost and accessibility. They constitute that models involving demographic variables, polygenic risk scores, and clinical assessments were the most accurate, with penalized LR and XG Boost being the top-performing algorithms. Polygenic risk scores and Olfactory function were singled out as the most significant predictors of PD risk. [19] developed an optimized preprocessing approach of data that increased forecasting accuracy to diagnose PD using a voice-recorded data set. They achieved 97.4% prediction accuracy using AdaBoost, with higher value of performance matrices. This

suggests that utilizing voice recordings with optimized machine learning techniques is a reliable method for predicting PD, with potential implications for cost-effective early-stage diagnosis. In their study, [3] developed the most efficient PD prediction method by applying the gradient boosting decision tree (GBDT) and the Hjorth parameter algorithms. They analyzed EEG signals from 41 PD patients and 41 healthy individuals who were in the control group, recorded at the University of New Mexico and the University of Iowa. Their best model performed an accuracy of 8. A study by [1, 27] highlighted the use of speech impairments as an early indicator for PD diagnosis. A DNN classifier with a stacked autoencoder and softmax classifier was made acquainted by them. Through simulations on two databases, they demonstrated the effectiveness of this classifier compared to traditional methods, showing high efficiency in diagnosing PD (9.3%), outperforming previous works and even surpassing pathologic examination-based diagnoses. [11, 20] introduced a new ANN approach considering data dependence in replicated measure-based designs. They conducted an audio replication-based experiment differentiating healthy individuals from PD patients. The proposed system achieved 94.93% accuracy in picking out PD patients from healthy individuals with fewer subjects. A study by [21] developed an anatomically partitioned artificial neural network (APANN) model to predict clinical scores at the individual level from MRI data related to AD. The model integrated data from cortical thickness and hippocampal segmentations, demonstrating accurate inference of clinical severity in AD using 10-fold cross-validation with cohorts from the Alzheimer's Disease Neuroimaging Initiative (ADNI). [15] discussed the use of DNN classification for AD detection, demonstrating a 96.6% accuracy rate and minimal error rate by implementing data segmentation and attribute selection. A model was created by [24, 26, 29] by employing DT for diagnosing AD by applying cerebrospinal fluid biomarkers. The tree outperformed previous cut-offs, showing higher diagnostic accuracy in validation cohorts. [34] developed a classification of features model for AD applying KPCA and AdaBoost algorithms. They selected 21 AD patients, including 9 with LAD, 11 with EAD, and 10 healthy individuals. The method showed promising classification results using these algorithms on AD. [16, 25] studied to make use of DNN and LSTM-based models to predict Parkinson's disease from voice samples. Results show high accuracy (97.12% for DNN and 99.03% for LSTM, indicating their efficiency in PD detection). [22] critiqued the ML techniques for PD using Cochrane's seven phases. They searched multiple databases with specific keywords.

10.2.1 Organization of the chapter

The reviewed studies provide a foundation for developing techniques such as decision tree (DT), ANNs, DNNs, DTANN, DTDNN, other boosting algorithm ML models, and TabNet model for diagnosing the two neurodegenerative disorders namely AD and PD at early prediction of the patients. The rest of the chapter is organized into six sections. The Section 10.3 data sets include prerequisite data analysis and the performance assessment metrics. Section 10.4 discusses the detailed conceptualization of the decision tree analysis, ANN, DNN, and boosting algorithm-based machine learning and "TabNet" models. The experimental evaluation and outcomes of all the models are shown in Section 10.5 and Section 10.6 thoroughly discusses the results, their' practical significance along with concluding remarks.

10.3 Data and Preliminary Analysis

There are 32 predictors to diagnose AD and PD in patients. Table 10.1 presents the descriptive statistics of different variables related to AD of patients and Table 10.2 shows the descriptive statistics of the different variables related to the PD of patients.

10.3.1 Performance measurement metrics

The "root mean square error" (RMSE) is applied for measuring performance for various forecasting models with hydrodynamic data sets [33]. For these two performance evaluation metrics, the formulae are expressed as follows:

$$\text{RMSE} = \sqrt{\frac{1}{n}\sum_{i=1}^{n}(w_{\text{i}} - \hat{w}_{\text{i}})^2}, \tag{10.1}$$

where n represents the number of data points in the time series, w_{i} is true value, while $\hat{w}_{\text{i}}$ is the estimated value. The performance metric's minimum value shows the better performance of the model.

10.4 Methodology

TabNet [31] is a state-of-the-art deep learning model specifically designed for tabular data, making it a strong candidate for binary classification tasks like differentiating between Alzheimer's and Parkinson's diseases. By merging

Table 10.1 Descriptive statistics of the variables of AD.

Sl. No.	Variables	Variable types	Minimum	Q1	Median	Mean	Q3	Standard deviation	Maximum	Skewness	Kurtosis
1	Age	Integer	60.00	67.00	75.00	74.91	83.00	8.99	90.00	0.05	1.81
2	Gender	Integer	0.0000	0.00	1.0000	0.5063	1.0000	0.50	1.0000	−0.03	1.00
3	Ethnicity	Integer	0.0000	0.00	0.0000	0.6975	1.0000	0.99	3.0000	1.23	3.23
4	Education level	Integer	0.000	1.000	1.000	1.287	2.000	0.90	3.000	0.21	2.25
5	BMI	Numeric	15.01	21.61	27.82	27.66	33.87	7.22	39.99	−0.03	1.82
6	Smoking	Integer	0.0000	0.00	0.0000	0.2885	1.0000	0.45	1.0000	0.94	1.87
7	Alchohol consumption	Numeric	0.002003	5.14	9.934412	10.039442	15.157931	5.76	19.989293	0.02	1.80
8	Physical activity	Numeric	0.003616	2.57	4.766424	4.920202	7.427899	2.86	9.987429	0.04	1.82
9	Diet quality	Numeric	0.009385	2.46	5.076087	4.993138	7.558625	2.91	9.998346	−0.01	1.77
10	Sleep quality	Numeric	4.003	5.48	7.116	7.051	8.563	1.76	10.000	−0.07	1.79
11	Family history of Alzheimer's	Integer	0.0000	0.00	0.0000	0.2522	1.0000	0.43	1.0000	1.14	2.30
12	Cardiovascular disease	Integer	0.0000	0.00	0.0000	0.1443	0.0000	0.35	1.0000	2.03	5.10
13	Diabetes	Integer	0.0000	0.00	0.0000	0.1508	0.0000	0.36	1.0000	1.95	4.81
14	Depression	Integer	0.0000	0.00	0.0000	0.2006	0.0000	0.40	1.0000	1.49	3.24
15	Head injury	Integer	0.0000	0.00	0.0000	0.0926	0.0000	0.29	1.0000	2.81	8.90
16	Hypertension	Integer	0.0000	0.00	0.0000	0.1489	0.0000	0.36	1.0000	1.97	4.89
17	Systolic BP	Integer	90.0	112.0	134.0	157.0		25.95	179.0	0.01	1.80
18	Diastolic BP	Integer	60.00	74.00	91.00	89.85	105.00	17.59	119.00	−0.05	1.77

Table 10.1 *Continued.*

Sl. No.	Variables	Variable types	Minimum	Q1	Median	Mean	Q3	Standard deviation	Maximum	Skewness	Kurtosis
19	Cholesterol total	Numeric	150.1	190.3	225.1	225.2	262.0	42.54	300.0	−0.02	1.84
20	Cholesterol LDL	Numeric	50.23	87.20	123.34	124.34	161.73	43.37	199.97	0.04	1.79
21	Cholesterol HDL	Numeric	20.00	39.10	59.77	59.46	78.94	23.14	99.98	0.04	1.78
22	Cholesterol triglycerides	Numeric	50.41	137.58	230.3	228.28	314.84	101.99	399.94	−0.03	1.78
23	MMSE	Numeric	0.005312	7.17	14.441660	14.755132	22.161028	8.61	29.991381	0.03	1.77
24	Functional assessment	Numeric	0.00046	2.57	5.09444	5.08005	7.54698	2.89	9.99647	−0.03	1.82
25	Memory complain	Integer	0.000	0.00	0.000	0.208	0.000	0.41	1.000	1.44	3.07
26	Behavior problem	Integer	0.000	0.00	0.0000	0.1568	0.0000	0.37	1.0000	1.89	4.56
27	ADL	Numeric	0.001288	2.34	5.038973	4.982958	7.581490	2.95	9.999747	−0.03	1.75
28	Confusion	Integer	0.000	0.00	0.0000	0.2052	0.0000	0.40	1.0000	1.46	3.13
29	Disorientation	Integer	0.0000	0.00	0.0000	0.1582	0.0000	0.37	1.0000	1.87	4.51
30	Personality change	Integer	0.0000	0.00	0.0000	0.1508	0.0000	0.36	1.0000	1.95	4.81
31	Difficulty completing task	Integer	0.0000	0.00	0.0000	0.1587	0.0000	0.37	1.0000	1.87	4.49
32	Forgetfulness	Integer	0.0000	0.00	0.0000	0.3015	1.0000	0.46	1.0000	0.86	1.75
33	Diagnosis	Integer	0.0000	0.00	0.0000	0.3537	1.0000	0.48	1.0000	0.61	1.37

Table 10.2 Descriptive statistics of the variables of PD.

Sl. No.	Variables	Variable types	Minimum	Q1	Median	Mean	Q3	Standard deviation	Maximum	Skewness	Kurtosis
1	Age	Integer	50.0	60.0	70.0	69.6	80.0	11.59	89.0	−0.03	1.82
2	Gender	Integer	0.0000	0.0000	0.0000	0.4926	1.0000	0.50	1.0000	0.03	1.00
3	Ethnicity	Integer	0.0000	0.0000	0.0000	0.6926	1.0000	1.00	3.0000	1.24	3.24
4	Education level	Integer	0.000	1.000	1.000	1.337	2.000	0.89	3.000	0.16	2.26
5	BMI	Numeric	15.01	20.78	27.18	27.21	33.46	7.21	40.00	0.04	1.78
6	Smoking	Integer	0.0000	0.0000	0.0000	0.2964	1.0000	0.46	1.00000	0.89	1.79
7	Alcohol consumption	Numeric	0.002228	5.150287	10.070337	10.004134	14.829565	5.69	19.988866	−0.02	1.82
8	Physical activity	Numeric	0.004157	2.455703	5.031550	5.016674	7.512795	2.89	9.995255	0.03	1.77
9	Diet quality	Numeric	0.00001	2.47850	4.82519	4.91290	7.3819	2.87	9.99586	0.03	1.82
10	Sleep quality	Numeric	4.000	5.489	6.930	6.997	8.559	1.75	10.000	0.01	1.77
11	Family History of Parkinson's	Integer	0.0000	0.0000	0.0000	0.1458	0.0000	0.35	1.0000	2.01	5.03
12	Traumatic brain injury	Integer	0.0000	0.0000	0.0000	0.1064	0.0000	0.31	1.0000	2.55	7.52
13	Diabetes	Integer	0.0000	0.0000	0.0000	0.1482	0.0000	0.35	1.0000	2.01	5.03
14	Depression	Integer	0.0000	0.0000	0.0000	0.2052	0.0000	0.36	1.0000	1.98	4.93
15	Stroke	Integer	0.0000	0.0000	0.0000	0.04893	0.0000	0.40	1.0000	1.46	3.13
16	Hypertension	Integer	0.0000	0.0000	0.0000	0.1458	0.0000	0.22	1.0000	4.18	15.49
17	Systolic BP	Integer	90.0	110.0	133.0	133.7	157.0	26.50	179.0	0.03	1.76
18	Diastolic BP	Integer	60.00	75.00	91.00	90.25	105.00	17.06	119.00	−0.06	1.83

Table 10.2 *Continued.*

Sl. No.	Variables	Variable types	Minimum	Q1	Median	Mean	Q3	Standard deviation	Maximum	Skewness	Kurtosis
19	Cholesterol total	Numeric	150.1	189.4	228.5	226.9	264.6	43.59	300.0	−0.05	1.80
20	Cholesterol LDL	Numeric	50.02	88.84	126.88	126.15	163.91	43.41	199.99	−0.02	1.80
21	Cholesterol HDL	Numeric	20.03	39.54	59.34	59.67	79.37	23.37	99.98	0.00	1.82
22	Cholesterol triglycerides	Numeric	50.11	132.52	222.80	222.94	311.70	101.89	399.98	0.02	1.79
23	UPDRS	Numeric	0.02844	53.04815	102.56102	101.41532	149.83168	56.59	198.95360	−0.05	1.84
24	MOCA	Numeric	0.02119	7.51716	14.96357	15.09431	22.60836	8.64	29.97011	−0.02	1.78
25	Functional assessment	Numeric	0.001505	2.415890	4.983227	4.989694	7.484220	2.94	9.992697	0.01	1.79
26	Tremor	Integer	0.0000	0.0000	0.0000	0.4318	1.0000	0.49	1.0000	0.28	1.08
27	Rigidity	Integer	0.0000	0.0000	0.0000	0.2527	1.0000	0.43	1.0000	1.14	2.29
28	Bradykinesia	Integer	0.0000	0.0000	0.0000	0.2076	0.0000	0.41	1.0000	1.44	3.07
29	Postural instability	Integer	0.0000	0.0000	0.0000	0.1387	0.0000	0.35	1.0000	2.09	5.37
30	Speech problem	Integer	0.0000	0.0000	0.0000	0.295	1.000	0.46	1.000	0.89	1.81
31	Sleep disorders	Integer	0.0000	0.0000	0.0000	0.2451	0.0000	0.43	1.0000	1.18	2.40
32	Constipation	Integer	0.0000	0.0000	0.0000	0.2969	1.0000	0.46	1.0000	0.89	1.79
33	Diagnosis	Integer	0.0000	0.0000	1.0000	0.6195	1.0000	0.49	1.0000	−0.49	1.24

the interpretability of decision trees with the capabilities of deep learning, TabNet can efficiently manage complex data sets. TabNet's capability to offer insights into feature importance further enhances the interpretability of classification results, making it an important tool for medical data analysis and decision-making. We have employed various machine learning models like decision tree, ANN, DNN, hybrid decision tree and ANN (DTANN), decision tree and DNN (DTDNN), boosting algorithm based, and TabNet. The suggested TabNet models outperform all the studied models.

10.4.1 Decision tree analysis

Decision trees are widely used tools for classification and prediction tasks. They function by recursively dividing the instance space or variable set. A decision tree is represented as a tree structure, consisting of nodes categorized as either decision nodes or leaf nodes. The leaf nodes indicate the value of the target attributes, while decision nodes specify rules based on attribute values. Each decision node divides the instance space into multiple subspaces based on a discrete function of the input attributes' values. For numeric attributes, this condition often involves a range. After applying the rule at a decision node, the resulting subtree represents one possible outcome. Leaf nodes then generate a probability vector that indicates the likelihood of the target attribute taking on various values. To classify instances, one navigates from the tree's root to a leaf, following the decisions made at each node along the path. A major advantage of decision tree algorithms is that their flowchart-like structure is often presented in a human-readable format after the model is built. This transparency offers valuable insights into the model's functioning and helps explain why it performs well or poorly for a given task.

10.4.2 Artificial neural network

One of the well-known supervised ML approaches for complex nonlinear time series forecasting is the "artificial neural network" (ANN). Neural nets, which are based on straightforward mathematical models of the brain, are utilized for complex nonlinear predictions. The architecture of any neural network may be envisioned as a network of the "neurons" organized into different layers, including input, hidden, and output layers, [33] using the weights that are chosen with a "learning algorithm" based on the risk minimization, where information is passed from the one layer to another layer.

10.4.3 Deep neural network

"Deep neural networks" (DNNs) are a special type of ANN characterized by having a multiple number of hidden layers placed between the input and output layers, allowing them to model with complex patterns in data sets. They excel at handling large volumes of data. By leveraging multiple hidden layers, DNNs can master data that is represented hierarchically, from low-level features to higher-level abstractions. This deep architecture allows them to capture complex relationships and subtleties within the data.

10.4.4 Boosting algorithm-based machine learning models

Generally, disease classification data sets are imbalanced. A few individuals only are found positive for the disease while most people are found negative for the tests. Hence there is generally a smaller proportion of positive labels. However, the data sets in this study are slightly imbalanced. The Alzheimer's data set has 35.4% of data points with positive labels and 64.6% of data points with nonpositive labels. Parkinson's data set has 38.1% of data points with positive labels and 61.9% of data points with nonpositive labels. Boosting techniques are known to perform well on imbalanced data sets as they aim to enhance the performance of the ML models on data points that are generally misclassified. In imbalanced data sets such as disease classification, the positive labels are generally misclassified especially as false negatives which can be detrimental to a person's health. Hence, boosting can help to improve the classification of positive labels.

10.4.5 TabNet deep learning model

TabNet is a state-of-the-art machine learning approach designed for data in tabular form, offering notable improvements in interpretability and performance over traditional methods. Developed by Google Cloud AI researchers, TabNet leverages a novel architecture that combines decision trees and deep learning to handle complex data structures efficiently. Unlike standard neural networks that rely on dense layers, TabNet employs attention mechanisms and decision steps to concentrate on the most relevant features, enhancing its ability to learn effective representations of the data.

The core mechanism of TabNet involves a series of decision trees combined with a DL approach that learns to interpret the output of these trees. The model utilizes a "sparse attention" mechanism where only a subset of features is considered at each decision step, which helps in reducing computational complexity and enhancing interpretability. This attention mechanism is crucial as it allows TabNet to prioritize important features while disregarding less relevant ones. The sparse attention also improves the model's capability to handle high-dimensional data efficiently.

In the context of binary classification tasks, like identifying AD and PD, TabNet offers significant advantages. Both these two diseases have complex along with subtle differences in clinical and biomarker data. TabNet's ability to focus on the most relevant features for each classification decision can be particularly beneficial for distinguishing between these two conditions, as it allows learning the model with the nuanced patterns that differentiate them. This can lead to enhanced accuracy in predictions when compared with the traditional models.

Furthermore, TabNet's interpretability features are beneficial in the medical domain, where understanding the reasoning behind predictions is crucial. By providing insights into which features are most influential for the classification decision, TabNet can help clinicians understand the model's predictions and make more informed decisions about patient diagnosis and treatment. This transparency can also assist in validating the model's performance and ensuring that it aligns with clinical knowledge.

TabNet is built upon a novel combination of decision trees and neural networks, integrating attention mechanisms to efficiently handle tabular data. The core components of TabNet's architecture include:

- Feature transformer: this module utilizes a sequence of fully connected layers to convert the input key features into a space with high-dimension. It effectively preprocesses data, enabling the model to make interactions among features and to capture complex patterns.
- Decision steps: TabNet employs a sequence of decision steps where each step consists of a decision tree followed by a deep learning network. The decision trees guide the model by selecting the most prominent features, while the neural network refines the representation of these features.
- Sparse attention mechanism: at each decision step, TabNet uses a sparse attention mechanism to find the most relevant features. This mechanism allows the model to assign different levels of importance to features, making it more efficient in learning and reducing computational overhead.
- Feature selection and aggregation: the output of decision steps is combined and aggregated to produce the final prediction. This process

involves weighting and summing the contributions of different features based on their relevance determined during the decision steps.

We have trained TabNet for 100 epochs using adam optimizer and used 10-fold cross-validation while training.

10.5 Experimental Evaluation and Results of Neurodegenerative Disorders

Identifying the characteristics and features of the health care data sets is a challenging task. The current study concentrates on diagnosing two neurodegenerative disorder diseases namely AD and PD using DT, ANN, DNN, ML-based boosting algorithm, and TabNet models. The models of TabNet deep learning models outperformed in comparison to other related models for the prediction and classification of these two neurodegenerative diseases. It is best to notify scientific experts and government or public policymakers to manage and control neurodegenerative diseases. Table 10.1 and Table 10.2 show descriptions of different predictors of the diagnosis of these two diseases.

10.5.1 Decision tree analysis

"Decision tree" (DT) models are influential classifiers that use a tree data structure to represent the relationships among potential outcomes and key features. When the final choice can be reached, the tree is concluded with leaf nodes (or terminal nodes) that indicate the action to be taken based on the sequence of decisions. For predictive models, these leaf nodes offer the anticipated outcome given the series of events processed through the tree.

10.5.1.1 Decision tree analysis for diagnosing AD

The decision to use a decision tree model for identifying significant input variables from 32 variables namely "age," "gender," "ethnicity," "educational level," "BMI," "smoking," "alcohol consumption," "physical activity," "diet quality," "sleep quality," "family history of Alzheimer's," "cardiovascular disease," "diabetes," "depression," "head injury," "hypertension," "systolic BP," "diastolic BP," "cholesterol total," "cholesterol LDL," "cholesterol HDL," "cholesterol triglycerides," "MMSE," "functional assessment," "memory complaints," "behavioral problems," "ADL," "confusion," "disorientation," "personality changes," "difficulty completing tasks," and "forgetfulness" for diagnosing AD stems from the model's simplicity, ease of interpretability, and high accuracy. We applied an optimal decision tree model to a data set comprising 2149 patient data points to identify potential causal variables associated with AD prediction. The DT was applied using the "rpart" package in R software, with a control parameter "minsplit" set to 10% of the total data. We evaluated the model's predictive performance evaluation using RMSE. The optimal DT, built with five input variables and a "minsplit" of five was created with the same costs for each variable. Figure 10.1 presents the fitted tree and Figure 10.2 shows the variable importance list. From the decision tree analysis, it is concluded that 5 out of the 32 potential input variables were found to be highly significant. But captivatingly, we captured five essential causal variables like functional assessment, memory complaints, behavioral problems, ADL, and MMSE can be managed to diagnose patients with AD.

By using the "rpart" package, we can evaluate the range of cost complexities. For comparing the errors for each of the cost complexity values, rpart performs cross-validation with 10-fold by computing the errors on the validation data. Figure 10.1 displays the optimal decision tree, which has 12 internal and 13 terminal nodes, respectively, and partitions the data based on five variables to develop its model. This tree can be expanded to a full tree with 13 terminal nodes by setting CP = 0 as shown in Figure 10.1. In Figure 10.3, the y-axis represents cross-validation error, the upper x-axis indicates the number of terminal nodes and the lower x-axis displays

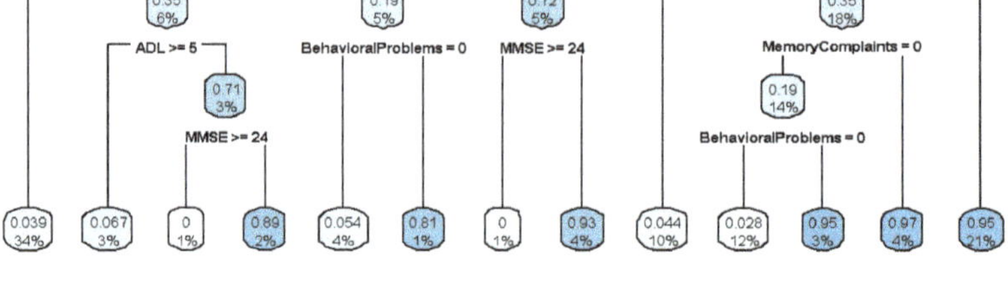

Figure 10.1 Decision tree for classification of AD.

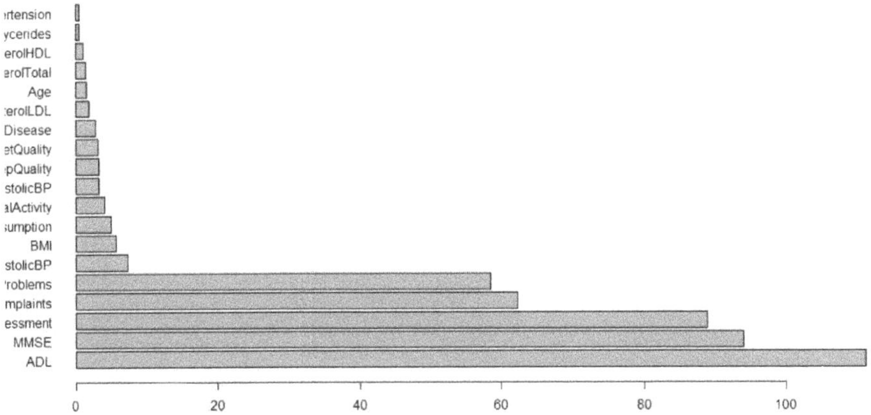

Figure 10.2 Variable importance for classification of AD.

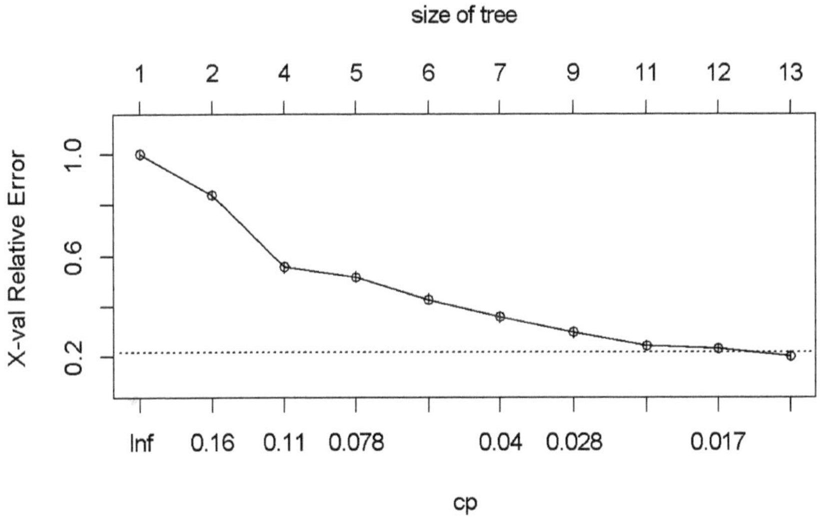

Figure 10.3 Complex parameter for classification of AD.

cost complexity values. Beyond 13 terminal nodes, the reduction in error becomes less significant as the tree grows deeper. For predicting AD, the decision tree identified 5 key variables out of the 32 variables: functional assessment, memory complaints, behavioral problems, ADL, and MMSE.

All 2149 patients' data points across 32 variables are processed through the decision tree as illustrated in Figure 10.1, where each data point is evaluated at a node, proceeding left for a "Yes" answer and right for a "No" answer.

First, 2149 data points of diagnosis of AD in comparison to all data points of 32 variables where functional assessment is greater than or equal to 5 go to the left branch, all other data points of diagnosing AD patients proceed to the right branch. The chance of being diagnosed as AD or no AD among patients having functional assessment (FA) ≥ 5 and less than 5 are presented. How the presence or absence of variables like memory complaints and behavioral problems, and different scores of ADL and MMSE influence the diagnosis of AD are described. At the outset, the chance of not being diagnosed as AD among all the patients having functional assessment ≥ 5 with the following variations in the other three or four variables are narrated. When such patients have no memory complaints and behavioral problems but with ADL greater than 5, then the chance of not being diagnosed as AD becomes 3%. Patients with no memory complaints, ADL less than 5, and behavioral problems will have a 4% chance of being diagnosed with no AD. When patients have the same variable but have no behavioral problems, then their chance of being diagnosed with AD is 1%. Patients with the same three variables but with MSME less than 24 will have a 1% chance of being diagnosed with no AD. However, the chance of these patients being diagnosed with AD is 2% when their ADL and MMSE are less than 5 and 24, respectively. For patients having FA ≥ 5, no memory complaints, ADL ≥ 5, and MMSE less than 24%, the chance to be diagnosed with no AD disease becomes 1%. When MMSE becomes greater than or equal to 24 in patients with the above-mentioned criteria, their chance of being diagnosed with AD is 4%. All the patients having memory complaints, behavioral problems, and ADL ≥ 5 will have a 1% chance of becoming diagnosed with AD. All the patients with memory complaints and with ADL less than 5 and MMSE less than 24, their chance of being diagnosed with AD is 4%. In the case of patients having functional, all the patients of functional assessment less than 5 have MMSE less than 24, ADL greater than or equal to 5.1, having no memory complaints and no behavioral problems is 12% chance to be diagnosed with no AD. All the patients with functional assessment less than 5 have MMSE less than 24, ADL greater than or equal to 5.1, have no memory complaints and behavioral problems is a 3% chance to be diagnosed with AD. When these patients have MMSE less than 24, ADL $\geq$ 5.1, and memory complaints, their chance of being diagnosed with AD is 4%. When all the variables remain the same as stated above, only ADL becomes less than 5.1, and the chance of a diagnosis of AD is 21%. Continuing the splitting process, evaluating all the variables with each split, until the data points of AD are divided into 13 partitions. The predicted diagnosis of AD in the patients is (0, 0, 0, 1, 0, 1, 0, 1, 0, 0, 1, 1, 1), based solely on five variables. The RMSE result of this tree model for evaluating predictive performance is 0.2055216.

10.5.1.2 Decision tree analysis for diagnosing PD

The decision to use a decision tree model for identifying significant input variables from 32 variables namely "age," "gender," "ethnicity," "educational level," "BMI," "smoking," "alcohol consumption," "physical activity," "diet quality," "sleep quality," "family history of Parkinson's," "traumatic brain injury," "hypertension," "diabetes," "depression," "stroke," "systolic BP," "diastolic BP," "cholesterol total," "cholesterol LDL," "cholesterol HDL," "cholesterol triglycerides," "UPDRS," "MoCA," "functional assessment," "tremor," "rigidity," "Bradykinesia," "postural instability," "speech problems," "sleep disorders," "constipation" for diagnosing PD stems from the model's simplicity, ease of interpretability, and high accuracy. We applied an optimal decision tree model to a data set comprising 2105 patient data points to identify potential causal variables related to PD prediction. The decision tree was applied using the "rpart" package in R software, with a control parameter "minsplit" set to 10% of the total data. We evaluated the model's predictive performance evaluation using RMSE. The optimal decision tree, built with eight input variables and a "minsplit" of five was created with the same costs for each variable. Figure 10.4 presents the fitted tree and Figure 10.5 shows the variable importance list. From the decision tree analysis, it is concluded that 8 out of the 32 potential input variables were found to be highly significant. But captivatingly, we captured seven essential causal variables like UPDRS, postural instability, tremor, functional assessment, Bradykinesia, rigidity, and MoCA, which can be managed to diagnose patients with PD.

By utilizing the "rpart" package, we can evaluate the range of cost complexities. For comparing the errors for each of the cost complexity values, rpart performs cross-validation with 10-fold by computing the errors on the validation data. Figure 10.4 displays the optimal decision tree, which has 10 internal and 11 terminal nodes, respectively, and partitions the data based on seven variables to develop its model. This tree can be expanded to a full tree with 11 terminal nodes by setting $CP = 0$ as shown in Figure 10.4. In Figure 10.6, the y-axis represents cross-validation error, the upper x-axis indicates the number of terminal nodes and the lower x-axis displays cost.

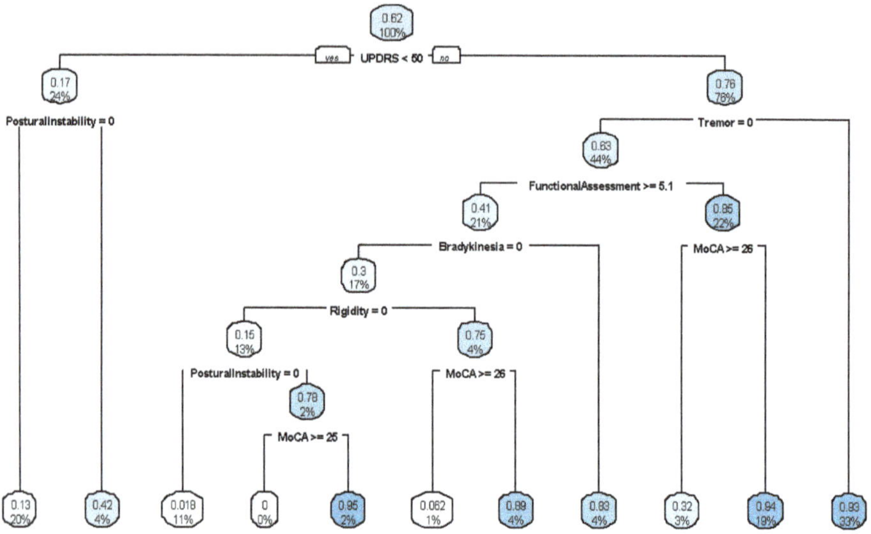

Figure 10.4 Decision tree for classification of PD.

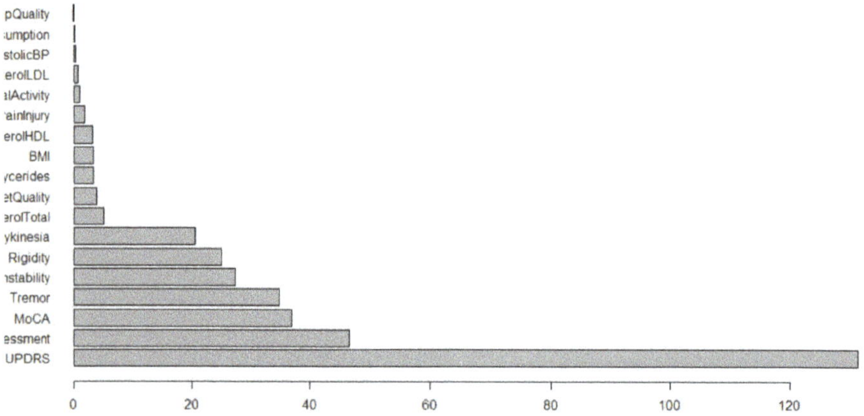

Figure 10.5 Variable importance for classification of PD.

Beyond 11 terminal nodes, the reduction in error becomes less significant as the tree grows deeper. For predicting the PD, the decision tree identified seven key variables out of the 32 variables: UPDRS, postural instability, tremor, functional assessment, Bradykinesia, rigidity, and MoCA. All 2105 patient data points across 32 variables are processed through the decision tree depicted as depicted in Figure 10.4, where each data point is evaluated at a node, moving left for a "Yes" answer and right for a "No" answer. First, 2105 data points of diagnosis of PD as compared to all data points of 32 variables where UPDRS is less than 50 go to the left branch, all other data points of diagnosing PD of the patients proceed to the right branch. Hence, patients with UPDRS less than 50 and no postural instability have a 20% chance of being diagnosed without PD, and in the presence of postural instability, the chance goes down to 4%. For all patients with UPDRS $\geq$ 50, FA$\geq$ 5.1 not showing any tremor, Bradykinesia, rigidity, and postural instability, the chance of being diagnosed without PD is 11%. The chance for the same becomes 0% for those patients having the above criteria but with MoCA $\geq$ 25 and postural instability. When MoCA is less than 25 among these patients, the zero chance of being diagnosed with PD increases to 2%. When patients with the same UPDRS and FA, no tremor, and Bradykinesia have MoCA greater than or equal to 26, and present signs of rigidity, their chance of being diagnosed with no PD is 1%. When MoCA is less than 26 in these patients with other parameters remaining the same, their chance of being diagnosed with PD becomes 4%. All patients with UPDRS $\geq$ 50, FA$\geq$ 5.1, and absence of tremor have Bradykinesia, their chance of being diagnosed as PD is 4%. For all the patients with UPDRS $\geq$ 50, FA $\geq$ 5.1, not showing any tremor, and MoCA $\geq$ 26, there is a 3% chance of being diagnosed without PD. MoCA less than 26 in these patients' chance to be diagnosed with PD becomes 19%. All patients of UPDRS $\geq$ 50 showing signs of tremor, there is a 33% chance to be diagnosed with PD.

With the continuing splitting process, evaluating all the variables with each split, until the data points of PD are divided into 11 partitions. The predicted diagnosis of PD in the patients is (0, 0, 0, 0, 1, 0, 1, 1, 0, 1, 1), based solely on seven variables. The RMSE result of this tree model for evaluating predictive performance is 0.2895523.

10.5.2 Neural networks and boosting algorithm-based machine learning models for diagnosing AD and PD

Analysis is conducted to diagnose two neurodegenerative disorders of the patients. In the first ANN model, 32 input variables are fed into a three-layered feed-forward neural network having 16 hidden neurons and one output neuron. Similarly, the second ANN model uses 32 input variables in a four-layered feed-forward neural network; it includes two hidden layers with 16 and 8 hidden neurons, respectively, and with one output neuron. The

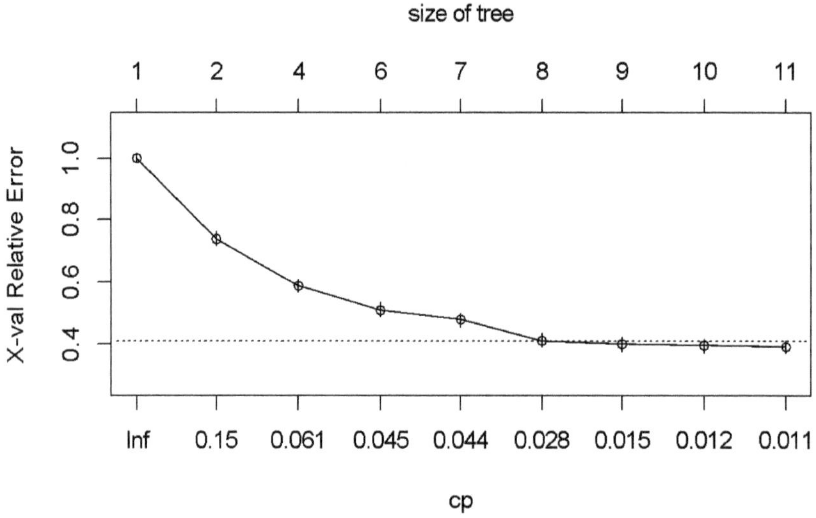

Figure 10.6 Complex parameter for classification of PD.

third hybrid decision tree and ANN (DTANN) model uses DT and five input variables in a three-layer feed-forward neural network, it includes one hidden layer with four neurons for diagnosing AD, and similarly, the hybrid decision tree and ANN (DTANN) model uses DT and seven input variables in a three-layered feed-forward neural network, includes one hidden layer with four neurons for diagnosing PD. Five different DNNs, hybrid decision tree and DNN (DTDNN) models, boosting algorithm-based ML models, and TabNet DL model are also developed to diagnose these two diseases.

10.5.2.1 ANN models for diagnosing AD and PD

ANN disease prediction models can diagnose the AD and PD of the patients. The entire data set is split into 70% and 30% to train and test the models, respectively. Two ANN models are developed: one with a single hidden layer of 16 neurons and another with two hidden layers of 16 and 8 hidden neurons, respectively. Figures 10.7, 10.8, 10.9, and 10.10 show the ANN models with single and two hidden layers for diagnosing two neurodegenerative disorders of the patients with respect to the 32 inputs, respectively. Similarly, a hybrid model with a single layer of four layers of the predicted value of the decision tree model and five identified risk factors namely functional assessment, memory complaints, behavioral problems, ADL, and MMSE constituted

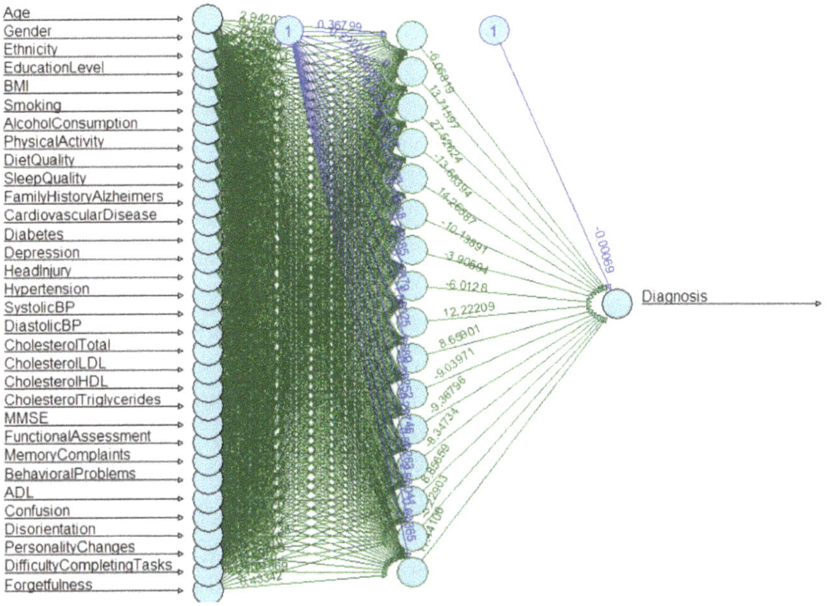

Figure 10.7 ANN with single-hidden layer model to diagnose AD of the patients.

decision tree and ANN (DTANN) prediction models can diagnose the AD and hybrid model with a single layer of four neurons of the predicted value of decision tree model and seven identified risk factors namely UPDRS, postural instability, tremor, functional assessment, Bradykinesia, rigidity, and MoCA constituted decision tree and ANN (DTANN) prediction models can diagnose the PD diseases of the patients, respectively. Table 10.3 shows the accuracy level for both train and test data to diagnose AD and PD of the patients. It is investigated that the fifth DTANN model shows better accuracy results with [0.958028 and 0.9537037] and [0.9585879 and 0.9129747] for train and test data of AD and PD, respectively, to diagnose both the neurodegenerative disorders of the patients. Figures 10.11 and 10.12 DTANN models with single hidden layers for diagnosing AD and PD of the patients respectively.

10.5.3 DNN models for diagnosing AD and PD

Deep neural network (DNN) disease prediction models can diagnose the AD and PD of the patients. We create five instances of the model so one can diagnose both diseases accurately. 70% of the total data set is used for training this model, while the remaining 30% is used for testing it. Activation

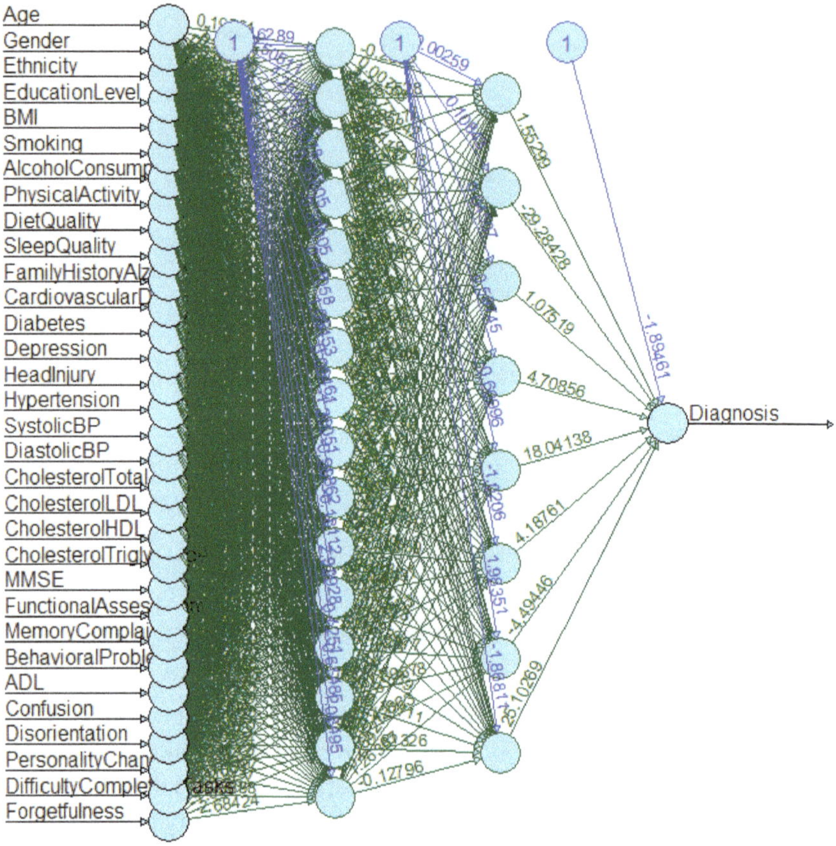

Figure 10.8 ANN with two-hidden layers model to diagnose AD of the patients.

functions namely ReLU and Sigmoid are used for hidden layer and output, respectively. Adam optimizer and binary cross entropy loss are applied as the matrix to train this hybrid model. The architecture of the five different DNN models are with [16, 2], [16, 8, 2], [32, 2], [50, 2], and [100-0.4, 50-0.3, 20-0.1, 2] hidden layers and output, respectively, with respect to 32 inputs. Table 10.3 shows the accuracy level for both train and test data to diagnose AD and PD of the patients. It is investigated that the fifth DNN model shows better accuracy results with [0.9474026 and 0.0.8505747] and [0.9548473 and 0.8297162] for train and test data of AD and PD, respectively, to diagnose both the neurodegenerative disorders of the patients. Similarly, the hybrid model of the predicted value of the decision tree model and five identified risk factors namely functional assessment, memory complaints, behavioral

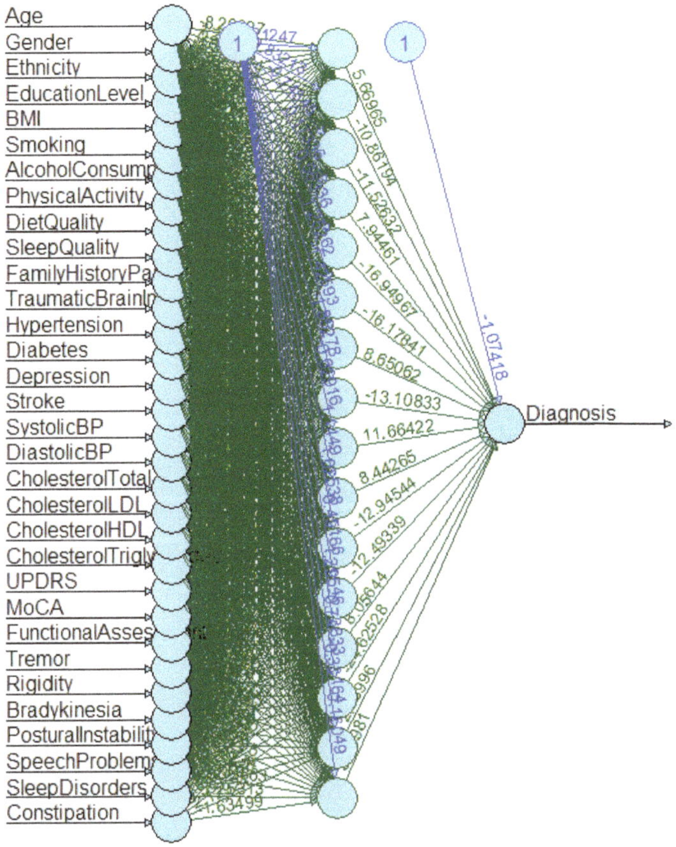

Figure 10.9 ANN with single-hidden layer model to diagnose PD of the patients.

problems, ADL, and MMSE constituted decision tree and DNN (DTDNN) prediction models can diagnose the AD and hybrid model of predicted value of decision tree model and seven identified risk factors namely UPDRS, postural instability, tremor, functional assessment, Bradykinesia, rigidity, and MoCA constituted decision tree and DNN (DTDNN) prediction models can diagnose the PD diseases of the patients, respectively. 70% of the total data set is used for training this model, while the remaining 30% is used for testing it. Activation functions namely ReLU and Sigmoid are used for hidden layer and output, respectively. Adam optimizer and binary cross entropy loss are applied as the matrix to train this hybrid model. The architecture of the five different DTDNN models are with [16, 2], [16, 8, 2], [32, 2], [50, 2], and [100-0.4, 50-0.3, 20-0.1, 2] hidden layers and output, respectively. Table 10.3

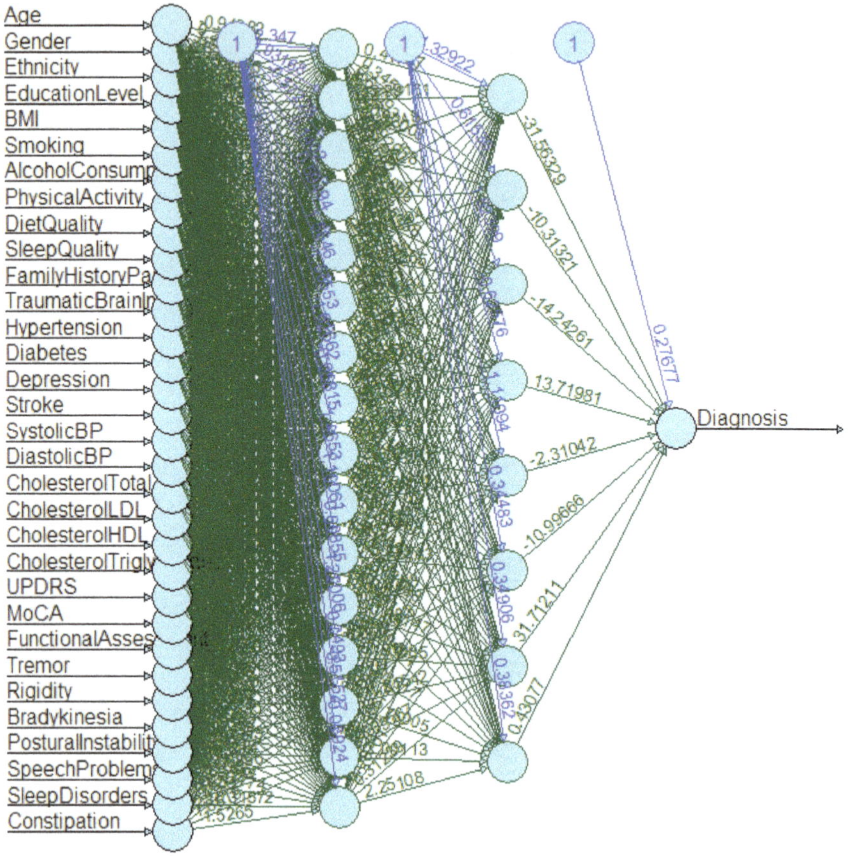

Figure 10.10 ANN with two-hidden layers model to diagnose PD of the patients.

shows the accuracy level for both train and test data to diagnose AD and PD of the patients. It is investigated that the fifth DTDNN model shows better accuracy results with [0.9571428 and 0.9589490] and [0.9482072 and 0.9415693] for train and test data of AD and PD, respectively, to diagnose both the neurodegenerative disorders of the patients.

10.5.4 Boosting algorithm-based machine learning models for diagnosing AD and PD

Generally, disease classification data sets are imbalanced. A few individuals only are found positive for the disease while most people are found negative for the tests. Hence, there is generally a smaller proportion of positive labels.

Table 10.3 Performance measure of different models for diagnosing AD and PD of the patients.

Model	Neurons in hidden layers	Diseases	Predictors	Accuracy	
				Training	**Testing**
ANN	16	Alzemier's	32	0.9791807	0.7696970
		Parkinson's	32	0.9871012	0.8053797
ANN	16-8	Alzemier's	32	0.9720187	0.7993827
		Parkinson's	32	0.9830278	0.7974684
DTANN	4	Alzemier's	6	0.958028	0.9537037
		Parkinson's	8	0.9585879	0.9129747
DNN	16-2/200-32-0.2	Alzemier's	32	0.9461039	0.8160920
		Parkinson's	32	0.9541833	0.803005
DNN	16-8-2/200-32-0.2	Alzemier's	32	0.9493507	0.8111659
		Parkinson's	32	0.9515272	0.8080134
DNN	32-2/200-32-0.2	Alzemier's	32	0.9487013	0.8325123
		Parkinson's	32	0.9541833	0.8063439
DNN	50-2/200-32-0.2	Alzemier's	32	0.9480519	0.8259442
		Parkinson's	32	0.9521912	0.8130217
DNN	100-0.4, 50-0.3, 20-0.1, 2/200-32-0.2	Alzemier's	32	0.9474026	0.8505747
		Parkinson's	32	0.9548473	0.8297162
DTDNN	16/2-200/32/0.2	Alzemier's	6	0.9538961	0.952381
		Parkinson's	8	0.9316069	0.9365609
DTDNN	16-8-2/200/32/0.2	Alzemier's	6	0.9558442	0.9556651
		Parkinson's	8	0.9395750	0.9398999
DTDNN	32-2/200/32/0.2	Alzemier's	6	0.9551948	0.9540230
		Parkinson's	8	0.9395750	0.9449082
DTDNN	50-2/200-32-0.2	Alzemier's	6	0.9545454	0.9573070
		Parkinson's	8	0.9409031	0.9465776
DTDNN	100-0.4, 50-0.3, 20-0.1, 2/200-32-0.2	Alzemier's	6	0.9571428	0.9589490
		Parkinson's	8	0.9482072	0.9415693
Cat Boost	–	Alzemier's	32	–	0.94
	–	Parkinson's	32	–	0.94
Ada Boost	–	Alzemier's	32	–	0.91
		Parkinson's	32	–	0.92
Random Forest	–	Alzemier's	32	–	0.91
		Parkinson's	32	–	0.91
Gradient Boost	–	Alzemier's	32	–	0.94
		Parkinson's	32	–	0.91
MLP Classifier	–	Alzemier's	32	–	0.81
		Parkinson's	32	–	0.83
TabNet Deep Learning	–	Alzemier's	32	**99.7**	**0.996**
		Parkinson's	32	**99.7**	**0.997**

However, the data sets in this study are slightly imbalanced. The Alzheimer's data set has 35.4% of data points with positive labels and 64.6% of data points with nonpositive labels. Parkinson's data set has 38.1% of data points with positive labels and 61.9% of data points with nonpositive labels. Boosting techniques are known to perform well on imbalanced data sets as they aim to enhance the model's performance on data points that are generally misclassified. In imbalanced data sets such as disease classification, the positive labels are generally misclassified, especially as false negatives, which can be detrimental to a person's health. Hence, boosting can help improve the classification of positive labels.

We experiment with a variety of boosting algorithms and a neural multilayer perceptron (MLP) that performs binary classification. For each of the methods, the best hyperparameter is chosen by a grid search across potential values. Random forest (RF) creates a forest of decision trees that each provides a single prediction on the input. An RF is generated from a random subset of the training data set for each tree. It is designed to prevent overfitting of the decision tree method on the training data by introducing randomness. The number of trees generated for both the Alzheimer's and Parkinson's data set is 250.

The boosting technique improves the prediction by creating an ensemble of weak learners. At each step, the technique creates a random sample of the training data set and trains a model of the given algorithm. Each subsequent model is trained by improving upon the weakness of the previous model. This training of the weak learners is done sequentially and their ensemble is used for final prediction. AdaBoost algorithm extends the binary classification into a multiclass by using an additive model in a forward stage-wise fashion, optimizing over an exponential loss function for multiclass usage. The ensemble of weak learners in AdaBoost is done by giving the highest weightage to the learner with high accuracy. The AdaBoost technique selectively picks those training samples where the previous model does misclassification, by increasing the weight of picking the samples. The best hyperparameters for AdaBoost are 0.1 for the learning rate and 200 estimators for both data sets. In contrast, the GradientBoost model trains each subsequent learner using residual errors of the predecessor. It uses a regression tree by considering the previous residual errors as the output. This process fits weak learners to the negative gradient of the loss function. The best learning rate was 0.1 for both data sets while the estimators were 100 for Parkinson's and 200 for Alzheimer's data set.

A multilayer perceptron (MLP) model was also used with three hidden layer sizes of sizes 200, 200, and 100 for each layer for both data sets. This was the best-hidden layer configuration that was found through grid search.

The number of iterations for Alzheimer's was 2000 while for Parkinson's was 1500. The ReLU activation function was used for each neuron with an adaptive learning rate. For each of the models described in this section, they do not handle the categorical feature well. Each feature is considered as a numeric value which will have certain implications such as treating the values as greater than or less than. This does not work well with categorical features where numbers like 1, 2, ..., can represent different categorical types rather than comparative values. Hence, for such discrete features, we perform one-hot encoding that creates separate features with values 0 and 1 indicating if the type is present or not. This new feature can be used as a numeric feature and normalized as required. On the other hand, the model CatBoost, internally converts such categorical features and does not require any explicit conversion. The output class in each model is 0 or 1 indicating the presence of the disease. We do a 70/30 split of the training/test data. The hyperparameters are tuned using the cross-validation approach. Figures 10.13 and 10.14 shows ROC curve for boosting-based algorithm machine learning models to diagnose the AD and PD respectivley where false-positive rate on the x-axis and true-positive rate on the y-axis.

10.5.5 TabNet DL model for diagnosing AD and PD

Disease classification data sets are often imbalanced, with fewer positive cases compared to negative ones, which can lead to challenges in accurate classification. Given the high risk of misclassifying positive cases as false negatives – a critical issue in medical diagnostics handling these imbalances effectively is crucial. TabNet is a DL model specifically intended for tabular data, and provides an effective approach for handling imbalanced data sets. Unlike conventional models, it leverages a unique architecture that allows for improved feature selection and interpretation, making it particularly well-suited for this type of data. TabNet can focus on the most relevant features and adaptively handle various types of data, including imbalanced classes. Its attention-based mechanism allows it to give more importance to difficult cases, which helps in better distinguishing between positive and negative labels.

By leveraging TabNet's ability to learn from imbalances and its sophisticated feature selection process, we can improve classification performance on minority classes, addressing the specific challenges posed by the imbalance in disease classification data sets. This makes TabNet a valuable tool for enhancing accuracy in detecting conditions like Alzheimer's and Parkinson's, where correctly identifying positive cases is crucial.

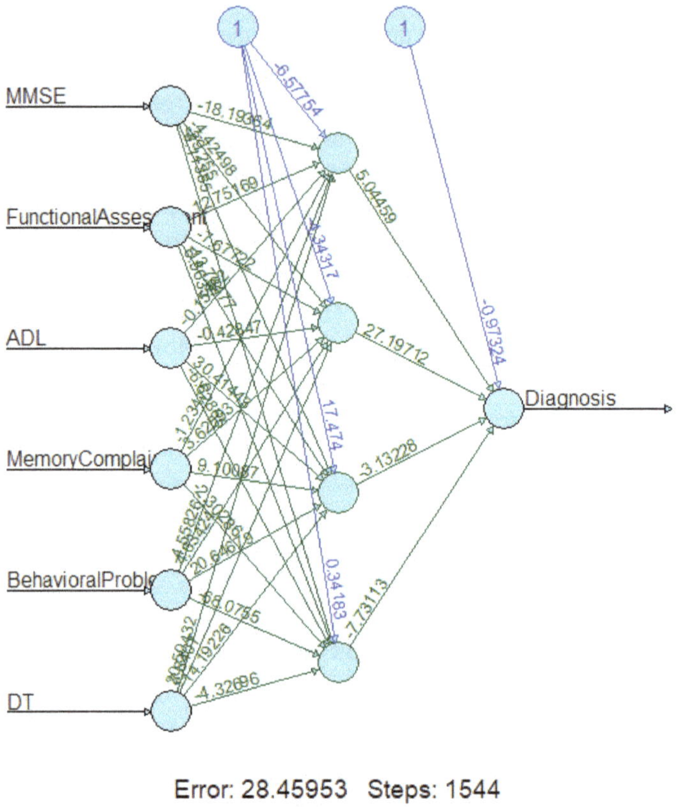

Figure 10.11 DTANN with single-hidden layer model to diagnose AD of the patients.

At the heart of TabNet's architecture are the decision transformer and feature transformer. The feature transformer performs a sequence of transformations with nonlinearity on the input features, allowing the model to capture interactions within the data and complex patterns. The decision transformer, on the other hand, utilizes an attention mechanism to selectively focus on different subsets of features at each decision step, allowing the model to refine its predictions progressively.

The model operates through a series of decision steps, where each step generates a decision mask that determines which features are used in that particular step. This feature masking is essential for minimizing overfitting and directing the model's attention to the most informative aspects of the data. Key hyperparameters that impact TabNet's performance include the number

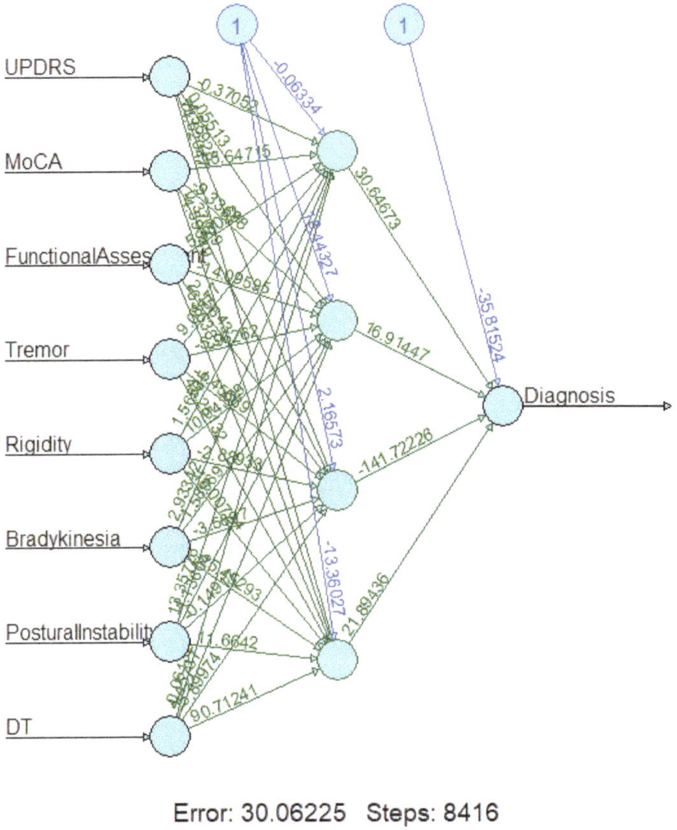

Figure 10.12 DTANN with single-hidden layer model to diagnose PD of the patients.

of decision steps (n_steps) and the dimensions of the decision (n_d) and attention (n_a) steps. Typically, n_d and n_a values are set between 64 and 256, balancing model complexity and computational efficiency. The number of decision steps determines how many iterations of feature refinement the model undergoes, usually ranging from 3 to 10 steps.

TabNet's attention-based mechanism enhances its performance on imbalanced data sets by allowing the model to focus on misclassified examples, which are particularly prevalent in binary classification tasks where one class is rare. This focus is achieved through an adaptive feature selection process that prioritizes challenging cases, enhancing the model's capability to correctly identify the alternative class. Key hyperparameters such as the learning rate, often set between 0.01 and 0.2, and batch size, which can range

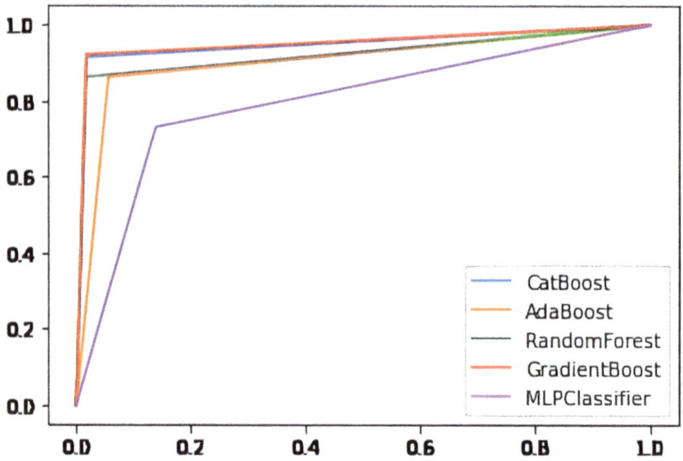

Figure 10.13 ROC curve for boosting-based algorithm machine learning models to diagnose the AD of the patients: false-positive rate on the x-axis and true-positive rate on the y-axis.

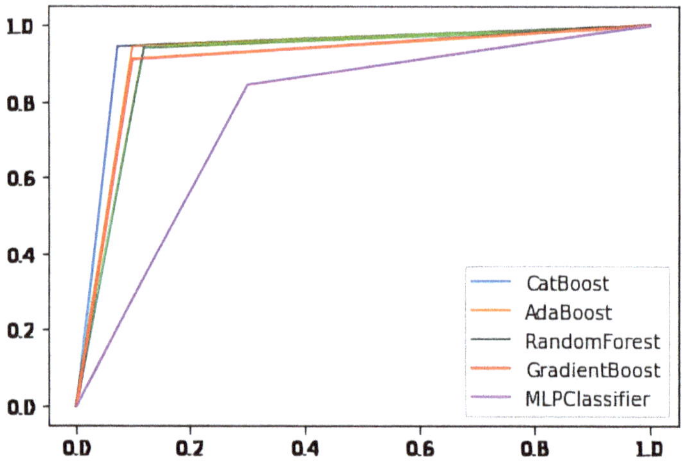

Figure 10.14 ROC curve for boosting-based algorithm machine learning models to diagnose the PD of the Patients: false-positive rate on the x-axis and true-positive rate on the y-axis.

from 32 to 256, are crucial for optimizing the training process. The choice of optimizer, typically Adam or AdamW, and learning rate schedulers like StepLR, further aid in fine-tuning the model's convergence and generalization capabilities.

In practical implementations, TabNet's ability to handle class imbalances and complex feature interactions makes it a valuable tool for binary classification problems, such as distinguishing between diseases in medical data sets. For instance, in a binary classification task with imbalanced classes, TabNet's attention mechanism can effectively prioritize the minority class, leading to improved classification performance. Through hyperparameter tuning and careful configuration of the model's architecture, together with the number of decision steps and the choice of activation functions, TabNet can be optimized to deliver accurate and reliable predictions, making it a powerful alternative to traditional machine learning methods for tabular data.

In our binary classification tasks for distinguishing between Alzheimer's and Parkinson's diseases, TabNet's hyperparameters play a crucial role in optimizing performance. For this application, the model was configured with 64 dimensions for both decision and attention steps (n_d = 64, n_a = 64), and five decision steps (n_steps = 5) to balance intricacy and computational efficiency. A learning rate of 0.02 was chosen to ensure stable convergence, while a batch size of 128 was used to manage memory usage effectively. The model's attention mechanism was configured with the sparsemax mask type to enhance feature selection, and the optimizer used was Adam with a learning rate scheduler, StepLR, then set to reduce the learning rate by a factor of 0.9 every 10 epochs. These settings were selected through grid search to handle class imbalances effectively and improve classification accuracy for the medical data sets. We have trained TabNet for 100 epochs and used 10-fold cross-validation while training.

The outcomes of all models are exhibited in Table 10.3. A TabNet deep learning model for two diseases shows higher values of accuracy both for training and testing than other models like ANNs, DNNs, DTANN, DTDNN, and boosting algorithm-based machine learning models.

10.6 Conclusion

This study presents our experimentation with different boosting algorithms that we use to classify AD and PD. Among the different models of boosting-based algorithm of machine learning models, we find CatBoost to perform more accurate predictions, especially with positive labels. It achieved 94% overall accuracy on both data sets while having a positive label f1-score of 0.92 and 0.94 on AD and PD data sets, respectively. It has around 0.01–0.03 difference in positive label f1-score in contrast to the second-best performing models. This might be due to their ability to handle categorical features.

Multilayer perceptrons were the worst-performing models in both cases with accuracy of 0.81 and 0.83. Albeit, experimenting with hidden layers with large numbers and hidden layer neurons. The TabNet deep learning-based prediction and classification for diagnosing the two neurodegenerative diseases offers a promising approach to the patients. The system enhances prediction accuracy and operational efficiency. We use more than 2000 patients' worth of data using a random split of 70/30 for train/test using RMSE for performance in the DT model. From the decision tree analysis, it is concluded that 5 out of the 32 potential input variables were found to be highly significant. But captivatingly, we captured five essential causal variables like functional assessment, memory complaints, behavioral problems, ADL, and MMSE which may be applied to diagnose patients with AD. From the decision tree analysis, it is concluded that 8 out of the 32 potential input variables were found to be highly significant. But captivatingly, we captured seven essential causal variables like UPDRS, postural instability, tremor, functional assessment, Bradykinesia, rigidity, and MoCA, which may be applied to diagnose patients with PD. The efficiency of diagnosis of the two diseases is tested by decision tree, ANN having hidden layer of one, ANN with two layers hidden, hybrid ANN, five different DNN, boosted algorithm-based machine learning, and TabNet deep learning models. TabNet deep learning model has shown the finest results for the two diseases diagnosing with accuracy 0.997 and 0.996 and 0.997 and 0.997 with train and test data set, respectively, which outperforms other models. Results showed improved accuracy in the prediction and classification of the diagnosis of two diseases compared to all other models. The strategic diagnosis of neurodegenerative diseases ensured that the model received comprehensive data, enhancing its predictive capabilities. Challenges included managing communication overhead and ensuring consistent model updates. Adaptive algorithms and regular system checks addressed limitations such as data variability for feature identification.

References

[1] A. Caliskan, H. Badem, A. Baştürk, and E. M. Yuksel. "Diagnosis of the Parkinson Disease by Using Deep Neural Network Classifier". *In IU-JEEE*, vol. 17, no. 2, 2017.

[2] A. Dadu, V. Satone, R. Kaur, S. H. Hashemi, H. Leonard, H. Iwaki, M. B. Makarious, K. J. Billingsley, S. B. Ciga, L. J. Sargent, A. J. Noyce, A. Daneshmand, C. Blauwendraat, K. Marek, S. W. Scholz, A. B. Singleton, M. A. Nalls, H. C. Roy, and F. Faghri ,"Identification

and prediction of Parkinson's disease subtypes and progression using machine learning in two cohorts," *npj Parkinson's Disease*, vol. 8, no. 1, Dec. 2022, doi: https://doi.org/10.1038/s41531-022-00439-z.

[3] A. Samad and E. Samet Aydı, "Rapid Alzheimer's Disease Diagnosis Using Advanced Artificial Intelligence Algorithms," *International Journal of Innovative Science and Research Technology (IJISRT)*, vol. 9, no. DOI: 10.38124/ijisrt/IJISRT24JUN1915, pp. 1760–1768, Jul. 2024, doi: https://doi.org/10.38124/ijisrt/ijisrt24jun1915.

[4] B. Dubois, H. H. Feldman, C. Jacova, H. Hampel, J. L. Molinuevo and K. Blennow, "Advancing research diagnostic criteria for Alzheimer's disease: the IWG-2 criteria". *Lancet Neurol.* vol. 13, no. 6, pp. 614–29, 2014.

[5] C. Kavitha, V. Mani, S. R. Srividhya, O. I. Khalaf, and C. A. Tavera Romero, "Early-Stage Alzheimer's Disease Prediction Using Machine Learning Models," *Frontiers in Public Health*, vol. 10, no. 853294, Mar. 2022, doi: https://doi.org/10.3389/fpubh.2022.853294.

[6] C. Sudlow, J. Gallacher, N. Allen, V. Beral, P. Burton, J. Danesh, P. Downey, P. Elliott, J. Green, M. Landray, B. Liu, P. Matthews, G. Ong, J. Pell, A. Silman, A. Young, T. Sprosen, T. Peakman and R. Collin, "UK Biobank: An Open Access Resource for Identifying the Causes of a Wide Range of Complex Diseases of Middle and Old Age," *PLOS Medicine*, vol. 12, no. 3, p. e1001779, Mar. 2015, doi: https://doi.org/10.1371/journal.pmed.1001779.

[7] F. J. Martinez-Murcia, A. Ortiz, J.-M. Gorriz, J. Ramirez, and D. Castillo-Barnes, "Studying the Manifold Structure of Alzheimer's Disease: A Deep Learning Approach Using Convolutional Autoencoders," *IEEE Journal of Biomedical and Health Informatics*, vol. 24, no. 1, pp. 17–26, Jan. 2020, doi: https://doi.org/10.1109/jbhi.2019.2914970.

[8] G. A. Aguayo, L. Zhang, M. Vaillant, M. Ngari, M. Perquin, V. Moran, L. Huiart, R. Krüger, F. Azuaje, C. Ferdynus and G. Fagherazzi, "Machine learning for predicting neurodegenerative diseases in the general older population: a cohort study," *BMC Medical Research Methodology*, vol. 23, no. 1, Jan. 2023, doi: https://doi.org/10.1186/s12874-023-01837-4.

[9] G. Singh, M. Vadera, L. Samavedham, and E. C. H. Lim, "Machine Learning-Based Framework for Multi-Class Diagnosis of Neurodegenerative Diseases: A Study on Parkinson's Disease," *IFAC-PapersOnLine*, vol. 49, no. 7, pp. 990–995, 2016, doi: https://doi.org/10.1016/j.ifacol.2016.07.331.

[10] H. A. Helaly, M. Badawy and A. Y. Haikal, "Deep Learning Approach for Early Detection of Alzheimer's Disease," *Cognitive Computation*, vol. 14, no. 1711–1727, Nov. 2021, doi: https://doi.org/10.1007/s12559-021-09946-2.

[11] I. Yasar, M. A. Saritas, Sahman, and A. C. Cinar, "Classification of Parkinson disease data with artificial neural networks," *IOP Conference Series: Materials Science and Engineering*, vol. 675, no. 012031, p. 012031, Nov. 2019, doi: https://doi.org/10.1088/1757-899x/675/1/012031.

[12] J. D. Álvarez, J. A. Matias-Guiu, M. N. Cabrera-Martín, J. L. Risco-Martín, and J. L. Ayala, "An application of machine learning with feature selection to improve diagnosis and classification of neurodegenerative disorders," *BMC Bioinformatics*, vol. 20, no. 1, Oct. 2019, doi: https://doi.org/10.1186/s12859-019-3027-7.

[13] J. Mei, C. Desrosiers, and J. Frasnelli, "Machine Learning for the Diagnosis of Parkinson's Disease: A Review of Literature," *Frontiers in Aging Neuroscience*, vol. 13, no. 633752, May 2021, doi: https://doi.org/10.3389/fnagi.2021.633752.

[14] J. Zhang, W. Zhou, H. Yu, T. Wang, X. Wang, L. Liu, and Y. Wen, "Prediction of Parkinson's Disease Using Machine Learning Methods," *Biomolecules*, vol. 13, no. 12, pp. 1761–1761, Dec. 2023, doi: https://doi.org/10.3390/biom13121761.

[15] K. K. Gulhare, S. Shukla, and L. K. Sharma, "Deep Neural Network Classification method to Alzheimers Disease Detection," *International journal of advanced research in computer science and software engineering*, vol. 7, no. 6, pp. 1–4, Jun. 2017, doi: https://doi.org/10.23956/ijarcsse/v7i6/0259.

[16] L. Qian, X. Yang, J. Xu, Y. Guo, X. He, H. Hu and T. Lyu, "Early prediction of Alzheimer's disease and related dementias using real-world electronic health records." *Alzheimer's & Dementia*, vol. 19, no. 8, pp. 3506-3518, 2023.

[17] M. B. Makarious, H. L. Leonard, D. Vitale, H. Iwaki, L. Sargent, A. Dadu, I. Violich, E. Hutchins, D. Saffo, S. Bandres-Ciga, J. J. Kim, Y. Song, M. Maleknia, M. Bookman, W. Nojopranoto, R. H. Campbell, S. H. Hashemi, J. A. Botia, J. F. Carter, D. W. Craig, Kendall V. K. J., H. R. Morris, J. A. Hardy, C. Blauwendraat, A. B. Singleton, F. Faghri, and M. A. Nalls, "Multi-modality machine learning predicting Parkinson's disease," *npj Parkinson's Disease*, vol. 8, no. 1, Apr. 2022, doi: https://doi.org/10.1038/s41531-022-00288-w.

[18] M. Crous-Bou, C. Minguillón, N. Gramunt and J. L. Molinuevo. "Alzheimer's disease prevention: from risk factors to early intervention". *Alzheimers Res Ther.* vol. 9, no. 1, Dec 2017. http://alzres.biomedcentral.com/articles/10.1186/s13195-017-0297-z.

[19] M. Kundu, M. A. Nashiry, A. K. Dipongkor, S. Sarmin Sumi, and Md. A. Hossain, "An Optimized Machine Learning Approach for Predicting Parkinson's Disease," *International Journal of Modern Education and Computer Science*, vol. 13, no. 4, pp. 68–74, Aug. 2021, doi: https://doi.org/10.5815/ijmecs.2021.04.06.

[20] M. Mahmudul Hasan, J. Phu, A. Sowmya, E. Meijering, and M. Kalloniatis, "Artificial intelligence in the diagnosis of glaucoma and neurodegenerative diseases," *Clinical and Experimental Optometry*, vol. 130–146, no. 130–146, pp. 1–17, Sep. 2023, doi: https://doi.org/10.1080/08164622.2023.2235346.

[21] N. Bhagwat, J. Pipitone, A. N. Voineskos, and M. M. Chakravarty, "An artificial neural network model for clinical score prediction in Alzheimer disease using structural neuroimaging measures," *Journal of Psychiatry and Neuroscience*, vol. 44, no. 4, pp. 246–250, Jul. 2019, doi: https://doi.org/10.1503/jpn.180016.

[22] N. Salari, M. Kazeminia, H. Sagha, A. Daneshkhah, A. Ahmadi, and M. Mohammadi, "The performance of various machine learning methods for Parkinson's disease recognition: a systematic review," *Current Psychology*, Feb. 2022, doi: https://doi.org/10.1007/s12144-022-02949-8.

[23] N. Shusharina, D. Yukhnenko, S. Botman, V. Sapunov, V. Savinov, G. Kamyshov, D. Sayapin, and I. Voznyuk, "Modern Methods of Diagnostics and Treatment of Neurodegenerative Diseases and Depression," *Diagnostics,* vol. 13, no. 3, p. 573, Feb. 2023, doi: https://doi.org/10.3390/diagnostics13030573.

[24] P. K. Keserwani, S. Das, and N. Sarkar, "A comparative study: prediction of parkinson's disease using machine learning, deep learning and nature inspired algorithm," *Multimedia tools and applications*, vol. 83, no. 69393–69441, Jan. 2024, doi: https://doi.org/10.1007/s11042-024-18186-z.

[25] Q. D. Nam Nguyen, A. B. Liu, and C. W. Lin, "Development of a Neurodegenerative Disease Gait Classification Algorithm Using Multiscale Sample Entropy and Machine Learning Classifiers," *Entropy*, vol. 22, no. 12, p. 1340, Nov. 2020, doi: https://doi.org/10.3390/e22121340.

[26] R. B. Mofrad, N. S. M. Schoonenboom , Betty M Tijms , Philip Scheltens , Pieter Jelle Visser , Wiesje M van der Flier , and Charlotte E Teunissen , "Decision tree supports the interpretation of CSF biomarkers in Alzheimer's disease," Alzheimer's & Dementia: Diagnosis, Assessment & Disease Monitoring, vol. 11, no. 2352–8729/, pp. 1–9, Dec. 2019, doi: https://doi.org/10.1016/j.dadm.2018.10.004.
[27] R. Das, "A comparison of multiple classification methods for diagnosis of Parkinson disease," *Expert Systems with Applications*, vol. 37, no. 2, pp. 1568–1572, Mar. 2010, doi: https://doi.org/10.1016/j.eswa.2009.06.040.
[28] R. Prajapati, U. Khatri, and G. R. Kwon, "An Efficient Deep Neural Network Binary Classifier for Alzheimer's Disease Classification," *IEEE Xplore*, Apr. 01, 2021. https://ieeexplore.ieee.org/stamp/stamp.jsp?tp=&arnumber=9415212
[29] S. B. Lee , Y. J. Kim , S. Hwang , H. Son , S. K. Lee , K. Park, and Y. G. Kim , "Predicting Parkinson's disease using gradient boosting decision tree models with electroencephalography signals," *Parkinsonism & Related Disorders*, vol. 95, no. 1353–8020, pp. 77–85, Feb. 2022, doi: https://doi.org/10.1016/j.parkreldis.2022.01.011.
[30] S. Klöppel, C. M. Stonnington , C. Chu, B. Draganski, R. I. Scahill, J. D. Rohrer, N. C. Fox, C. R Jack Jr, J. Ashburner and R. S. J. Frackowiak, "Automatic classification of MR scans in Alzheimer's disease," *Brain*, vol. 131, no. 3, pp. 681–689, Feb. 2008, doi: https://doi.org/10.1093/brain/awm319.
[31] S. Ö. Arik and T. Pfister, "TabNet: Attentive Interpretable Tabular Learning," Proceedings of the AAAI Conference on Artificial Intelligence, vol. 35, no. 8, pp. 6679–6687, May 2021, doi: https://doi.org/10.1609/aaai.v35i8.16826.
[32] S. Srinivasan, P. Ramadass, S. K. Mathivanan, K. P. Selvam, B. D. Shivahare, and Mohd. A. Shah, "Detection of Parkinson disease using multiclass machine learning approach," *Scientific reports*, vol. 14, no. 1, Jun. 2024, doi: https://doi.org/10.1038/s41598-024-64004-9.
[33] T. Chakraborty, and I. Ghosh, "Real-time forecasts and risk assessment of novel coronavirus (COVID-19) cases: A data-driven analysis". Chaos, Solitons & Fractals. vol. 135, 109850. 2020.
[34] Z. Fan, F. Xu, C. Li, and L. Yao, "Application of KPCA and AdaBoost algorithm in classification of functional magnetic resonance imaging of Alzheimer's disease," *Neural Computing and Applications*, vol. 32, no. 10, pp. 5329–5338, Jan. 2020, doi: https://doi.org/10.1007/s00521-020-04707-y.

11

Advanced Fingerprint Authentication System and Neurodegenerative Disorder Multi-modal Pattern Recognition Techniques Using Deep Learning

Sajol Debnath[1], K. M. Danial Sadad[1], Md. Shamim Parvej[1], Shaik Abdul Kareem[2], Kaysun Molla[1], and Anindya Nag[1]

[1]Department of Computer Science and Engineering, Northern University of Business and Technology, Bangladesh
[2]Independent Researcher, USA
E-mail: superboysajol@gmail.com; danialsadad042@gmail.com; bd.shamim.cse@gmail.com; kaysun430@gmail.com; anindyanag@ieee.org; shaikcloud@outlook.com

Abstract

Biometric fingerprint identification systems are critical for improving security across a variety of businesses; nevertheless, single biometric approaches frequently have limits due to non-universality and noise, resulting in lower genuine acceptance rates (GAR) and greater false acceptance rates (FAR). To overcome these issues, this work investigates a multimodal biometric system that integrates fingerprint data with other biometric traits to improve accuracy and resistance to spoofing. We create a multimodal pattern recognition framework with deep learning models like EfficientNet (89%), WideResNet (94%), Xception (83%), DenseNet (91%), and CNN (88%), with WideResNet attaining the highest classification accuracy. Beyond security, generative AI applications within this framework have the potential to advance neurodegenerative illness research by allowing for the analysis of biometric data to diagnose and monitor cognitive decline early on. This method dramatically

DOI: 10.1201/9788743801764-11

improves biometric systems' resilience, security, and dependability, making it appropriate for both high-security situations and noninvasive neuropsychological examinations.

Keywords: Deep Learning, EfficientNet, WideResNet, Xception, DenseNet, CNN, FAR, GAI, Neurodegenerative, Biometric, Fingerprint.

11.1 Introduction

Unidiomatic systems use a single biometric source – such as a fingerprint, retina, finger vein, iris, DNA, voice recognition, or fingerprint – to identify an individual. Despite their widespread use, these systems have some significant drawbacks. For example, variable biometric data quality may be due to sensor inaccuracy or a user's unique biometric characteristics being of poor quality. Furthermore, uni biometric systems find it difficult to achieve the exact standards of accuracy required for high-security applications and comprehensive citizen recognition systems [1]. Multibiometric systems, which combine data from different biometric sources, are being investigated as a result of the inherent shortcomings of uni-biometric systems. The integration of different biometrics seeks to improve recognition accuracy, using the distinct advantages of each biometric feature. Because a subset of biometric data may be in flux due to aging, this technique is particularly helpful in addressing the shortcomings of single-source biometric systems such as noise, incompleteness, or aging. Multibiometric systems can solve these problems and offer more [2].

Reliable and accurate identification method by combining different biometric sources. The main advantage of multibiometric systems is that they can reduce the overlap between feature distributions of different individuals by increasing the dimensionality of the feature space. More accurate identification is made possible by this larger feature space, which reduces the likelihood of misclassifying individuals with comparable biometric characteristics. Additionally, the accuracy of the system is increased as the combination of different biometric attributes makes the identification process more unique to a particular individual. Apart from increased accuracy, multibiometric systems have several advantages over unidiomatic systems [3]. They can help with the problem of non-universality, which arises when certain people may not have a certain biometric characteristic that can be accurately measured. For example, certain individuals may have fingerprints that are too worn or may not have an identifiable iris pattern, making it difficult for unidiomatic devices to register correctly. By offering additional biometric features that can be used for identification, multibiometric systems reduce enrolment failures and increase the number of people who can be accurately identified. Multibiometric systems provide flexible user authentication. These systems are more adaptable than unidiomatic ones because they rely on several biometric sources, allowing them to accommodate different user preferences and types of situations. For example, the system can still verify the user using a different biometric feature, such as their voice or retina, even if their fingerprint is momentarily rendered useless by accident [4]. Large biometric database searches conducted using multibiometric systems are more efficient. These systems can more efficiently limit the search field, allowing faster and more accurate identification by combining numerous biometric features. Furthermore, the system's resistance to spoofing attacks increases when several biometric attributes are used because it becomes much more difficult for a fraudster to duplicate all the required biometric attributes at once. The paper discusses a proposed multibiometric system that combines biometric attributes from fingerprints, retina, and finger veins with an asymmetric cryptographic method called RSA to secure biometric templates [5]. Among several fusion techniques accessible, the fusion of these biometric attributes is implemented at the feature layer, which includes the sensor layer, score layer, decision layer, and rank layer. Because it enables the integration of the most discriminating features from each biometric source, feature-level fusion is particularly beneficial because it creates a detection process that is more reliable and accurate.

With improved accuracy, versatility, and security over conventional unidiomatic systems, multibiometric systems are a major improvement. These systems meet the requirements of large-scale identification systems and high-security applications while addressing the shortcomings of unidiomatic systems through the use of numerous biometric inputs and sophisticated fusion techniques.

Generative AI is increasingly being used in the context of neurodegenerative disorders through the analysis of biometric data such as fingerprints, speech, and facial recognition. These technologies can aid in the early detection, diagnosis and monitoring of conditions such as Alzheimer's and Parkinson's disease by detecting subtle changes that may indicate disease progression. The integration of AI increases accuracy and speed of diagnosis, potentially leading to more effective management plans.

11.1.1 Motivation

Compared to single-modal systems, multi-modal biometric authentication systems offer improved security, accuracy and robustness. These systems can reduce the risk of spoofing attacks, increase reliability in difficult situations, and support a larger user base by combining data from different biometric methods.

11.1.2 Objective

The key goals of this research are to create and test deep learning models for fingerprint-based multimodal biometric systems. The objective of combining various biometric modalities is to increase classification accuracy while also considering computing efficiency and model scalability for real-time applications. Furthermore, the research seeks to reduce overfitting, improve performance on huge datasets, and investigate techniques for strengthening security through multimodal biometric integration.

The remainder of the chapter is organized into the following sections. Section 11.2 provides a comprehensive overview of the existing literature related to our research area, highlighting the algorithms used in our study and their foundation. Section 11.3 delves into the methodology employed in this study, outlining the dataset used, its attributes, and preprocessing steps. Section 11.4 presents the results of our experiments using different models. We provide a comparative analysis of the model's performance. Section 11.5 concludes our findings and discusses potential future directions.

11.2 Literature Survey

Jagadiswary et al. [6] suggested a method that combines the fingerprint, retina, and finger vein biometric features into a multimodal biometric system that was created with MATLAB 2014. Techniques for feature extraction are used, including maximum curvature approaches for finger veins, blood vessel extraction for retinas, and minutiae extraction for fingerprints. RSA encryption is utilized to protect the feature-level fusion of these features. When compared to unimodal systems, the system's performance demonstrates a notable improvement in both false acceptance rate (FAR) and genuine acceptance rate (GAR). The multimodal system outperforms unimodal systems, which have issues with non-universality and noise, with a GAR of 95.3% and a FAR of 0.01%. The system is appropriate for high-security applications since it is made to improve accuracy, security, and resistance to spoofing.

Upcoming research attempts to improve feature extraction, improve database management, and explore different fusion levels to further enhance the system's performance.

Adami et al. [7] examined the application of biometric technologies in eHealth, with a particular emphasis on the SpeechXRays project, which improves accuracy and anti-spoofing capabilities by fusing video and face and voice biometrics. The chapter described an innovative user interface for safe access to eHealth systems, which allows medical professionals and patients to securely access clinical data. It presents a detailed review of the SpeechXRays system, taking into account both user experience and technological needs. The study also emphasized the significance of properly selecting biometric solutions for applications that handle sensitive data, notably in healthcare, to ensure security, ease, and accountability. Secure authentication relies on biometrics, which includes both physiological (e.g., fingerprints, iris) and behavioral aspects (e.g., voice, typing rhythm). It offers a user-friendly biometric platform that allows medical professionals and patients to securely access clinical and health data. This research is unique in that it collects extensive requirements and conducts formative evaluations of the SpeechXRays system's user interface using a user-centered design methodology. It discusses the important necessity for safe access to sensitive medical information and assesses the system's modular architecture. The platform has customizable security settings, which allow administrators to balance false acceptance and rejection rates based on data sensitivity. The findings seek to improve the design of biometric systems for eHealth by increasing security, convenience, and user experience.

Ayesha et al. [8] improved authentication and data security in remote applications by introducing an advanced multimodal biometric framework. Traditional biometric systems frequently rely on static characteristics and fixed features, which reduces their usefulness in dynamic contexts. To solve these constraints, the proposed architecture incorporates biometric characteristics such as iris, face, and fingerprint identification, as well as dynamically generated keys for each user. This technique improves data integrity and security, making it appropriate for huge datasets in open and closed set environments. The system incorporates a revolutionary integrity verification method and encryption mechanism, which are intended to provide strong security even in distributed applications. Experimental findings from real-time datasets stored on Amazon AWS servers reveal that the suggested methodology improves computational integrity by 7% and reduces runtime by 5% compared to existing methods. These findings demonstrate the framework's efficiency and efficacy in managing huge datasets. The report also indicates that future research might apply this approach to real-time IoT contexts, with an emphasis on safeguarding streams of pictures or video data using multimodal biometric security. This makes it a possible answer to emerging data security concerns in a variety of industries.

A. K. Jain et al. [9] presented a deep learning architecture for fingerprint identification that incorporates a feature extraction step utilizing histogram equalization, Gabor augmentation, and thinning. The model achieves 93.21% accuracy with a loss of 0.9, much higher than the previous 77% accuracy reported on the same dataset of 280 samples (196 for training and 84 for testing). The findings indicate the efficacy of sophisticated feature extraction approaches in biometric identification.

Minaee et al. [10] work described a deep learning approach for categorizing fingerprint characteristics in the Automatic Fingerprint Identification System (AFIS), with emphasis on left-right hand, sweat-pore, scratch, and finger type classifications. Five models were trained, with Yolo-v2 obtaining 90.98% accuracy for left-right hand and ResNet-50 at 91.29% for sweat-pore categorization. Both models processed photos in roughly 250.37 milliseconds apiece. The authors intend to create a unified model and increase the dataset to improve accuracy, with real-world applications in fingerprint recognition systems.

Shankar et al. [11] evaluated a multimodal biometric system based on Gabor imaginary part features, demonstrating greater reliability with larger sample numbers. For 25 samples, the FRR was 1.10%, the FAR was 3.0%, and the accuracy was 91.00%. With 125 samples, FRR dropped to 0.70%, FAR to 2.3%, and accuracy increased to 92.23%. The maximum sample size of 600 yielded an FRR of 0.02%, FAR of 1.3%, and an accuracy of 93.60%. These data show that bigger sample numbers greatly improve accuracy while lowering FRR and FAR.

Barham et al. [12] tackled security issues about fingerprint biometrics by using a deep convolutional neural network (CNN) as a pre-verification filter to improve identification accuracy. The suggested technique filters away low-quality fingerprints before subjecting them to minutiae-based verification, using Google's pre-trained inception model. This two-phase technique offers around 90% accuracy in fingerprint verification. The addition of the pre-filter CNN considerably decreases noise and lowers the FAR, hence boosting overall fingerprint authentication security. An overview of previous research is given in Table 11.1.

Table 11.1 Summary of literature review

Author	Model	Dataset	Accuracy
Jagadiswary et al. [6]	Multimodal biometric system (fingerprint, retina, finger vein)	Online Platform	GAR: 95.3%, FAR: 0.01%
Adami et al. [7]	SpeechXRays (video, face, and voice biometrics)	DEAP	Not specified
Ayesha et al. [8]	Multimodal biometric framework (iris, face, fingerprint)	Real-time datasets on AWS servers	7% improvement in integrity, 5% reduction in runtime
Jain et al. [9]	CNN	Self-collected	93.21%
Minaee et al. [10]	ResNet-50	AFIS Dataset	91.29%
Shankar et al. [11]	Multimodal biometric (gabor imaginary part features)	KAGGLE	93.60%
Barham et al. [12]	CNN	–	90%

11.3 Methodology

Biometric fingerprint authentication systems that use multi-modal pattern recognition go through several phases of data preprocessing to assure authentication accuracy, efficiency, and robustness.

The workflow diagram of the proposed system. The data preprocessing, missing value handling, encoding, data splitting, implementation of models, model training, testing, and evaluation. Figure 11.1 represents the flow diagram of our proposed work. Figure 11.1 represents the flow diagram of our proposed work.

This algorithm describes the categorization process with deep learning models. First, the picture data is imported, preprocessed, and separated into training and test sets. Models like as EfficientNet, Xception, WideResNet, DenseNet, and CNN are trained and assessed using precision, recall, and F1 scores. The model with the greatest F1 score is chosen and stored for deployment, resulting in an efficient method of picture categorization. It is shown in algorithm 11.1.

11.3.1 Data collection

We utilized a Kaggle dataset with 6,000 photos divided into three different classes. The dataset is well-structured, with each class representing a distinct category for training and testing [23]. It provides a broad set of samples that are appropriate for a variety of machine learning and deep learning applications. This dataset gives a robust foundation for classification tasks and model validation. Some sample images shown in Figure 11.2.

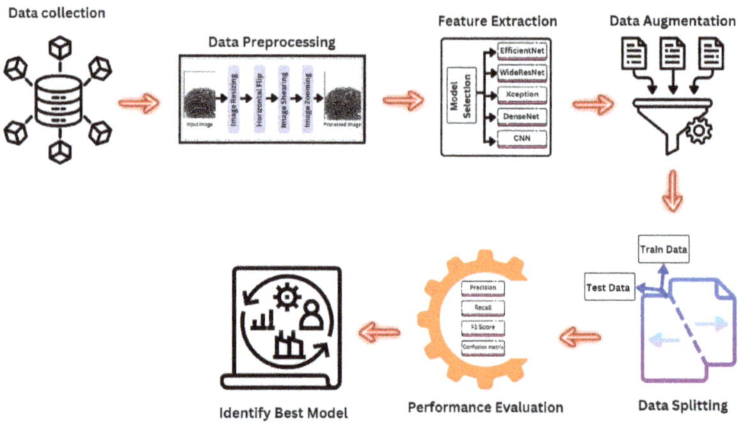

Figure 11.1 Flow diagram of our proposed work.

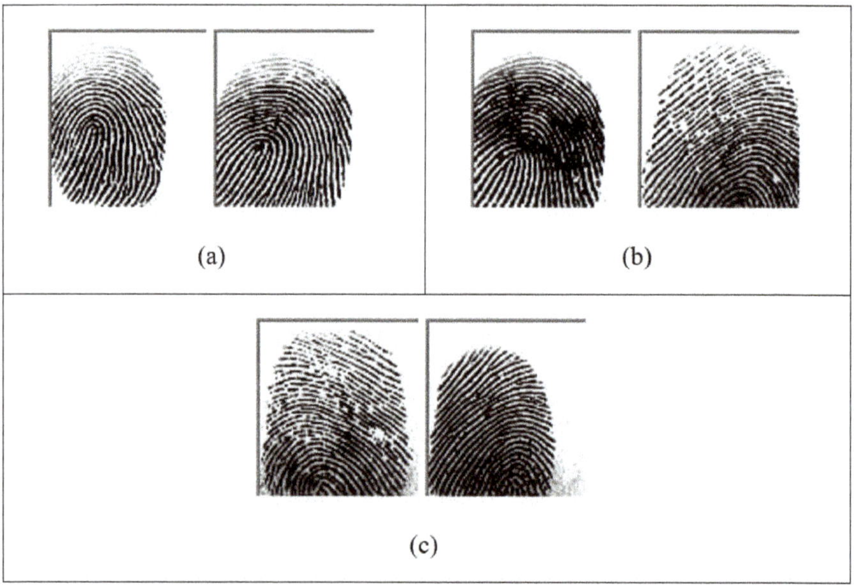

Figure 11.2 Image data (a) Whorl, (b) Loop, (c) Arch.

11.3.2 Data preprocessing

Data pretreatment is critical for ensuring accuracy and consistency across several biometric inputs. It includes noise reduction, image improvement, normalization, and feature extraction for fingerprints, iris scans, and facial recognition data. These preprocessing procedures align and standardize the various modalities to provide seamless integration. Effective preprocessing boosts the system's overall performance by improving the quality of the extracted biometric features.

- **Image resizing**

Image scaling is a critical data preprocessing technique that guarantees all photos are the same size. Adjusting the size of photographs to a preset width and height ensures consistency for subsequent processing and eliminates distortion. Important details are preserved while resizing by using interpolation methods such as bilinear and bicubic.

- **Perform horizontal clipping**

Horizontal clipping is a data preprocessing technique that removes undesired areas of an image or focuses on a specific region of interest (ROI). It removes superfluous regions from photographs by cutting them off horizontally, such as excess background in facial images or blank space around fingerprints. This method entails deciding which section to keep and using slicing or cropping functions to remove any undesirable parts.

- **Perform image scaling**

Image scaling standardizes pixel intensity levels, which improves model learning and convergence. It sets pixel values to a certain range (e.g., [0, 1] or [–1, 1]) to ensure consistency among images. This can be accomplished by normalizing data to the maximum pixel value (255 in 8-bit images) or by employing min-max scaling. The min-max scaling formula is as follows:

$$\text{Scaled Value} = \frac{\text{Original Value} - \text{Min}}{\text{Max} - \text{Min}}. \tag{11.1}$$

- **Perform image zooming**

Image zooming is a data augmentation technique that simulates different scales of the image to make the model more robust to variations in biometric data. It involves zooming in or out on the image, which can be performed uniformly or randomly. Interpolation techniques are used to maintain image quality during zooming. Zooming in simulates a closer sensor and zooming out simulates a further sensor.

11.3.3 Features extraction

- Ridge and valley patterns: The system extracts ridge flow, ridge direction, and minor details (such as bifurcations and ridge termination) from the fingerprint image. These patterns constitute the basis for fingerprint recognition.
- Frequency and directionality: Features such as local ridge frequency and orientation are examined for extra levels of recognition. These parameters enhance resistance to image noise and distortion.
- Texture and wavelet transformations**:** Textural features, such as Gabor filters or wavelet transforms, can enrich fingerprint data by emphasizing unique patterns in the image to aid classification.
- Multimodal integration: Multi-modal recognition combines features from other biometric data (e.g., palm print, finger geometry) with fingerprint features to generate a more comprehensive dataset for model training and pattern identification.

11.3.4 Data augmentation

Data augmentation in biometric fingerprint identification systems increases the diversity and volume of training data, which improves multi-modal pattern recognition models. Rotation, scaling, cropping, noise addition, and mirroring are examples of alterations that can be applied to existing fingerprint images. It improves model generalization by mimicking variations in real-world circumstances, such as changes in finger pressure, direction, or environmental variables. This technique is critical for developing robust biometric systems, particularly when the available dataset is small or imbalanced.

11.3.5 Data splitting

Data splitting is a vital stage in determining the model's performance. The dataset is often divided into three subsets:

- Training set: The data used to train the model. It is made up of the majority of the dataset (usually 70–80%), in which the model learns the patterns and properties of fingerprint photos.
- Validation set: A smaller subset (usually 10–15%) utilized during training to fine-tune the model's parameters and prevent overfitting. It aids in modifying the model hyperparameters.

- Test set: The final component (usually 10–15%) is used to assess the model's performance following training. It ensures that the model accurately generalizes to previously unseen data.
- Splitting can be random or class-based to guarantee that all subgroups are represented fairly.

11.3.6 Applied models

The purpose of this project is to create a model that minimizes the number of instances.

- EfficientNet

EfficientNet is a series of CNN created by Google AI for image categorisation. Introduced in 2019, it employs a compound scaling strategy to optimise depth, breadth, and resolution, resulting in cutting-edge accuracy with fewer parameters. Its blend of performance and efficiency has made it popular among the deep learning community [13].

$$\propto^{\emptyset} \bullet \beta^{\emptyset} \bullet \gamma^{\emptyset} \approx 2. \tag{11.2}$$

- Xception

Xception, or "Extreme Inception," is a deep learning architecture for image categorisation that employs depth wise separable convolutions to increase performance and minimise parameters. Its deep structure improves feature extraction, resulting in great accuracy on benchmarks like as ImageNet [14].

$$\mathrm{Z} = \mathrm{X} * (\mathrm{W_d} \cdot \mathrm{W_p}). \tag{11.3}$$

- DenseNet

Densely connected convolutional networks (DenseNet) are a CNN design in which each layer feeds information to the next layer. DenseNet has fewer parameters than typical CNNs but maintains good accuracy, making it suitable for image classification and other computer vision applications [15].

$$\mathrm{H_l} = \mathrm{H_{l-1}} + \mathrm{F}(\mathrm{H_{l-1}}, \mathrm{W_l}\ ). \tag{11.4}$$

- CNN

A CNN is a deep-learning model designed specifically for image processing. It uses convolutional layers to automatically learn features and pooling layers

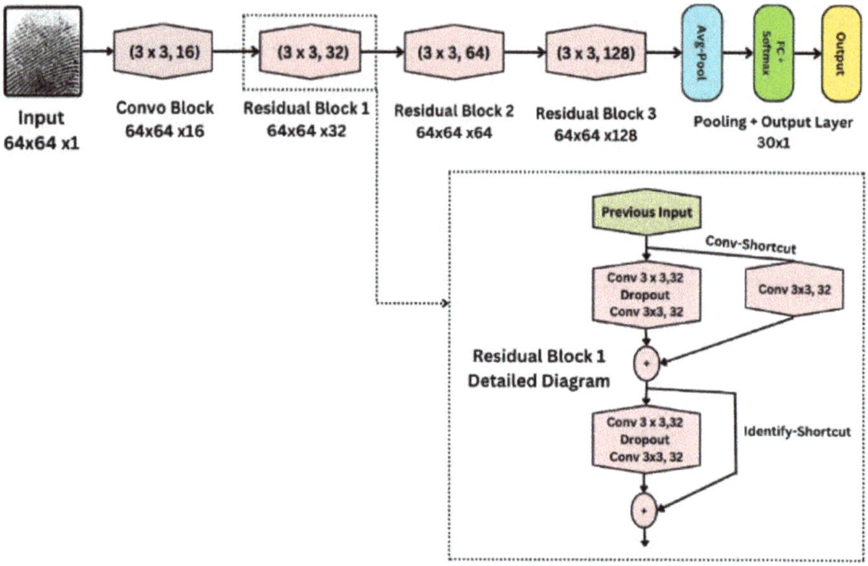

Figure 11.3 Proposed model architecture.

to minimise dimensionality. CNNs are extremely successful at tasks like as picture categorisation and object recognition because they capture spatial hierarchies through their layered architectures [16].

$$Y[i,j] = \sum_{mn} X[i+m,\ j+n] \cdot K[m,n]. \tag{11.5}$$

- WideResNet (proposed)

WideResNet is an improved variant of ResNet that focuses on expanding network width, hence enhancing capacity and performance for picture categorization. It reduces overfitting and disappearing gradients by employing bigger layers with more filters and residual connections, resulting in cutting-edge performance on datasets such as CIFAR-10 and CIFAR-100 [17]. The visual representation of the proposed model architecture is given in Figure 11.3.

11.3.7 Performance evaluation

Evaluation metrics are crucial tools for assessing the performance of deep learning models. They give quantitative assessments of a model's accuracy, precision, recall, and other essential performance characteristics [18].

Accuracy

It is the percentage of correctly classified cases out of all occurrences. It is best suited for balanced datasets and evenly distributed classes [19]. It is defined as:

$$\text{Accuracy}=\frac{\text{TP}+\text{TN}}{\text{TP}+\text{TN}+\text{FP}+\text{FN}}. \tag{11.6}$$

Precision

Precision measures the proportion of accurate positive predictions to all positive forecasts [20]. The equation for precision is:

$$\text{Precision}=\frac{\text{TP}}{\text{TP}+\text{FP}}. \tag{11.7}$$

Recall

Recall, often called sensitivity or true positive rate, is the ratio of accurate positive forecasts to positive instances [21]. The equation for the recall is:

$$\text{Recall}=\frac{\text{TP}}{\text{TP}+\text{FN}}. \tag{11.8}$$

F1 score

We can reduce feature space and improve model training speed and accuracy by identifying the primary prediction factors [22]. The equation for the F1 score is:

$$\text{F1 Score}=2\times\frac{\text{Precision}\times\text{Recall}}{\text{Precision}+\text{Recall}}. \tag{11.9}$$

11.4 Result and Discussion

This model compares the performance of five deep learning models (EfficientNet, WideResNet, Xception, DenseNet, and CNN) on a multi-class classification task with three classes (0, 1, and 2). These three classes are Class 0 name = Whorl, Class 1 name = Loop, Class 2 name = Arch. Models are evaluated based on precision, recall, and F1-score. A comparison of the performance of the models is provided in Table 11.2.

Table 11.2 Comparison of model performance.

Model	Accuracy	Class	Precision	Recall	F1 score
EfficientNet	89%	Whorl	0.914	0.890	0.902
		Loop	0.885	0.899	0.892
		Arch	0.856	0.890	0.873
WideResNet	94%	Whorl	0.940	0.953	0.946
		Loop	0.936	0.944	0.940
		Arch	0.922	0.940	0.931
Xception	83%	Whorl	0.830	0.867	0.848
		Loop	0.816	0.845	0.830
		Arch	0.783	0.814	0.798
DenseNet	91%	Whorl	0.922	0.929	0.926
		Loop	0.905	0.916	0.910
		Arch	0.888	0.910	0.899
CNN	88%	Whorl	0.880	0.907	0.893
		Loop	1	0.869	0.891
		Arch	0.842	0.867	0.854

Algorithm 11.1: Algorithm for Classification Using Deep Learning Models

Input:

- Image dataset (images and labels)
- Models MbaseM_{\text{base}}Mbase (e.g., EfficientNet, Xception, WideResNet, DenseNet, CNN)

Output:

- Best model MbestM_{\text{best}}Mbest
- Saved model file

Steps:

Step 1: Dataset Preparation

Load and preprocess data:

- Load images and labels from the dataset.
- Resize images to a consistent input shape (e.g., 224x224).
- Normalize pixel values to [0, 1] range.

Split data:

- Xtrain,Xtest,ytrain,ytest=traintestsplit(X,y,testsize=0.2,randomstate=42) X_{\text{train}}, X_{\text{test}}, y_{\text{train}}, y_{\text{test}} =

train_test_split(X, y, test_size=0.2, random_state=42)Xtrain,Xtest,ytrain, ytest=traintestsplit(X,y,testsize=0.2,randomstate=42)

Step 2: Model Creation

Define and compile models using base models MbaseM_{\text{base}} Mbase:

- For each model (EfficientNet, Xception, WideResNet, DenseNet, CNN):
  - Initialize model with an appropriate architecture.
  - Compile model with Adam optimizer and categorical crossentropy loss for multi-class classification.

Step 3: Model Training

Train each model:

- For each model:
  - model.fit(X_train, y_train, epochs=10, batch_size=32, validation_split=0.2)

Step 4: Model Evaluation

Evaluate models:

- For each model:
  - Calculate precision, recall, F1 score and plot performance using:
    - y_pred = model.predict(X_test)
    - f1_score(y_test, y_pred.argmax(axis=1), average='weighted')
  - Plot performance metrics (e.g., confusion matrix, ROC curve).

Step 5: Identify Best Model

Select a model with the highest F1 score as MbestM_{\text{best}} Mbest

Step 6: Model Deployment

Save the best model:

- Save the model file using:
  - model.save('best_model.h5')

We used a confusion matrix to test the performance of several models, including CNN, DenseNet, Xception, WideResNet, EfficientNet. WideResNet model outperformed the others, achieving 94% accuracy while maintaining good precision and recall. DenseNet (91%) performed second best. EfficientNet and CNN are fairly similar in performance, though EfficientNet edges out in terms of overall metrics. Xception is the least effective model in this comparison, with notably lower scores in both precision and recall across all classes. It is defined in Figure 11.4.

The accuracy and loss curves indicate how the model performed at each epoch. The WideResNet achieved 94% accuracy, and the accuracy curve climbs while the loss curve lowers, demonstrating efficient learning. Compared to CNN, Xception, DenseNet, and EfficientNet, the WideResNet

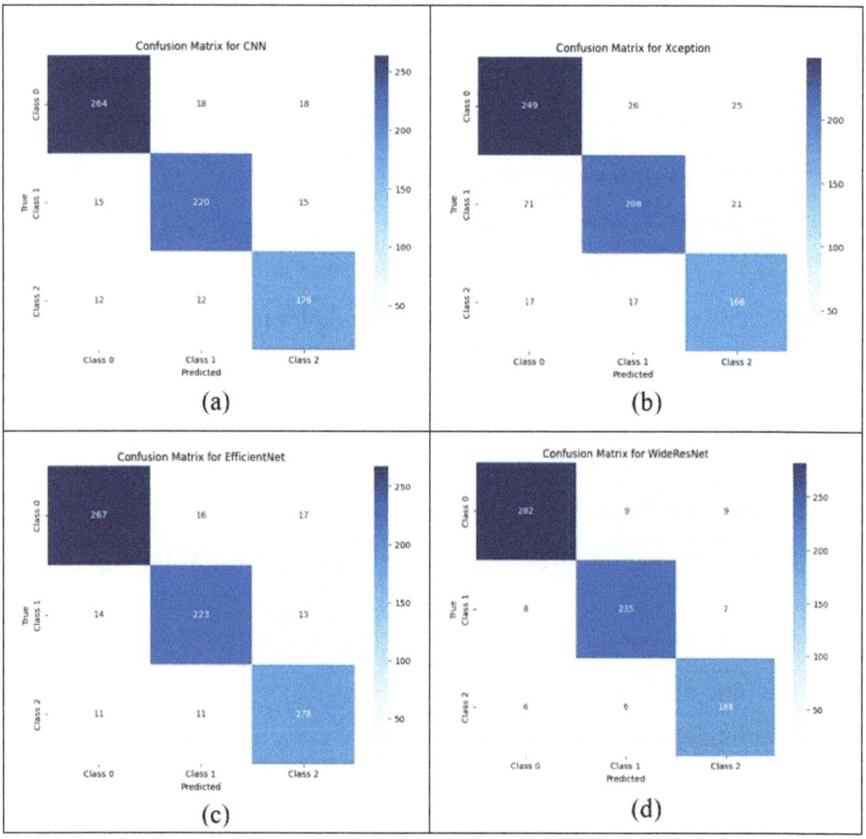

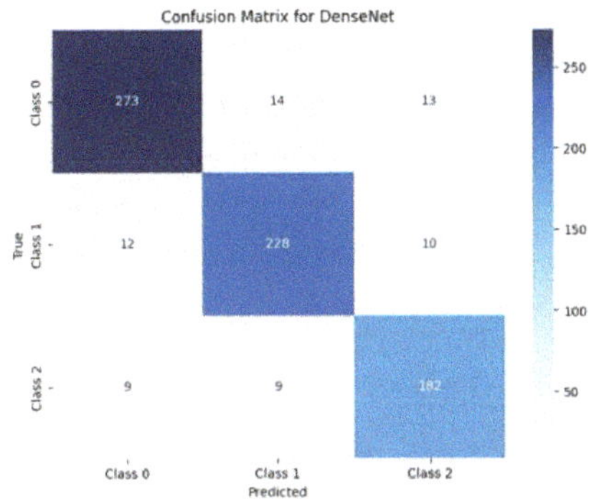

(e)

Figure 11.4 Confusion matrix of all models: (a) CNN, (b) DenseNet, (c) Xception, (d) WideResNet, (e) EfficientNet.

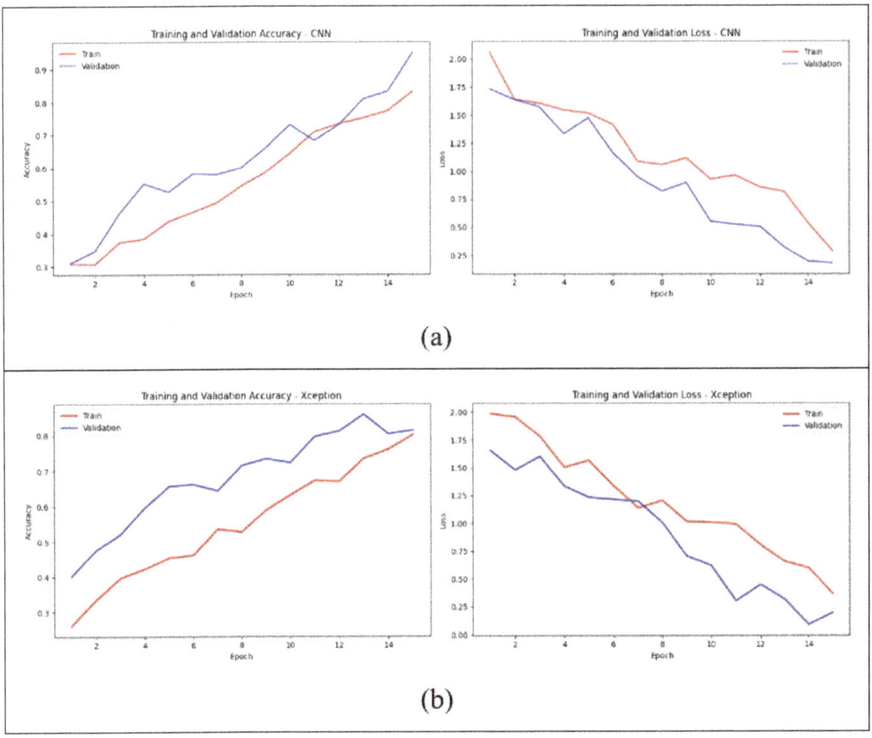

Figure 11.5 *Continued.*

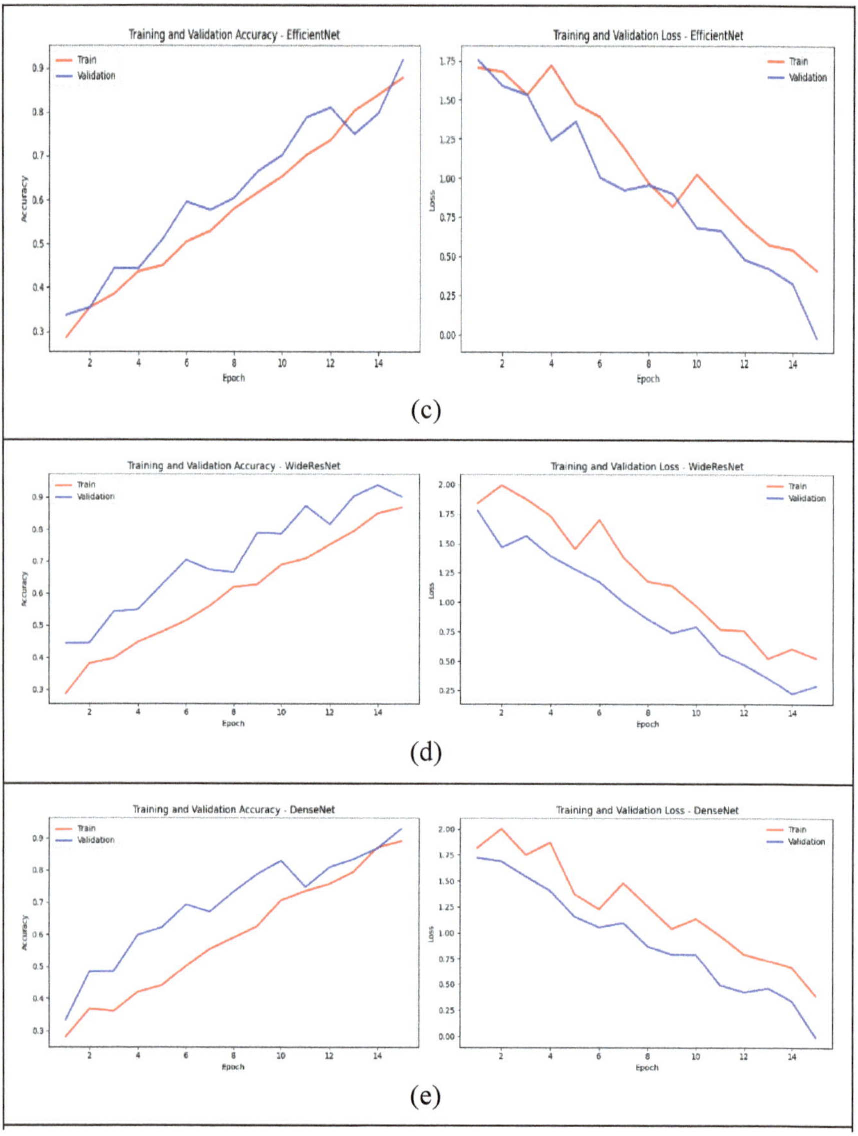

Figure 11.5 Accuracy and loss curve of all models: (a) CNN, (b) DenseNet, (c) Xception, (d) WideResNet, (e) EfficientNet.

regularly outperforms them all in terms of accuracy and loss. It is defined in Figure 11.5.

WideResNet appears to be the best model for this particular multi-class classification problem, achieving high accuracy and excellent performance on all three classes; however, the choice of the best model may be determined by the application's specific requirements, such as the relative importance of precision and recall for different classes.

11.5 Comparison with State-of-the-Art Techniques

The chart compares multiple models used for fingerprint pattern recognition with the related papers.

The primary limits of our work include the high computational needs for training complicated models such as EfficientNet, Xception, and WideResNet, as well as the reliance on big, high-quality datasets to avoid overfitting. The system's scalability may be limited by these models' processing and memory requirements, especially in real-time applications. Furthermore, the emphasis on fingerprint-based multimodal biometrics restricts the incorporation of other modalities, and deep learning models lack explainability, making decision processes difficult to comprehend.

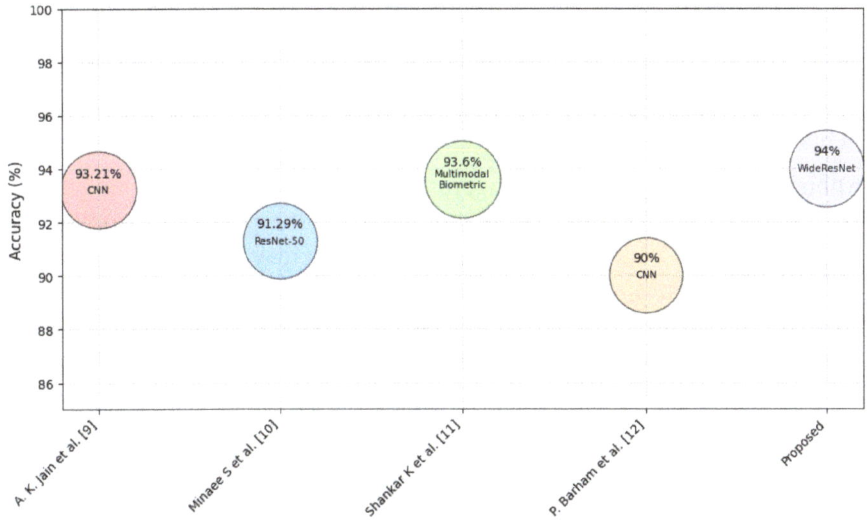

Figure 11.6 Model comparison with related works.

11.6 Using GAI for Neurodegenerative Disorder in Biometric Fingerprint

Biometric fingerprint detection can be integrated with Generative AI to monitor and diagnose neurodegenerative conditions like Alzheimer's and Parkinson's disease. This is achieved by analyzing biometric data, such as fingerprints, to identify unique patterns that may correlate with cognitive decline. Generative AI can enhance this process by generating digital biomarkers from the collected data, which allows for remote neurocognitive assessments and can potentially distinguish between different conditions non-invasively. The high-dimensional data from biometric fingerprints, combined with machine learning algorithms, helps in recognizing subtle changes that may indicate the onset or progression of these diseases.

However, generative AI (GAI) can indirectly contribute to the understanding and management of neurodegenerative diseases in various ways:

1. Drug discovery: GAI can accelerate drug discovery by simulating molecular interactions and predicting potential drug candidates. This could lead to the development of treatments for neurodegenerative diseases.
2. Medical image analysis: GAI can examine medical images such as MRIs and CT scans to detect early signs of neurodegeneration. This can help in early diagnosis and intervention.
3. Patient monitoring and care: Wearable devices powered by GAI can track patient behavior and vital signs to detect early disease progression. This may allow for more appropriate care and interventions.

Although GAI and biometric fingerprint analysis are useful techniques, their applications are different. Although GAI has the potential to revolutionize the study of neurodegenerative diseases, it may not have a direct impact on fingerprint analysis. Instead, the emphasis should be on using GAI to address the root causes of these disorders, such as better understanding disease mechanisms, developing effective drugs, and improving patient care.

11.7 Conclusion and Future Works

In this paper, we created a multimodal biometric fingerprint authentication system using sophisticated deep learning models such as EfficientNet, WideResNet, Xception, DenseNet, and CNN. We addressed the constraints of single biometric systems by merging several biometric qualities, such as fingerprints, retinal scans, and finger vein patterns, with the goal of increasing GAR and decreasing FAR. WideResNet performed the best, with 94% accuracy, demonstrating the usefulness of the multimodal method. The combination of biometric data with deep learning algorithms improves the security, accuracy, and robustness of biometric authentication systems, providing a more dependable solution for crucial security applications.

Future research will focus on increasing the scalability and efficiency of the multimodal biometric system. This involves looking at other biometric modalities, such as voice and facial recognition, to improve security. In addition, we want to incorporate real-time processing capabilities and examine the usage of new deep learning architectures to minimise computing complexity while retaining excellent accuracy. Finally, resolving privacy problems with more advanced encryption and privacy-preserving mechanisms will be an important topic of future study.

Future research combining biometric fingerprint identification with biometric fingerprint identification for neurodegenerative disorders seeks to increase diagnostic accuracy, accessibility, and ethical standards. Key goals include increasing data collection by generating larger datasets from diverse populations and ensuring privacy using methods such as differential privacy. Refinement of generative models to simulate realistic disease progression may improve detection accuracy by better understanding how motor deficits develop.

Combining fingerprint data with other biometrics, such as voice, gait, or handwriting, will provide a more complete picture of neurodegenerative symptoms, allowing for more precise identification. Furthermore, clinical trials are important to test the accuracy of the model in a real-world context, therefore increasing confidence in clinical adoption. The development of wearable or mobile devices can enable continuous, real-time monitoring, making diagnostics more accessible. Finally, adopting ethical norms for data protection and transparency will promote responsible management of sensitive biometric data, facilitating widespread adoption and deployment.

Acknowledgments

We would like to express our gratitude to our team members and instructors for the help and support they have given us during this project, including their valuable suggestions, ideas and encouragement. Your insightful conversations and useful criticisms have been really beneficial.

Data Availability Statement

The image dataset utilized in this work is publicly available and accessible via Kaggle. All relevant data were taken from https://www.kaggle.com/datasets/ruizgara/socofing dataset repository and are freely available for research use [22]. The dataset is subject to the terms and restrictions set out by Kaggle.

References

[1] Nagar, Abhishek, Karthik Nandakumar, and Anil K. Jain. "Multibiometric cryptosystems based on feature-level fusion." IEEE transactions on information forensics and security 7.1 (2011): 255-268.

[2] Rathod, Hiral, Mahendra Singh Sisodia, and Sanjay Kumar Sharma. "Design and implementation of image encryption algorithm by using block based symmetric transformation algorithm (hyper image encryption algorithm)." International Journal of Computer Technology and Electronics Engineering (IJCTEE) 1.3 (2011): 7-13.

[3] Fu, Bo, et al. "Multibiometric cryptosystem: Model structure and performance analysis." IEEE Transactions on information forensics and security 4.4 (2009): 867-882.

[4] Simoens, Koen, et al. "A framework for analyzing template security and privacy in biometric authentication systems." IEEE Transactions on Information forensics and security 7.2 (2012): 833-841.

[5] Sim, Terence, et al. "Continuous verification using multimodal biometrics." IEEE transactions on pattern analysis and machine intelligence 29.4 (2007): 687-700.

[6] Jain, Anil K., and Jianjiang Feng. "Latent fingerprint matching." IEEE Transactions on pattern analysis and machine intelligence 33.1 (2010): 88-100.

[7] Marín, Diego, et al. "A new supervised method for blood vessel segmentation in retinal images by using gray-level and moment invariants-based features." IEEE Transactions on medical imaging 30.1 (2010): 146-158.

[8] Upmanyu, Maneesh, et al. "Blind authentication: a secure crypto-biometric verification protocol." IEEE transactions on information forensics and security 5.2 (2010): 255-268.

[9] Kumar, Ajay, and Yingbo Zhou. "Human identification using finger images." IEEE Transactions on image processing 21.4 (2011): 2228-2244.

[10] Trewin, Shari, et al. "Biometric authentication on a mobile device: a study of user effort, error and task disruption." Proceedings of the 28th Annual Computer Security Applications Conference. 2012.

[11] Nandakumar, Karthik, and Anil K. Jain. "Biometric template protection: Bridging the performance gap between theory and practice." IEEE Signal Processing Magazine 32.5 (2015): 88-100.

[12] Chingovska, Ivana, Andre Rabello Dos Anjos, and Sebastien Marcel. "Biometrics evaluation under spoofing attacks." IEEE transactions on Information Forensics and Security 9.12 (2014): 2264-2276.

[13] Bhagavatula, Rasekhar, et al. "Biometric authentication on iphone and android: Usability, perceptions, and influences on adoption." (2015): 1.

[14] Miltgen, Caroline Lancelot, Aleš Popovič, and Tiago Oliveira. "Determinants of end-user acceptance of biometrics: Integrating the "Big 3" of technology acceptance with privacy context." Decision support systems 56 (2013): 103-114.

[15] Ali, Zulfiqar, et al. "Edge-centric multimodal authentication system using encrypted biometric templates." Future Generation Computer Systems 85 (2018): 76-87.

[16] Chen, Yarui, et al. "Multimodal biometrics recognition based on local fusion visual features and variational Bayesian extreme learning machine." Expert Systems with Applications 64 (2016): 93-103.

[17] Sarier, Neyire Deniz. "Multimodal biometric identity based encryption." Future Generation Computer Systems 80 (2018): 112-125.

[18] Walia, Gurjit Singh, et al. "Robust multimodal biometric system based on optimal score level fusion model." Expert Systems with Applications 116 (2019): 364-376.

[19] Xin, Ma, and Jing Xiaojun. "Correlation-based identification approach for multimodal biometric fusion." The Journal of China Universities of Posts and Telecommunications 24.4 (2017): 34-50.

[20] Jain, A. K. "Handbook of biometrics." Springer google schola 2 (2007): 114-116.

[21] Minaee, Shervin, et al. "Biometrics recognition using deep learning: A survey." Artificial Intelligence Review 56.8 (2023): 8647-8695.

[22] Fingerprint Dataset https://www.kaggle.com/datasets/ruizgara/socofing

[23] Shankar, K., et al. "RETRACTED ARTICLE: Secret image sharing scheme with encrypted shadow images using optimal homomorphic

encryption technique." Journal of Ambient Intelligence and Humanized Computing 11.5 (2020): 1821-1833.

[24] Abadi, Martín, et al. "{TensorFlow}: a system for {Large-Scale} machine learning." 12th USENIX symposium on operating systems design and implementation (OSDI 16). 2016.

12

A Convolutional Neural Network Based Biomarkers for Alzheimer's Diagnosis and Prognosis

Meenal H.[1], Kishor Kumar Reddy C.[2], Reddaboina Rajini[3], Pendyala Loka Priya[4], and Marlia Mohd Hanafiah[5]

[1]Department of Computer Science & Engineering, Methodist College of Engineering and Technology, India
[2]Department of Computer Science & Engineering, Stanley College of Engineering & Technology for Women, India
[3,4]Department of Computer Science & Engineering, Keshav Memorial Institute of Technology, India
[5]Faculty of Science and Technology, Universi Kebangasaan Malaysia, Malaysia
E-mail: hmeenal0891@gmail.com; drckkreddy@gmail.com; rajinireddaboina35@gmail.com; lokapriya7852@gmail.com; mhmarlia@ukm.edu.my

Abstract

Convolutional neural network are used by biomarkers to diagnose Alzheimer's disease. To enable prompt intervention and improve patient outcomes, the project aims to improve early identification and precise prediction of disease development. With the help of Open Access Series of Imaging Studies (OASIS) the data is prepared for the model testing for prediction. The model train consists of few steps like preprocessing included standardizing and augmenting imaging data. Functional and structural biomarkers suggestive of AD were trained into the CNN. Different metrices like accuracy, Roc curve is used for predicting model performance. To make sure the findings could be applied to a wider audience, cross-validation methods were used. When it came to differentiating between AD, MCI, and healthy

DOI: 10.1201/9788743801764-12

control participants, the CNN model showed excellent accuracy. The model found distinct patterns of hippocampal shrinkage and alterations in cortical thickness as key biomarkers. By monitoring the course of the disease in MCI patients, the model's predictive abilities were confirmed and those who converted to AD were correctly predicted. The accuracy of CNN model is 99.95%. This work opens the door for the prediction of Alzheimer's disease using CNN model. The model's strong predictive abilities and high accuracy demonstrate its usefulness for early AD detection and monitoring in clinical settings. To further improve the model's therapeutic applicability, future studies should concentrate on integrating multimodal data and testing it across bigger and more diverse populations.

Keywords: Alzheimer's Disease, Biomarkers, Prognosis, Neuroimaging, Early Detection, Precision Medicine, Neurodegenerative Disorders, Diagnostics Cognitive Decline.

12.1 Introduction

Alzheimer's is basically a neurodegenerative disease that affects memory loss, behaviour change, and as well as lowering brain health overall [1]. It is the most prevalent cause of dementia in the early stage and is distinguished by a steadily declining ability to think [2]. The illness progresses gradually, starting with mild memory loss and possibly leading to major impairment in day-to-day activities and fundamental physiological functions [4]. Alzheimer's disease can cause a wide range of symptoms, but the most typical ones include memory loss, confusion, difficulty making decisions and solving problems, disorientation in time and space, and linguistic difficulties. People may find it difficult to remember recent discussions or occurrences in the early stages [6]. They may have behavioural and emotional changes as the illness worsens, such as increased agitation, anxiety, or depression. Severe memory loss develops in later stages, accompanied by a reduction in cognitive function, an inability to recognize loved ones, and a decline in motor functions like walking and swallowing.

Alzheimer's disease is more common in older age groups; hence elderly people are more vulnerable to it. Another important factor is genetics; people who have a family history of Alzheimer's disease are more vulnerable [8]. Some genetic factors, such the APOE ε4 allele, are linked to an increased risk of acquiring the illness. Understanding these genetic predispositions is critical to identifying at-risk individuals and initiating early therapy [10]. Alzheimer's disease risk also increases with other cardiovascular disorders such as diabetes, high blood pressure, and high cholesterol. This risk is further increased by lifestyle choices such as low cognitive engagement, poor eating habits, and physical inactivity. These elements emphasize the significance of preventing Alzheimer's disease holistically, addressing lifestyle and genetic variables to slow the illness's start and progression. Through deep learning-based biomarkers, the prediction of Alzheimer's may be efficient and accurate, allowing for earlier intervention and better patient outcomes [19]. In order to create these markers, which will eventually help with Alzheimer's disease early detection and therapy, it is critical to understand how genetic, cardiovascular, and lifestyle variables interact.

Table 12.1 provides a breakdown of all fatalities by year from 2010 to 2023, including numbers specific to men and women. The overall death toll has risen over this time, rising from 500,000 in 2010 to 760,000 in 2023. The data shows a steady trend wherein each year, there are more deaths among women than among men. 2010 saw 300,000 fatalities among women and 200,000 deaths among men. These numbers increased to 304,000 for males and 456,000 for women by 2023, continuing the long-term trend of women dying at a higher rate than men, graphically shown in Figure 12.1.

Table 12.2 shows number of deaths from 2010 to 2023, along with a breakdown by gender. The overall death toll has steadily increased during this time, going from 10,000 in 2010 to 17,500 in 2023. The statistics regularly indicates that there are more deaths among women than among men each year. 2010 saw 6,000 fatalities among women and 4,000 deaths among men. These figures rose to 10,500 deaths for women and 7000 deaths for men by

Table 12.1 Death rate for Alzheimer's disease in 2010–2023 across the globe.

S.no	Year	Total deaths	Men	Women
1	2010	500,000	200,000	300,000
2	2011	520,000	208,000	312,000
3	2012	540,000	216,000	324,000
4	2013	560,000	224,000	336,000
5	2014	580,000	232,000	348,000
6	2015	600,000	240,000	360,000
7	2016	620,000	248,000	372,000
8	2017	640,000	256,000	384,000
9	2018	660,000	264,000	396,000
10	2019	680,000	272,000	408,000
11	2020	700,000	280,000	420,000
12	2021	720,000	288,000	432,000
13	2022	740,000	296,000	444,000
14	2023	760,000	304,000	456,000

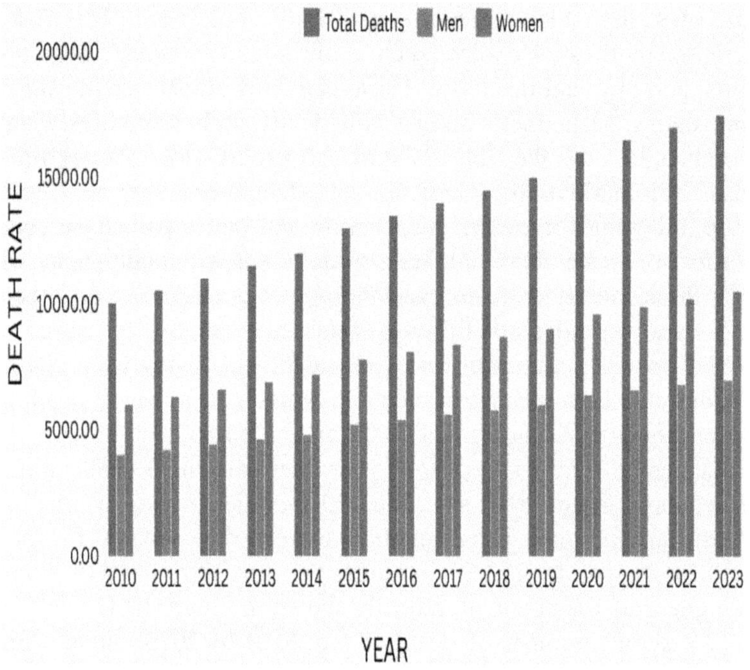

Figure 12.1 Mortality rates for Alzheimer's disease across the World from 2010 to 2023.

Table 12.2 Death rate for Alzheimer's disease in 2010–2023 across India.

S.no	Year	Total deaths	Men	Women
1	2010	10,000	4000	6000
2	2011	10,500	4200	6300
3	2012	11,000	4400	6600
4	2013	11,500	4600	6900
5	2014	12,000	4800	7200
6	2015	13,000	5200	7800
7	2016	13,500	5400	8100
8	2017	14,000	5600	8400
9	2018	14,500	5800	8700
10	2019	15,000	6000	9000
11	2020	16,000	6400	9600
12	2021	16,500	6600	9900
13	2022	17,000	6800	10,200
14	2023	17,500	7000	10,500

2023. This trend shows a persistent increase in mortality rates for both sexes throughout the course of the measured years, with a larger frequency among women, graphically shown in Figure 12.2.

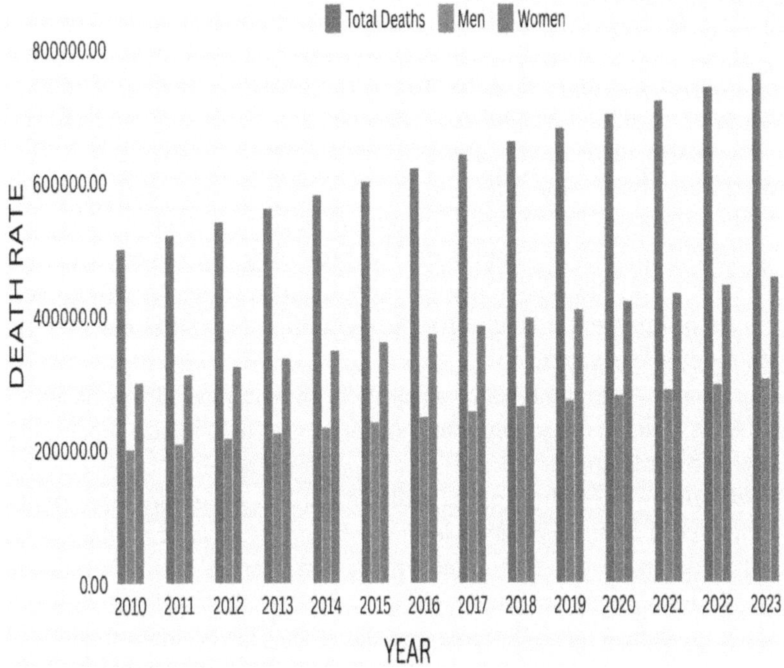

Figure 12.2 Mortality rates for Alzheimer's disease across the world from 2010 to 2023.

Numerous techniques, including deep learning and machine learning techniques, are put forth. These are the random forest classifiers [1], decision tree classifiers [1], support vector machine (SVM) [1], artificial neural network [3], generative adversarial network (GAN) [3], stacked auto-encoder (SAE) [4], deep neural network (DNN), and recurrent neural network (RNN) [6], bidirectional encoder [6], single value decomposition (SVD) [7], principal component analysis (PCA) [8], logistic regression [9], stochastic gradient descent (SGD) [14], gradient boosting classifier (GBC) [14], K-nearest neighbors (KNN) [14], multilayer perception (MLP) [14], PRISMA [17], NeAE-Eye [18], transfer learning and the Grad-CAM technique [29].

Existing approaches to Alzheimer's disease diagnosis and prognosis face several significant limitations. The sensitivity and precision required by current approaches, including neuroimaging and biomarker assays, are sometimes lacking, especially in the early phases when treatments could have the greatest potential impact. The cost and discomfort of invasive treatments such as PET scans and cerebrospinal fluid (CSF) analysis prevents widespread usage. Subjective clinical evaluations can cause inconsistent diagnosis, which makes it more difficult to provide patients with consistent and trustworthy care. Furthermore, these methods might not be able to accurately anticipate the course of a disease or customize a course of therapy for a given patient, which emphasizes the need for more sophisticated and accurate diagnostic instruments. Integrating deep-learning-based biomarkers could address these problems and enhance patient care and outcomes in Alzheimer's disease by offering increased accuracy, non-invasiveness, and the potential for early diagnosis. By providing improved accuracy, non-invasiveness, and the possibility of early identification, by using deep-learning-based biomarkers it is easy for the prediction of Alzheimer's for the patient treatment at early stage.

Table 12.3 shows the analysis of several diagnostic procedures based on important factors such as cost, accuracy, simplicity of use, intrusiveness, and creative use of biomarkers.

The Alzheimer's convolutional neural network is the main topic of the proposed chapter. The field of deep learning-based biomarkers, which have revolutionized determining Alzheimer's disease diagnosis and prognosis, is led by convolutional neural networks (CNNs). CNNs' unparalleled ability to analyse and comprehend complex imaging data has allowed them to analysis and detecting indications of Alzheimer's disease through PET and MRI images from the dataset. Through automation of the feature extraction process, CNNs are able to detect minute but significant alterations to the brain's composition and capabilities that may occur before the clinical symptoms. This deep learning method increases diagnosis accuracy and aids in prognostic assessments by predicting the disease's trajectory. The proposed chapter's primary focus is the Alzheimer's convolutional neural network. The field of deep learning-based biomarkers, which have revolutionized the diagnosis and

Table 12.3 Comparison of diagnostic methods for Alzheimer's disease.

Diagnostic method	Invasiveness	Cost	Accuracy	Accessibility	Novel biomarkers
Clinical assessments	Low	Low	Moderate	High	No
Neuroimaging	Moderate	High	High	Moderate	Limited
CSF biomarkers	High	High	High	Low	Yes
Genetic testing	Low	Moderate	Moderate	High	No
Deep learning-based	Low	Low	High	High	Yes

prognosis of Alzheimer's disease, is led by convolutional neural networks (CNNs). Because of CNN decipher and evaluation of image data it became easier to predict Alzheimer's using PET and MRI data. CNN is able to detect minute but significant alterations in the composition and functioning of the brain that take place prior than the clinical symptoms by the model extraction. By forecasting the course of the illness, this deep learning technique improves prognostic assessments and raises diagnosis accuracy.

12.2 Literature Survey

The author of [1] used phosphorylated-tau (CP-13) pictures, CBD, and PSD databases. They suggested a model for Alzheimer's disease that obtained performance values higher than 92% using decision tree class classifiers and random forest classifiers. These results show the adaptability of the model for predicting Alzheimer's disease diagnosis across various datasets. The Alzheimer's disease neuroimaging initiative (ADNI) and the Open Access Series of Imaging Studies (OASIS) were two of the numerous datasets that the authors used in [2]. They proposed convolutional neural networks (CNN), recurrent neural networks (RNN), and artificial neural networks (ANN) with the following accuracies: SVM-85.71%, CNN-98.6%, and RNN-91.2%. These results demonstrate the adaptability and potential of deep learning models for accurate Alzheimer's disease diagnosis across a range of datasets. The Alzheimer's disease Neuroimaging Initiative (ADNI) and the Open Access Series of Imaging Studies (OASIS) were two of the few datasets that the authors used in [3]. They suggested utilizing convolutional neural networks (CNN), artificial neural networks (ANN), and radio frequency (RF), which produced a wide range of accuracy of 90.3%.

Many datasets like Alzheimer's disease neuroimaging initiative (ADNI) are used by the authors in [4]. They suggested employing deep learning techniques, which produced a wide range of results, including 88.2% accuracy, 88.64% precision rate, 88.39% F1-score, and 11.84% false negative rate (FNR). Error rate: 0.12% and area under the curve (AUC): 0.92%. These findings highlight the deep learning models' versatility and promise for precise Alzheimer's disease diagnosis on a variety of datasets. In [5], the authors utilized multiple datasets including microarray gene expression. They proposed using preprocessing gene selection (SVD, CNN, PCA) which resulted in an accuracy of 96.09% and an error rate of less than 1%. These findings highlight the deep learning models' versatility and promise for precise Alzheimer's disease diagnosis on a variety of datasets. Numerous datasets like ADNI are used by the authors in [6]. They suggested a deep learning method known as variational Bayesian network, which produced results with an error rate of less than 1% and an accuracy of 98.57%. These findings highlight the deep learning models' versatility and promise for precise Alzheimer's disease identification across many datasets. Magnetic resonance imaging and the open access series of imaging studies datasets were among the most used datasets that the authors used [7]. They proposed a classification approach that yielded results with an error rate of less than 6% and 94% accuracy rate, 93% precision, 98% recall, and 96% accuracy, along with AUC values of 94.8%, 93%, 97.75%, and 99.7%.

Datasets like the author used the ADNI in [8]. They recommended deep learning (DL) techniques that produced a performance metric of 91.8% and an error rate of less than 9%. These findings highlight the deep learning models' versatility and promise for precise Alzheimer's on a variety of datasets. [9]'s author used datasets such pet photographs from MRI and the ADNI. They recommended deep learning (DL) techniques, which produced results with a 73.90% accuracy rate and a 26.1% error rate. These findings highlight the deep learning models' versatility and promise for precise Alzheimer's disease diagnosis on a variety of datasets. The MRI report is one of the datasets that the author of [10] used. They recommended deep learning (DL) techniques, which produced precision: Genetic algorithms with SVM: 96.80 SVM with 93.30 image processing; Fisher: 96.32 SVM: 92.48 95 Procedures for image processing and weight extraction; 91.40 Multimodal Neuroimaging arbitrary. Stochastic forest: 93 PCA using SVM: 95 CNN with various architectures: 98.08, less than 7.52% error rate on average. These findings show how versatile and promising deep learning models are for providing precise diagnoses of Alzheimer's across a variety of datasets. The author of [11] employed datasets, including the Training cum-validation dataset and the independent test dataset. They suggested machine learning (DL) methods that yielded results with less than 1% error rate and 0.9799% accuracy. These findings highlight the deep learning model's versatility and promise for precise Alzheimer's disease on the various datasets.

Korean based aging study for the diagnosis initiated the prediction of Alzheimer's disease (KBASE; kbase.kr) dataset was one of the datasets used by the author of [12] from the Severance Hospital. They recommended applying deep learning (DL) techniques, the results produced are accuracy with 78.05, sensitivity with 76.0, and F1-score with 74.0, respectively, with an error rate of 10–20%. These findings show how adaptable and efficient deep learning models are for predicting Alzheimer's disease using datasets. The dataset OASIS was utilized by the author of [13]. It was suggested to SVM SGD GBC KNN DT RF MLP. CNN provided accuracy of 94.61% for CNN and 92.12% for MLP with a 5.39 error rate range. The data collecting and preparation methods suggested by the author of [14] yielded an accuracy of 85% and an error rate of 15%. These findings highlight the deep learning models' versatility and promise for precise Alzheimer's disease diagnosis on various datasets. The authors of [15] used the OASIS dataset. CNN was suggested by them, and it produced results with an accuracy rate of 80% and an error rate of less than 20%. These findings highlight the deep learning models' versatility and promise for precise Alzheimer's disease diagnosis on various datasets. The authors of [16] used datasets from OASIS, ADNI, IXI, AIBL, MIRIAD, and MILAN. They advised using the PRISMA approach, which produced results with an error rate of less than 8.30% and an accuracy of 91.30%. These findings highlight the deep learning models' versatility and promise for precise Alzheimer's disease diagnosis on various datasets. The authors of [17] used eye tracking data. It was advised to use the NeAE-Eye approach, which produced results with an accuracy of 85% and an error rate of 15%. These findings highlight the deep learning models' versatility and promise for precise Alzheimer's disease diagnosis on various datasets.

The writers of [18] received information from the (AFAC) daycare centre. They suggested using CNN, which produced results with an error rate of less than 9% and an accuracy of 90.91%. These findings highlight the deep learning models' versatility and promise for precise Alzheimer's disease diagnosis on various datasets. The authors of [19] employed two-dimensional coronal view MRI image slices that they obtained from Kaggle. They suggested using transfer learning in conjunction with the Grad-CAM approach, which produced results with a 1% error rate and 99% accuracy. These findings highlight the deep learning models' versatility and promise for precise Alzheimer's disease diagnosis on various datasets. Table 12.4 shows the approaches for predicting Alzheimer's disease using different dataset and models. These works leverage the MRI, ADNI, and OASIS datasets in addition to machine learning and deep learning methods including CNN, RNN, SVM, and GAN. Performance evaluations demonstrate how well these techniques work to achieve high accuracy. Results are greatly enhanced by methods like data augmentation and transfer learning. The below tables show the approaches to Alzheimer's disease prediction.

Table 12.4 *Continued.*

Reference No	Dataset used	Algorithm proposed	Demerits
[1]	Images of phosphorylated-tau (CP13), (PSP), (CBD)	DT, RF	A lone researcher trained the diagnostic model using data from a single neuropathology laboratory, which may affect generalization.
[2]	ANDI, OASIS	CNN, SVM, RNN	Significant overlap high cost of acquiring fMRI data and restricted access to other datasets.
[3]	ADNI	CNN, SVM, RF	The datasets in the AD sector are still small compared to datasets in computer vision tasks since medical data privacy is an issue. Due to the complexity of AD-related tasks, researchers need a large-scale dataset in order to develop more powerful and efficient models.
[4]	ADNI	RNN, NM, MRI Biomarkers MLP	Complexity in feature learning, data dependency
[5]	Microarray gene expression data	Preprocessing Gene Selection (SVD, CNN, PCA)	High-dimensional data
[6]	ADNI	VBN, CNN, RNN, LR	Over-fitting ML is less effective than deep learning.
[7]	OASIS ,MRI Data	SVM, DT, RF, KNN	Susceptibility to over-fitting, high computational cost for prediction.
[8]	ADNI, NIFD	SGD	In the losser datasets the multiclassification performance is not up to the par.
[9]	MRI and PET images ADNI	DL methods	Lower sensitivity, complex architecture
[10]	MRI reports	SVM, CNN, PCA	Lower sensitivity, higher specificity, complex processes.
[11]	Training cum-validation on dataset Independent test dataset	ML methods	Obtaining all of these biomarkers for multiple marker examinations from a single patient is both costly and impractical. Our novel CSF protein combination offers the unique advantage of being economical, as it can precisely classify patients with AD in its early stages by profiling.
[12]	The Alzheimer's disease neuroimaging initiative includes the Korean brain aging study for the early diagnosis and prediction of Alzheimer's disease (KBASE; kbase.kr) dataset from Severance Hospital.	Deep learning framework technique	Large datasets 10% of false negative instances can be attributed to amyloid PET sensitivity.
[13]	The Imaging Studies Open Access Series (OASIS)	MLP, CNN	MLP gives less accuracy than CNN.

Table 12.4 Analysis of the existing approaches to Alzheimer's prediction.

Reference No	Dataset used	Algorithm proposed	Demerits
[14]	3D T1-weighted structural MRI data collected from two open accessible databases: NIFD and ADNI	CNN, SGD	Sensitivity to feature scaling, Computational Cost.
[15]	(OASIS-3) dataset	CNN	Early stopping of the model at the 80th iteration out of 100 epochs.
[16]	ADNI, OASIS, IXI, AIBL, MIRIAD, MILAN	PRISMA methodology	Data heterogeneity, Variability in pre-processing, Limited generalizability techniques.
[17]	Eye-tracking datasets	NeAE-Eye	Lack of large-scale eye-tracking datasets, current models and algorithms are mostly applied to 2D displays.
[18]	Data from (AFAC) daycare centre	CNN	Few sequences are obtained for each patient, seek to increase the size of the original dataset.
[19]	Two-dimensional MRI image slices in the coronal view, sourced from Kaggle	Transfer learning and the Grad-CAM technique	Limited dataset, over-fitting risk.

12.3 Materials and Methods

12.3.1 Dataset

The Washington University Knight Alzheimer Disease Research Center collected clinical data on MRI and PET imaging results from 1098 people over a 15-year period. This data is known as the OASIS dataset. The ages of the participants range from 42 to 95 years old and comprise 493 persons in varying stages of cognitive decline and 605 adults with full cognitive functioning. The OASIS collection contains around 2000 MR Sessions with different functional and structural sequences. Together with raw imaging scans from the PET metabolic and amyloid imaging, about 1500 images from the PET Unified pipelines (PUP) are viewable. Another benefit provided by OASIS is access to imaging data which was post-processed, including 3D image analysis and positron emission tomography investigations. The imaging data includes APOE, mental state, and long-term thinking, and behavioural effects. The OASIS dataset is made available to the scientific community for use in studying dementia and healthy aging-related topics. In addition to its longitudinal dataset, OASIS also contains a cross-sectional dataset.

Researchers and other interested parties can access brain imaging data from the organization OASIS dataset. The OASIS longitudinal [6] and OASIS cross-sectional [5] datasets were obtained using MRI image neuroanatomical atlases. OASIS is a neuroimaging biomarker that can be used in both healthy individuals and AD patients, both cross-sectionally and longitudinally. Clinical and demographic data are supplied in the file in XML format. Data obtained from magnetic resonance imaging scans. For additional details on the picture properties and terminology, visit http://www.oasisbrains.org/longitudinal_facts.html (accessed on May 25, 2021). Fifteen features from 374 patients – of whom 37 are converted, 190 are demented, and 147 are not included in the oasis longitudinal dataset. The age range of the patients is sixty to ninety years old.

12.3.2 Data preprocessing

There are several data pre-processing techniques utilized to create a clean data collection for the investigations. To increase the precision and caliber of the analytical findings, clinical datasets related to Alzheimer's disease can be pre-processed using a variety of techniques. Pre-processing techniques that researchers most frequently employ include data cleaning which is the process of eliminating and rectifying any erroneous, faulty, or absent information from a dataset. This method normally starts with looking for anomalies, discrepancies, and missing values in the data thereafter altering or getting rid of them. Feature selection is the process of choosing the most important features that are expected to have a considerable influence on the analysis' findings from the dataset. This can be accomplished using a variety of statistical methods, including principal component analysis, mutual information, and correlation analysis. The process of transforming the data into an analysis-ready format is called as data transformation. Applying techniques like normalization, logarithmic transformation, and standardization will help achieve this.

Imputation entails substituting approximated values for the blanks. Many imputation techniques, including mean imputation, regression imputation, and multiple imputations, can be used to achieve this. Imaging datasets for Alzheimer's disease include PET and MRI scans. The following pre-processing techniques were applied to the research articles that this review article reviewed. The practice of aligning each intensity value in an image with every other image is known as image normalization. To do this, techniques including histogram equalization, contrast stretching, and normalization can be leveraged to enhance the images' visual presentation. Cropping and resizing images include resizing the photos to a uniform size and removing any extraneous components from the picture. This could increase the approaches' efficiency and lower the analysis's computing complexity. Enhancement of images This technique uses a number of modifications, including rotation, flipping, and scaling, to generate additional images from the original dataset. By doing so, the dataset may be increased and the analysis's resilience can be strengthened. Extraction of features during this stage, i.e., pertinent features from the photos that can be utilized for analysis are extracted. Techniques like edge detection, texture analysis, and form analysis can be used for this.

An important step in data mining is data cleaning, which entails replacing missing values and eliminating anomalies. We now analysed the distribution of categorical and numerical columns to determine which features align with our research goals; these attributes should not have a substantial relationship with the target trait. In order to eliminate them, we also looked at characteristics with distinct values. Missing values and incorrect data types were the next topics we covered. No correlation was observed between the Subject ID, MRI ID, and the target feature. The hand feature was also non-informative, having a constant value of R. Therefore, these columns were removed from the dataset to reduce dimensionality.

Processing the unbalance of the OASIS dataset

Three imbalanced classes make up the 373 rows in the Open Access Series of Imaging Studies dataset. Three classifications, representing changing frequencies within the dataset, are non-demented (190 instances, or 51% of the dataset), demented (147 instances, or 39%), and converted (37 occurrences, or 10%). In this study, we applied the SMOTE algorithm to reduce the impact of class imbalance. SMOTE is a useful method for achieving dataset equilibrium. The SMOTE technique finds the minority class's nearest neighbors, creates new samples for the minority class at random intervals, and chooses the minority class ranks at random.

The performance of classification is significantly impacted by the size of the training set. In each of the previously described datasets, there is a cap on the quantity of imaging scans that were recovered from individuals suffering from AD and MCI. Pre-processing is usually required in investigations before data tampering. Pre-processing is the term used to describe a set of image processing processes carried out on the resulting image scans. Many MRI software packages, such statistical parametric mapping (SPM), computational anatomy toolbox (CAT12), FMRIB Software Library (FSL) (Jenkinson et al., 2012), Free Surfer (Fischl, 2012), ANTS (Avants et al.,

2009), etc., have well-encapsulated pre-processing approaches accessible for them. Temporal filtering, covariates removal, registration, normalization, smoothing, segmentation, skull-stripping, and noise reduction are preprocessing techniques that are commonly used. This review will address intensity normalization, registration, tissue segmentation, skull-stripping, and class balancing.

When dealing with datasets that exhibit significant range variability, normalization is essential to the data preparation phase. This is especially true after turning nominal values (1 and 2) into real numbers. Due to a lack of standardization, some traits might be more prevalent than others with smaller numerical ranges, which could induce biases in the analysis. Normalization not only minimizes these biases but also facilitates algorithm performance by restricting the use of broad datasets. This guarantees a more exhaustive and unbiased inquiry, supporting the overall stability of the ensuing data-driven procedures. Here, values are kept between 0 and 1, in accordance with eqn (12.1), by data scaling. Min a denotes the attribute's lowest value, whereas max a denotes its highest value, the scaled value by x normalized, and the attribute's initial value by x in this equation. By transforming the values of each characteristic into a predetermined range, this scaling method facilitates consistency and comparison across the various features in the dataset. The normalization method ensures that the initial scale of the attributes will not affect later research, allowing for a more thorough and precise analysis of the data.

$$X_{\text{Normalized}} = \frac{\mathrm{x} - \min}{\max - \min}. \tag{12.1}$$

12.4 CNN for Alzheimer's Prediction

To address complex learning tasks, a specialized subset of machine learning called deep learning uses a hierarchical architecture made up of several layers. Deep learning techniques have acquired a lot of popularity in recent years and are now frequently used in different brain research projects. Convolutional neural networks (CNNs) are particularly popular among these techniques. CNNs can effectively recognize and analyze patterns in input data by extracting pertinent features through the use of convolutional procedures. The field has rapidly grown and extended as a result of CNN's outstanding performance in a variety of applications, including object identification, classification, and segmentation. CNNs are closely watched by researchers because they have yielded state-of-the-art results in various domains like as medical imaging, natural language processing, and computer vision. The remarkable efficiency of CNN in classifying and dividing reality-based photos utilized in application development.

The input layer provides data to the network. The input for image data in this layer is a multi-dimensional array representing the image. Convolutional layers perform convolution operations to the input data through a sequence of learnable filters to extract features such as edges, shapes, and textures. It is made up of filters and kernels: Little matrices are slid over the input image to build feature maps. For example, a 3×3 filter only captures a small percentage of the input image. The mechanism of activation ReLU (rectified linear unit) is usually added after the convolution procedure to add non-linearity. By keeping only the most important data, the pooling layer – more especially, the max pooling technique –down samples the feature maps. Through this procedure, the spatial dimensions are lowered, which lowers the number of factors and processing demands. Max pooling is a useful technique for capturing the most prominent features in a feature map by choosing the maximum value from each patch. Dense layer performs higher-level reasoning and classification using the features that have been gathered by the convolutional and pooling layers. Neurons in a dense layer in a neural network are connected to all other neurons in the layer above it. This allows the network to learn complex representations. Activation function: Common activation functions (in classification issues) are SoftMax for the output layer and ReLU complex for hidden layers. The output layer, which normally consists of as many neurons as there are classes in a classification issue, produces final predictions.

Algorithm for Alzheimer's prediction using CNN

1. Input, dataset, dataset true labels,word2vec matrix
2. Find the output score for the model using test dataset
3. Set 3d matrix using f as feature
4. For j in i
5. Set feature set matrix for sample i
6. For j in i
7. Vectorize vj
8. Append f from fi
9. Set ftrain, ftest, ltrain into train and test subsets
10. Evaluate score using ftrain and ltrain
11. At last return score for the model

After multiplying two Maricely represented images, a new matrix is created from which a convolutional network retrieves attributes. Two stages are carried out by Convolutional Neural Networks (CNNs): first, they automatically extract pertinent characteristics from the input data, and then they classify these features into predetermined categories. CNNs' capacity to learn and generalize characteristics from big datasets is one of their main advantages. Using the set of input image, the convolution operation creates a series of feature maps that highlight significant structures and patterns. A pooling layer is used to minimize the dimensions of these feature maps and highlight the most significant features, allowing the model to concentrate on the most pertinent data. The offsets of the subregion in the x and y directions are indicated by the variables "a" and "b," respectively. The bottom-right corner of the subregion is indicated by these offsets, which are binary numbers (0 or 1) that represent its location in relation to the origin ($2x$, $2y$).

$$fx_1(s) = \max, b = 0s2x + 2y + b \tag{12.2}$$

Convolutional architectures are used by CNNs, a class of feed-forward neural networks, to extract features from input automatically and without the need for human involvement. On the other hand, manual feature engineering is the foundation of conventional feature extraction techniques. The CNN's activation functions mimic the biological neurons' threshold-based signal propagation mechanism, while the CNN's kernels represent a variety of receptors with varying patterns and features recognition abilities. CNN outperforms other generic artificial neural network. Local connectivity in CNNs helps reduce the number of parameters, as each neuron is only connected to a small region of the input, rather than the entire layer. This significantly reduces computational complexity and speeds up training. Additionally, weight sharing across the network further minimizes the number of parameters by reusing the same filter across different parts of the image. Downsampling, typically done through pooling layers, reduces the spatial dimensions of feature maps while preserving the most important information. This procedure lowers the model's parameter count while simultaneously increasing its effectiveness. Convolution is a crucial step in feature extraction that is highly relied upon by convolutional neural networks (CNNs), the foundation of deep learning, to produce feature maps that effectively capture the essence of the input image. The size of the convolution kernel, however, needs to be carefully considered since it can result in information loss at the image borders, highlighting the necessity of wise kernel selection.

12.5 Result and Discussion

Accuracy is the degree to which a diagnostic test correctly finds or excludes a condition. A high true positive rate indicates that a test is accurate; a high true negative rate indicates that it is not accurate in identifying those who do not have the ailment. It is necessary for precise diagnosis and therapy planning. A few elements that impact accuracy are the caliber of the test, the technology used, and the experience of the healthcare professionals. Achieving high diagnosis accuracy in medicine is essential to patient safety and effective treatment outcomes. The accuracy of several current models is displayed in Table 12.4. The benchmark for performance Table 12.5 illustrates the accuracy. The graphical depiction of the different current model accuracy rates is shown in Figure 12.3.

$$\text{Accuracy} = \frac{\text{TP} + \text{TN}}{(\text{TP} + \text{TN} + \text{FP} + \text{FN}) * 100}. \tag{12.3}$$

Table 12.5 shows the accuracy of various existing models compared with proposed model. From the below table CNN has high accuracy compared to other existing models that is 99.95%. The graphical representation of accuracy for different models is shown in Figure 12.4.

One essential statistic in machine learning that 'is used to assess a classification model's performance is its error rate. It shows the percentage of inaccurate predictions the model produced out of all the predictions. The error rate directly measures how frequently the model predictions do not match the actual labels in the dataset. Understanding the error rate is essential to determining how effective a machine learning model is. Better performance,

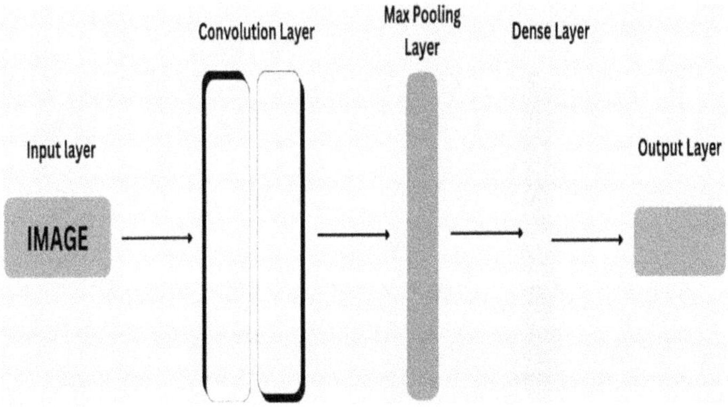

Figure 12.3 Convolutional neural network for Alzheimer's prediction.

Table 12.5 Comparision of accuracy of proposed models on various existing models.

S.no	Model name	Accuracy(%)
1	CNN	99.95
2	DTRF	95
3	SVM	85.71
4	RF	90.3
5	RNN	88.24
6	Preprocessing gene selection (SVD)	96.09
7	VBN	98.57
8	KNN	99.7
9	SGD	91.83
10	DL methods	73.9
11	PCA	95
12	ML methods	97
13	Deep learning model technique	75
14	MLP	92.12
15	SGD	85
16	GBC	80
17	PRISMA methodology	91.30
18	NeAE-Eye	85
19	PCA	90.91
20	Transfer learning and the Grad-CAM technique	99

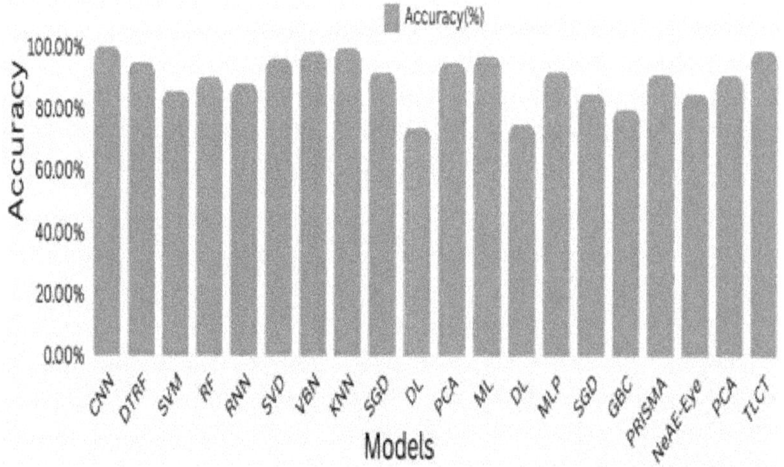

Figure 12.4 Comparision of accuracy of proposed model with various existing models.

or fewer errors made by the model, is indicated by a lower error rate. On the other hand, if the error rate is more the model prediction are not accurate.

$$\text{Error Rate} = \frac{\text{No of incorrect Predictions}}{\text{Total no of Predictions}}. \tag{12.4}$$

Another popular indicator for assessing model performance is accuracy, which has a tight relationship with the error rate. The percentage of accurate forecasts among all predictions is known as accuracy. There is a clear correlation between accuracy and mistake rate. Table 12.6 shows the error rate of various models, from the below table we conclude that the least error rate model is CNN compared with other existing models. The graphical representation of error rates with various existing models are shown in Figure 12.5.

Recall is the proportion of true positives that a diagnostic test or model correctly detects. The other name of recall is true positive. Recall is calculated as shown in eqn (12.5). When a test or model has a high recall rate, it reduces the frequency of false negatives by accurately capturing the bulk of positive occurrences. In order to ensure that potentially harmful illnesses are not missed and to enable early diagnosis and treatment, high recall is crucial in medical diagnostics. Optimal recall often requires balancing precision and memory to provide the best overall diagnostic performance.

Table 12.6 Comparisons of error rate of proposed model with various existing models.

S.no	Model name	Error rate (%)
1	CNN	0.05
2	DTRF	5
3	SVM	14.26
4	RF	9.7
5	RNN	11.76
6	Preprocessing gene selection (SVD)	3.91
7	VBN	1.43
8	KNN	0.3
9	SGD	8.17
10	DL methods	26.1
11	PCA	5
12	ML methods	3
13	Deep learning model technique	25
14	MLP	7.88
15	SGD	15
16	GBC	20
17	PRISMA methodology	8.7
18	NeAE-Eye	15
19	PCA	9.09
20	Transfer learning and the Grad-CAM technique	1

$$\text{Recall} = \frac{\text{True Positive}}{\text{True Positive} + \text{False Negative}}. \tag{12.5}$$

Table 12.7 shows the recall rate of various existing models. From the below table results CNN model has recall value of 96.30, which is higher

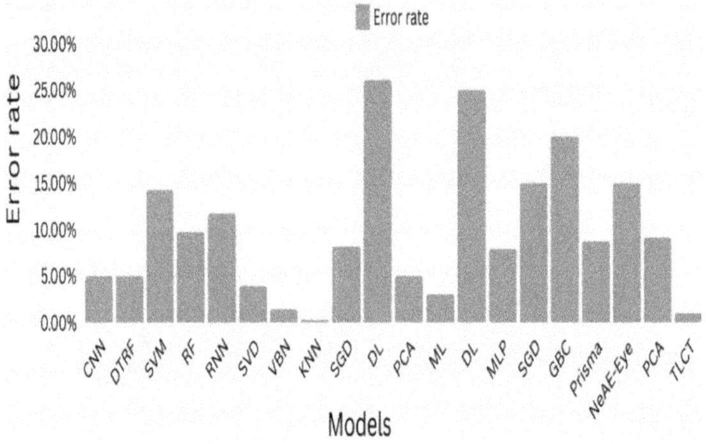

Figure 12.5 Comparisons of error rate of proposed model on various existing model.

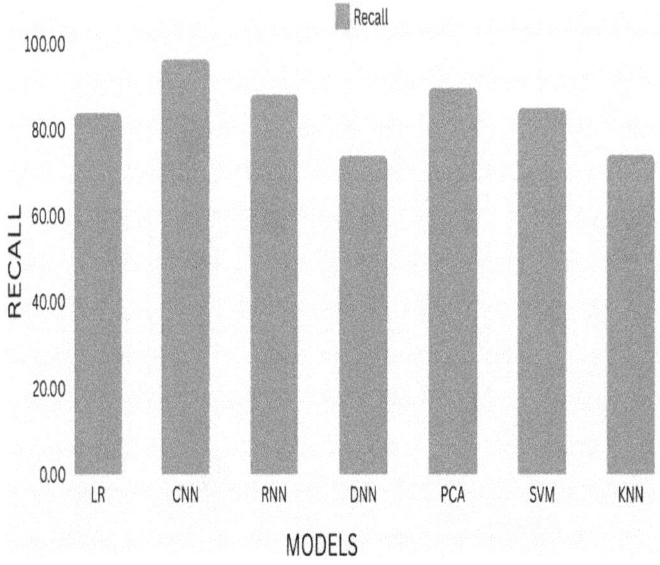

Figure 12.6 Comparing the proposed model's recall rates with several other model.

than the other models. A graphical representation of recall value with other existing models is shown in Figure 12.6.

Precision is an important metric to consider when evaluating classification algorithms, especially where false positives can have a big financial impact, as in spam, fraud, and medical diagnosis. Precision is calculated as shown in eqn (12.6). When the model has low false positive value then we say that positive predictions are accurate. This is the trade-off between precision and recall. Recall is usually sacrificed for precision. Precision is a critical factor in the creation of reliable and trustworthy classification models for a variety of real-world applications since the area under this curve Table 12.8, shows the precision value of the proposed model on various existing models. Figure 12.5 shows the graphical representation of various existing models for precision value.

$$\text{Precision} = \frac{\text{True Positive}}{\text{True Positive} + \text{False Positive}}. \tag{12.6}$$

Table 12.8 shows the precision values for the various models. From the table we conclude that CNN model has high precision value that is 93.80 among the other existing models. Graphical representation of precision valve for the models is shown in Figure 12.7.

Table 12.7 Comparison of recall of proposed model with various existing models.

S.no	Model name	Recall
1	LR	83.90
2	CNN	96.30
3	RNN	88.16
4	DNN	73.90
5	PCA	89.61
6	SVM	85.05
7	KNN	74.04

Table 12.8 Comparision of precision of proposed model on various existing models.

S.No	Model name	Precision
1	CNN	93.80
2	LR	82.49
3	RNN	88.24
4	GAN	72.12
5	PCA	93.01
6	SVM	91
7	KNN	72

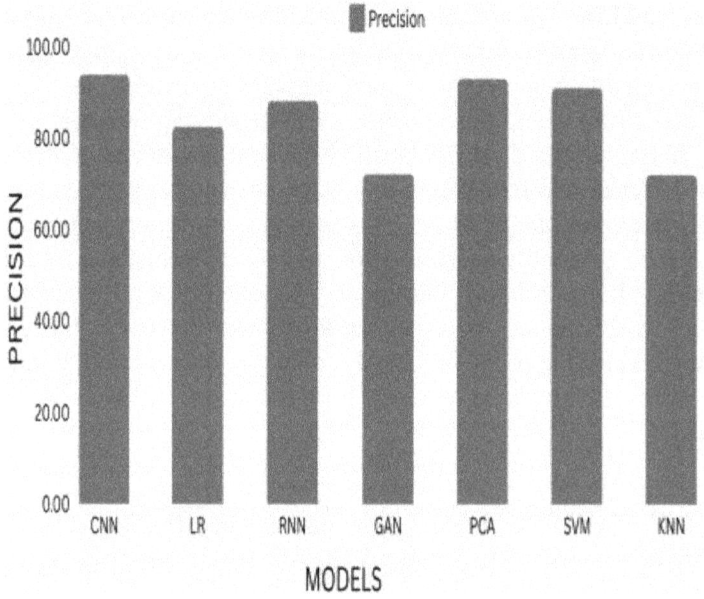

Figure 12.7 Comparing the proposed model's precision rates with several other models.

12.6 Conclusion

Alzheimer's disease is dangerous neurological condition that progressively goes worst over time, affecting cognitive function, leading to severe memory loss and the inability to do even basic tasks. It is a common cause of dementia that affects millions of people globally, especially the elderly. Alzheimer's disease places a tremendous strain on all those involved, including family members and caregivers. In this study, we concentrate on applying cutting-edge machine learning methods to enhance Alzheimer's disease diagnosis and prognosis. To be more precise, we use a convolutional neural network (CNN) in conjunction with the extensive brain imaging dataset from OASIS to find and examine disease-related biomarkers. Using this dataset, we train the CNN and compare its results with those of other available methods.

The research utilized a range of assessment criteria, including accuracy, recall, error rate, precision, and several other elements that are critical to assessing the performance of diagnostic models. Comprehensive testing and analysis show that CNN outperforms traditional methods in each and every one of these characteristics. The CNN model shows great potential as a powerful tool for early diagnosis and prognosis as it has been demonstrated to be a highly accurate and reliable way of identifying biomarkers associated with dementia. A proficient way for timely diagnosis of Alzheimer's disease can lead to improved management and treatment strategies, thereby shortening the illness's course and improving patients' quality of life. Furthermore, the use of CNNs in medical imaging and diagnostics creates new opportunities in clinical and research uses, which makes this a noteworthy advancement in the medical field. The study concludes by demonstrating how well convolutional neural networks can diagnose and prognosticate Alzheimer's disease. Our work highlights the possible use of these machine learning techniques in the fight against Alzheimer's disease by showing the superiority of CNNs over traditional methods using the OASIS dataset.

References

[1] Shunsuke Koga, Akihiro Ikeda, Dennis W Dickson,"Deep learning-based model for diagnosing Alzheimer's disease and tauopathies", WILEY British Neuropathological Society,2021.

[2] Akhilesh Deep Arya, Sourabh Singh Verma, Prasun Chakarabarti, Tulika Chakrabarti, Ahmed A. Elngar, Ali-Mohammad Kamali, and Mohammad Nami, "A systematic review on machine learning and deep learning techniques in the effective diagnosis of Alzheimer's disease", Springer Brain Informatics 2023.

[3] Zhen Zhao, Joon Huang Chuah, Khin Wee Lai, Chee-Onn Chow, MunkhjargalGochoo, Samiappan Dhanalakshmi, Na Wang, Wei Bao, and Xiang Wu, "Conventional machine learning and deep learning in Alzheimer's disease diagnosis using neuroimaging", Frontiers Computational Neuroscience 2023.

[4] Anza Aqeel, Ali Hassan, Muhammad Attique Khan, Saad Rehman, Usman Tariq, Seifedine Kadry, Arnab Majumdar, and OrawitThinnukool, "A Long Short-Term Memory Biomarker-Based Prediction Framework for Alzheimer's Disease", MDPI Sensors 2022.

[5] Mahmoud M. Abdelwahab, Khamis A. Al-Karawi, and Hatem E. Semary, "Deep Learning-Based Prediction of Alzheimer's Disease Using Microarray Gene Expression Data", MDPI Biomedicines 2023.

[6] SuganyadeviSellappan, Shiny Pershiya Anand, Finney Daniel Shadrach, Balasamy Krishnasamy, Renu Karra, Umamaheshwari Annamalai, "A Survey of Alzheimer's disease diagnosis using deep learning approaches", frontiers Autonomous Intelligence 2024.

[7] BadieaAbdulkarem Mohammed, Ebrahim Mohammed Senan, Taha H. Rassem, Nasrin M. Makbol, AdwanAlownie Alanazi, Zeyad Ghaleb Al-Mekhlafi, Tariq S. Almurayziq, and Fuad A. Ghaleb, "MultiMethod Analysis of Medical Records and MRI Images for Early Diagnosis of Dementia and Alzheimer's Disease Based on Deep Learning and Hybrid Methods", MDPI Electronics 2021.

[8] Jingjing Hu1, Zhao Qing, Renyuan Liu, Xin Zhang, Pin Lv, Maoxue Wang, Yang Wang, Kelei He1, Yang Gao, Bing Zhang, "Deep Learning based Classification", Frontiers in Neuroscience 2021.

[9] Modupe Odusami, Rytis Maskeliūnas, Robertas Damasevicius, Sanjay Misra, "Deep-Learning-Based Diagnosis of Alzheimer's Disease Using Multimodal Input Fusion of PET and MRI Images", Springer Medical and Biological Engineering 2023.

[10] Omer Asghar Dara, Jose Manuel Lopez-Guede, Hasan Issa Raheem, Javad Rahebi, Ekaitz Zulueta, and Unai Fernandez-Gamiz, "Alzheimer's Disease Diagnosis Using Machine Learning", MDPI Applied Sciences 2023.

[11] Asif Hassan Syed, Tabrej Khan, Atif Hassan, Nashwan Alromema, Muhammad Binsawad, "An EnsembleLearning Based Application to Predict the Earlier Stages of Alzheimer's Disease", IEEE 2020

[12] Suhong Kim, Peter Lee, Kyeong Taek Oh, Min Soo Byun, Daehyun Yi, Jun Ho Lee, Yu Kyeong Kim, Byoung Seok Ye, Mi Jin Yun, Dong Young Lee, and Yong Jeong, "Deep learning-based amyloid PET positivity classification model in the Alzheimer's disease continuum by using 2-FDG PET", Springer EJNMMI research 2021.

[13] Waqas Haider Bangyal, Najeeb Ur Rehman, Asma Nawaz, Kashif Nisar, Ag. Asri Ag. Ibrahim, Rabia Shakir, and Danda B. Rawat, "Constructing Domain Ontology for Alzheimer Disease Using Deep Learning Based Approach", MDPI Electronics 2022.

[14] Jinglin Sun, Yu Liu, Hao Wu, Peiguang Jing, and Yong Ji, "A novel deep learning approach for diagnosing Alzheimer's disease based on eye-tracking data", Frontiers in Human Neuroscience 2022.

[15] Gopi Battineni, Nalini Chintalapudi, Francesco Amenta, and Enea Traini, "Deep Learning Type Convolution Neural Network Architecture for Multiclass Classification of Alzheimer's Disease", Research gate 2021.

[16] Deevyankar Agarwal, Gonçalo Marques, Isabel de la Torre-Díez, Manuel A. Franco Martin 3, Begoña GarcíaZapiraín, and Francisco

Martín Rodríguez, "Transfer Learning for Alzheimer's Disease through Neuroimaging Biomarkers", MDPI Sensors 2021.

[17] Jinglin Sun, Yu Liu, Hao Wu, Peiguang Jing, and Yong Ji, "A novel deep learning approach for diagnosing Alzheimer's disease based on eye-tracking data", Frontiers in Human Neuroscience 2022.

[18] Santos Bringasa, Sergio Salomónb, Rafael Duquec, Carmen Laged, José Luis Montañac, "Alzheimer's Disease stage identification using deep learning models", Elsevier Biomedical Informatics 2020.

[19] Manu Raju, Thirupalani M, Vidhyabharathi S, and Thilagavathi S, "Deep Learning Based Multilevel Classification of Alzheimer's Disease using MRI Scans", ICCSSS 2020.

[20] Vijeeta Patil, Manohar Madgi, and Ajmeera Kiran, "Early Prediction of Alzheimer's disease using convolutional neural network", Springer 2022.

[21] Tausifa Jan Saleem, Syed Rameem Zahra, Fan Wu, Ahmed Alwakeel, Mohammed Alwakeel, Fathe Jeribi, and Mohammad Hijji,"Deep learning-based diagnosis of Alzheimer's disease",MDPI 2022.

[22] ChangxingQu, YinxiZou, YingqiaoMa, QinChen, JiaweiLuo, HuiyongFan, ZhiyunJia, Qiyong Gong, and Taolin Chen, "Diagnostic Performance of Generative Adversarial Network-Based Deep Learning Methods for Alzheimer's Disease", Frontiers 2022.

[23] DeevyankarAgarwal, Manuel Álvaro Berbís, Antonio Luna, VivianLipari, Julien Brito Ballester, and Isabel de la Torre-Díez1, "Automated Medical Diagnosis of AlzheimerÂt's Disease Using an Efficient Net Convolutional Neural Network", Springer 2023.

[24] GowharMohiud din dar, Avinash Bhagat, Syed Immamul Ansarullah, Mohamed Tahar Ben Othman, Yasir Hamid, Hend Khalid Alkahtani, Inam Ullah and Habib Hamam, "A Novel Framework for Classification of Different Alzheimer's Disease Stages Using CNN Model", MDPI 2023.

[25] Anza Aqeel, Ali Hassan, Muhammad Attique Khan, Saad Rehman, Usman Tariq, Seifedine Kadry, Arnab Majumdar, and OrawitThinnukool, "A Long Short-Term Memory Biomarker-Based Prediction Framework for Alzheimer's Disease", MDPI 2022.

[26] Jenkinson, M., Beckmann, C. F., Behrens, T. E., Woolrich, M. W., & Smith, S. M. (2012). FSL. *NeuroImage*, 62(2), 782-790.

13

Generative AI Novel Drug Discovery Avenues

M. V. Vijaya Saradhi, Ch. Srivatsa Alivelu Mangatayi, N. Swathi, and K. Swathi

Department of Computer Science and Engineering,
ACE Engineering College, India
E-mail: meduri.vsd@gmail.com; srivatsajava@gmail.com;
swathippscse@gmail.com; swathi0990@gmail.com

Abstract

This chapter explores the utilization of generative AI in diagnosing and treating neurodegenerative diseases, aiming to enhance our understanding of these complex conditions and support the development of more effective treatment strategies. By reviewing the existing research methods, the chapter highlights how AI-driven models can process large-scale neurological data, identify patterns, and predict disease progression with greater accuracy than traditional approaches. The potential for generative AI to assist in creating personalized treatment plans, simulate disease scenarios, and explore novel drug discovery avenues is also examined. Insights from the recent studies demonstrate how AI can improve clinical decision-making and patient outcomes. In addition to discussing technological advancements, the chapter addresses significant challenges. These include ethical concerns surrounding data privacy, the potential for biased algorithms, and the limitations of current datasets, which may not be representative of diverse patient populations. The

DOI: 10.1201/9788743801764-13

chapter calls for more inclusive, transparent AI models that prioritize patient safety while maximizing the technology's potential. Drawing from the latest research, the objective is to provide a comprehensive overview of current opportunities and future possibilities, with an emphasis on how generative AI can reshape the diagnosis and treatment of neurodegenerative diseases, ultimately contributing to improved patient care and clinical outcomes.

Keywords: Generative AI, Neurodegenerative Disorders, AI-driven Diagnostics, AI-Based Biomarkers, Brain Imaging Analysis, Automated Diagnostic Systems.

13.1 Introduction

Chronic neurological disorders, such as Alzheimer's and Parkinson's affect a significant portion of the global population. These conditions are marked by the gradual decline of neuronal function, leading to severe consequences that disrupt individuals' daily lives. Researchers are exploring various methods to tackle these challenges, with generative AI emerging as a promising tool. Understanding the value of AI in both research and patient care is crucial. This chapter aims to explore recent innovations in the field, professional perspectives, and the associated challenges.

Generative AI refers to systems that can create new content or data based on the input provided. In the context of neurodegenerative disorders, generative AI can analyze vast amounts of medical data, including genetics, patient histories, and medical imaging. This capability enables early disease diagnosis, prognosis, and even the discovery of new treatment strategies [1].

One of the primary benefits of AI is its ability to process data much faster than humans, which can lead to quicker diagnoses and more personalized treatment options. For example, AI is now being used to diagnose conditions like dementia at early stages by analyzing brain scans. These advancements have the potential to significantly improve patient care [2].

Additionally, generative AI can aid in drug discovery by predicting how newly developed compounds may interact with proteins associated with neurodegenerative diseases. This can streamline the drug development process, making it more efficient and cost-effective, ultimately leading to more accurate treatments for patients. The generative AI in neurodegenerative disorder approach is shown in Figure 13.1.

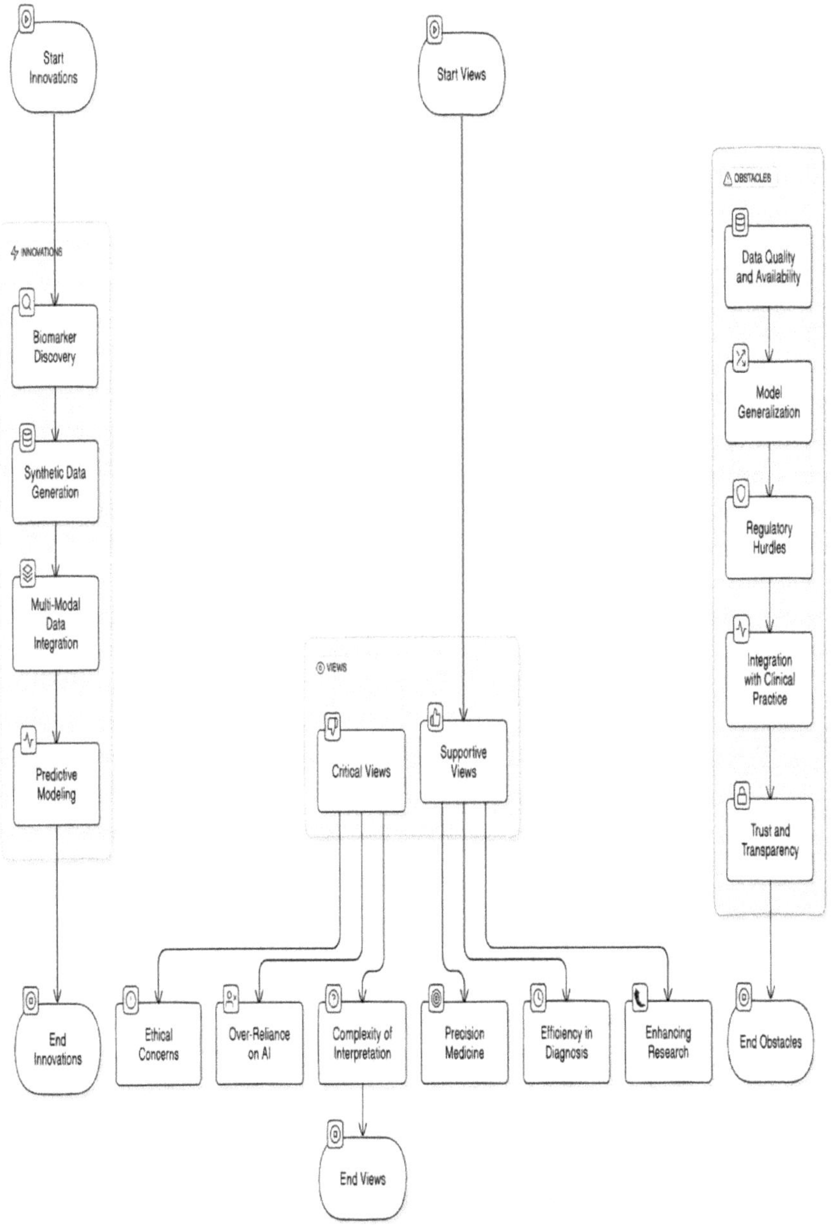

Figure 13.1 Generative AI in neurodegenerative disorder.

13.2 Applications and Use Cases

Early detection: AI systems can be leveraged to identify early signs of conditions like Alzheimer's by analyzing MRI scans and detecting patterns that may not be easily visible to human physicians. This capability enables earlier and more accurate diagnoses [3].

Drug development: AI can predict how different compounds will interact with biological markers, offering insights that can elevate the process of developing new medications, particularly for diseases like Parkinson's. This could lead to more effective and innovative drug solutions.

Personalized action plans: A major advancement achieved through AI is its ability to analyze patient-specific data and create customized treatment plans based on the individual's unique medical profile. This ensures that therapies are tailored to the specific needs and conditions of each patient.

Support for caregivers: AI-powered tools can also provide valuable assistance to caregivers, helping them perform their duties more efficiently and offering crucial support in their daily tasks, ultimately improving the quality of care provided to patients.

13.2.1 Challenges and limitations in applications and use cases

In [3], despite the vast potential of generative AI, several obstacles limit its widespread adoption in addressing neurodegenerative disorders:

1. Data privacy: Managing sensitive health information raises serious concerns regarding patient privacy. It is essential to ensure that patient data is protected at all times, and regulations must be strictly followed to prevent any breaches.
2. Bias in data: If the datasets used to train AI models are biased or incomplete, the resulting models may be ineffective or unrepresentative for different populations. This issue can lead to inaccurate diagnoses and treatments for diverse patient groups.
3. Ethical concerns: Ethical issues become particularly significant in healthcare, especially as AI increasingly influences treatment decisions. The use of AI in these critical areas requires clear guidelines to define its role and limitations, ensuring ethical decision-making processes.
4. Administrative and regulatory hurdles: Implementing AI tools in healthcare systems often faces bureaucratic challenges, slowing down the development and adoption of AI solutions due to organizational resistance and complex regulatory frameworks [11].

In light of these challenges, it is clear that while generative AI holds significant promise for research and treatment of neurodegenerative diseases, its application is not without limitations. Governance plays a crucial role in balancing innovation with ethical considerations. The pace of technological progress must be accompanied by ongoing dialogue between scientists, clinicians, and ethicists to ensure responsible deployment of AI in healthcare. Greater emphasis must be placed on solving data-related challenges, particularly regarding privacy and the need to build robust, diverse datasets. Additionally, there remains limited evidence on the long-term impact of AI solutions on patient care [3, 4].

Generative AI is increasingly being used to diagnose and understand neurodegenerative diseases such as Alzheimer's, Huntington's, and Parkinson's. Below is an overview of the current innovations, perspectives, and challenges in this rapidly evolving field.

13.3 Innovations in Modern Diagnosing Methods

13.3.1 AI-driven biomarker discovery in neurodegenerative diseases

Machine learning and artificial intelligence [4, 5] are advancing rapidly in the field of biomarker discovery, offering generative AI solutions to identify biomarkers – key indicators of disease presence, progression, and severity. Despite significant progress in recent years concerning neurodegenerative disorders, there remains a lack of universally recognized biomarkers for diagnosing all such diseases or creating precise treatment plans [23, 24, 25].

13.3.1.1 Role of generative AI in biomarker discovery

Generative AI models, including generative adversarial networks (GANs) and variational autoencoders (VAEs), show great promise in this area. These models are equipped to handle the vast volumes of data often involved in biomarker discovery.

Key sources of this data include:

Genetic data: Many neurodegenerative diseases are associated with genetic mutations and variations. Generative AI can analyze large genetic databases to identify patterns and mutations linked to specific diseases. These genetic biomarkers can offer insights into a person's susceptibility to neurodegenerative conditions, improving early detection and preventive strategies.

Brain imaging: Neuroimaging techniques such as MRI and PET scans generate substantial data reflecting the structural and functional changes in the brain. Generative AI can enhance these images, allowing for the detection of subtle differences that might otherwise go unnoticed. These imaging biomarkers can help identify early signs of neurodegeneration and track disease progression over time.

13.3.1.2 Advantages of AI-driven biomarker discovery

Early diagnosis: AI models have the capability to detect biomarkers that emerge early in the disease process. This ability is crucial for the early diagnosis of conditions, enabling timely interventions that may slow or prevent disease progression.

Accuracy and precision: AI models excel in sensitivity and specificity, leading to highly accurate identification of biomarkers. These models can detect minute differences with minimal delays, reducing the chances of false positives or negatives.

Personalized medicine: AI-driven biomarker discovery allows for the identification of biomarkers tailored to a patient's unique genetic and biological profile. This paves the way for personalized treatment plans, improving patient outcomes by aligning treatments with individual characteristics.

Uncovering hidden patterns: While traditional methods may overlook subtle patterns in data, AI can identify previously undetectable biomarkers. This capability allows for the discovery of new insights that were not accessible through conventional techniques [16, 17].

13.3.1.3 Challenges and considerations

Despite the promising advantages of using biomarkers identified through AI technologies, several challenges still need to be addressed. A key issue revolves around data quality and availability. Training deep neural networks requires well-structured, adequately labeled datasets, which are often scarce. This is particularly problematic when working with rare neurodegenerative disorders, where data may be limited or even nonexistent.

Another major challenge lies in model interpretability. In many cases, it is unclear how certain AI models reach their conclusions or decisions. This lack of transparency can make it difficult for clinicians and researchers to trust and adopt these AI-driven insights. Therefore, it is crucial to develop models that are interpretable, allowing clinicians to understand and confidently apply the AI-generated biomarkers in real-world medical scenarios.

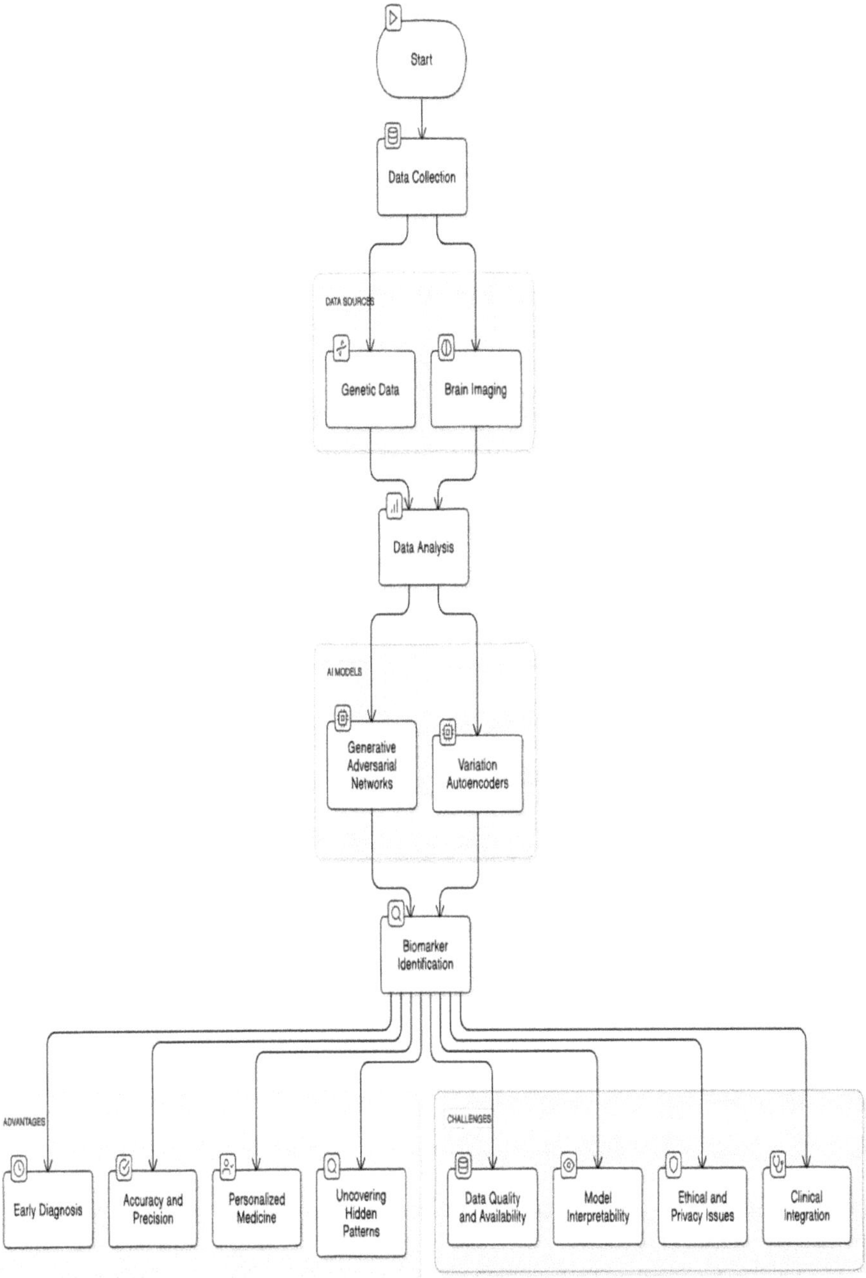

Figure 13.2 AI-driven biomarker discovery in neurodegenerative diseases.

Ethical and privacy issues are also of significant concern. The use of sensitive health information in AI research raises questions about data privacy and security. Ensuring that patient records are protected and that ethical standards are upheld is essential. Strong regulatory frameworks must be in place to address these concerns, offering proper safeguards for both data and ethical integrity in research.

Clinical integration is another critical factor. For AI-based biomarkers to be truly useful in clinical practice, they must be validated for accuracy and integrated into the patient management process. This requires close collaboration among AI developers, clinicians, and regulatory bodies to ensure compliance, safety, and effective implementation.

AI-powered biomarker discovery represents a revolutionary approach with enormous potential for the prognosis and early detection of neurodegenerative diseases. When large datasets are processed through generative AI, new biomarkers emerge that could transform diagnosis and treatment strategies for these debilitating conditions. As the demand for AI-driven technologies grows, addressing challenges related to data quality, model transparency, ethical concerns, and clinical adoption becomes more urgent. Figure 13.2 illustrates the AI-driven biomarker discovery process in neurodegenerative diseases [13, 14].

13.4 Imaging Techniques for Generative AI in Neurodegenerative Disorders

In recent studies [6, 7], neuroimaging techniques like MRI, PET, and CT scans can be significantly enhanced through the use of Generative Adversarial Networks (GANs) and other deep learning models [26, 27]. These models improve image resolution, define brain regions with greater precision, and track slow, progressive changes in spatiotemporal imaging sequences. This is achieved by simulating disease progression through virtual scans that reveal subtle structural changes in the brain.

Imaging techniques remain one of the most important methods for diagnosing and evaluating neurodegenerative diseases, providing highly detailed images of both brain structures and the cardiovascular system. Generative AI has made it possible to refine these processes, facilitating earlier diagnoses, more targeted treatments, and a deeper understanding of complex neurological conditions.

The current discussion focuses on how generative AI has advanced neuroimaging and the perspectives of medical professionals and researchers, while also highlighting the challenges that need to be overcome [21, 22].

13.4.1 Key imaging techniques enhanced by generative AI

13.4.1.1 Magnetic resonance imaging (MRI)

Structural MRI: This type of MRI generates high-resolution images of the brain, which are useful in detecting structural changes, such as brain shrinkage in conditions like Alzheimer's. Generative AI can enhance these images, making them sharper and clearer, allowing for more accurate assessments of different brain structures.

Functional MRI (fMRI): fMRI tracks brain activity by monitoring changes in blood flow. AI can enhance its efficiency, providing clearer insights into neural activity and cognitive function.

13.4.1.2 Positron emission tomography (PET)

PET scans measure metabolic processes in the brain, such as glucose consumption and amyloid plaque buildup – both indicators of neurodegeneration. Generative AI models can improve image reconstruction, reducing the need for radioactive tracers and shortening scan times, making PET scanning safer and more efficient.

13.4.1.3 Diffusion tensor imaging (DTI)

DTI maps the movement of water molecules in the brain, providing information about the condition of white matter tracts. Generative AI can enhance the precision of DTI, producing more accurate images that can aid in diagnosing conditions like multiple sclerosis and Parkinson's disease.

13.4.1.4 Computed tomography (CT)

Although CT scans are less detailed than MRIs, they are faster and more widely available. By applying generative AI, the quality of CT images can be improved to resemble MRI-like clarity in specific clinical situations, offering enhanced diagnostic capabilities.

13.4.2 Innovations in imaging techniques with Generative AI

Image enhancement and reconstruction: One key application of generative AI lies in improving image quality by minimizing noise and artifacts, and increasing the resolution of images derived from low-quality input data. This is particularly true when utilizing generative adversarial networks (GANs). Such advancements are crucial for achieving more precise diagnoses while reducing the need for invasive imaging equipment [8, 9].

Data augmentation: Generative AI can also generate synthetic datasets that simulate rare or hard-to-capture disease conditions, aiding in the

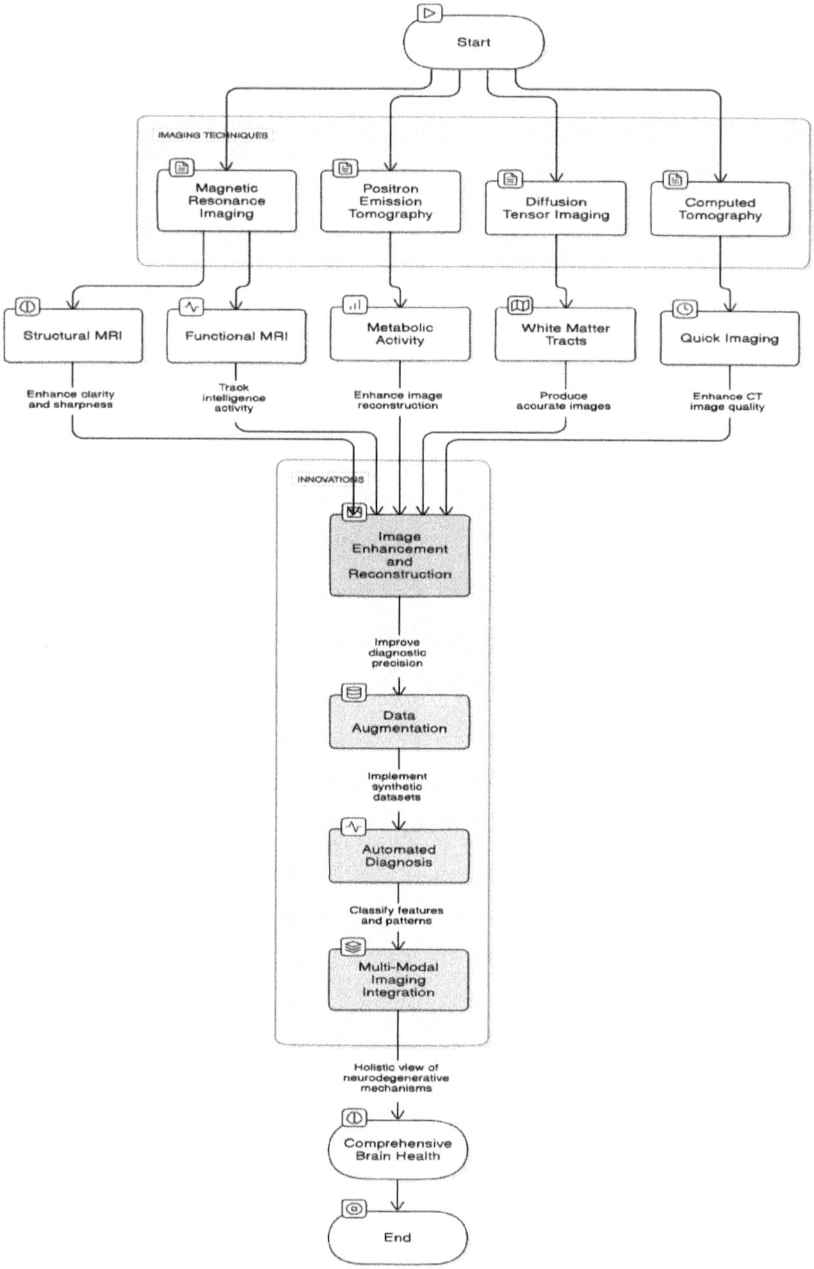

Figure 13.3 Imaging techniques for generative AI in neurodegenerative disorders.

development of more accurate diagnostic algorithms. This is particularly useful in fields like neurodegenerative disease research, where patient sample sizes are often limited. Synthetic data generation helps alleviate this issue by providing richer datasets for training.

Automated diagnosis: AI algorithms are now being integrated with imaging techniques to automatically classify features and patterns indicative of neurodegenerative diseases. These systems assist radiologists by highlighting areas of the image that require closer examination, ultimately speeding up the diagnostic process and improving accuracy [19, 20].

Multi-modal imaging integration: By combining data from various imaging methods, such as MRI, PET, and DTI, generative AI enables a more comprehensive understanding of brain health. This multi-modal approach offers a more holistic perspective on the mechanisms underlying neurodegenerative diseases, potentially identifying biomarkers that single imaging methods might miss.

As highlighted in sources [28, 29], generative AI shows significant promise for enhancing imaging techniques used in diagnosing neurodegenerative diseases. Its ability to detect early-stage conditions with greater accuracy, along with improved image quality and automated diagnostic processes, could revolutionize the field. However, challenges such as data quality, ethical concerns, regulatory hurdles, and model interpretability remain. Addressing these issues will require close collaboration between AI researchers, clinicians, and regulatory bodies to ensure these technologies can be fully realized and integrated into clinical practice. Figure 13.3 illustrates the imaging techniques for generative AI in neurodegenerative disorders.

13.5 Personalized Medicine for Generative AI in Neurodegenerative Disorders

Personalized medicine is revolutionizing traditional healthcare by offering tailored treatment strategies that are based on an individual's genetic makeup, lifestyle, and environmental factors. In the context of neurodegenerative diseases, this approach focuses on creating more effective and targeted therapies that not only enhance treatment outcomes but also slow the progression of these challenging conditions. The application of generative models in healthcare is playing a pivotal role in advancing this approach by analyzing complex data to design personalized treatment plans.

13.5.1 Innovations in personalized medicine with generative AI

Genomic analysis and precision therapies: Deep learning, particularly through models like generative AI and generative adversarial networks (GANs), is instrumental in processing large-scale genomic data. These models help detect genetic mutations and variations associated with neurodegenerative diseases, paving the way for precision therapies that target specific molecular signatures in individual patients.

Patient-specific disease modeling: Generative AI holds immense potential in medicine, particularly in creating personalized disease models. These models are tailored to a patient's unique genetic profile, radiographic images, and clinical history, allowing for predictions about disease progression and exploring the effectiveness of potential treatments. This ability to simulate outcomes enables more accurate and personalized treatment plans.

Drug discovery and repurposing: Generative AI is driving a transformative shift in drug discovery, identifying new molecules and finding novel uses for existing drugs in treating neurodegenerative diseases. By leveraging AI models, physicians can predict how different medications will interact with a patient's genetic makeup, allowing for the selection of the most effective treatment combination with minimal side effects.

Personalized treatment monitoring: Generative AI is also highly effective in tracking the success of treatment plans. It can monitor patient responses in real-time, identifying changes in data that signal whether the patient is improving or developing resistance to the therapy, allowing for timely adjustments before the condition worsens.

Multimodal data integration: By integrating genomic data, imaging results, biomarkers, and patient records, generative AI creates a comprehensive view of a patient's condition. This multimodal approach is particularly beneficial in identifying disease markers that may not be detectable through other diagnostic methods.

13.5.2 Obstacles and challenges

Data privacy and ethical concerns: Personalized medicine heavily depends on an individual's sensitive information, such as genetic data. Protecting the privacy and security of this data is a significant concern, especially as the use of AI in healthcare continues to expand globally. Safeguarding this information is crucial to ensuring trust and preventing misuse.

Complexity and interpretability of AI models: One of the major challenges with applying generative AI in personalized medicine is the

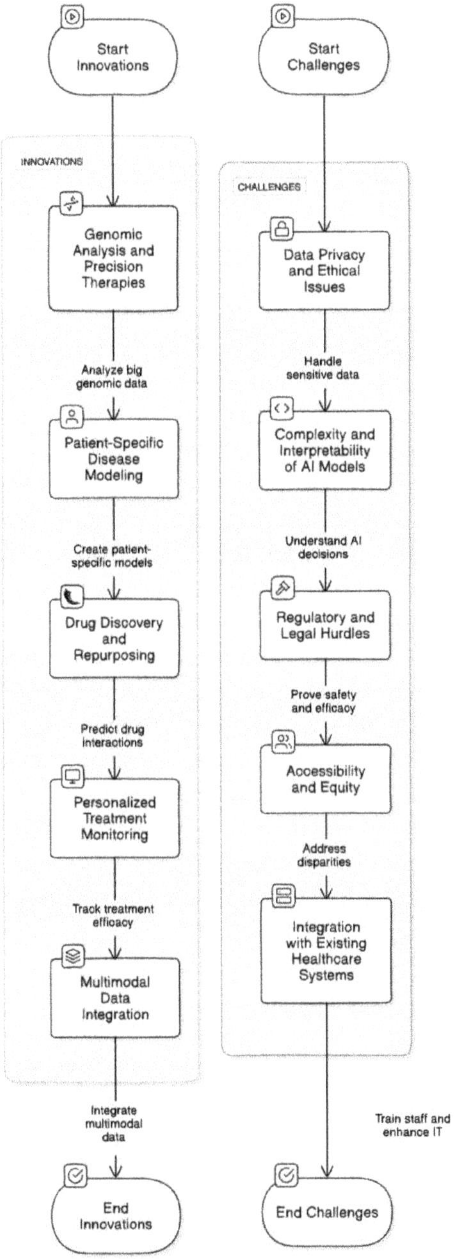

Figure 13.4 Personalized medicine for generative AI in neurodegenerative disorders.

complexity and opacity of these models. Clinicians need to fully understand how AI arrives at its conclusions in order to apply these results reliably in practice. Without clear interpretability, the clinical utility of AI decisions remains limited.

Regulatory and legal challenges: The use of AI in personalized medicine is subject to stringent regulatory oversight. Before being deployed in clinical settings, AI-driven treatments must prove their safety and efficacy. Navigating these regulatory frameworks can be time-consuming and costly, posing a barrier to wider adoption.

Accessibility and equity: There is a risk that the benefits of personalized AI-based treatments may not be equally available to all. Wealthier regions or individuals may have better access to these advancements, leaving others at a disadvantage. Ensuring that personalized medicine is accessible and equitable is essential to preventing disparities in healthcare outcomes.

Integration with existing healthcare systems: Implementing AI-driven personalized medicine also presents logistical and operational challenges. Healthcare providers will need to train their staff to work with AI tools, and existing IT infrastructure must be upgraded to handle the increased data load that comes with these technologies.

AI holds great promise in advancing personalized medicine, particularly in the management of neurological disorders. However, achieving this vision will require addressing significant challenges such as data privacy, model transparency, regulatory barriers, and equitable access. Overcoming these obstacles will depend on continued collaboration between AI researchers, clinicians, ethicists, and policymakers to ensure the efficient and ethical adoption of AI in personalized healthcare. Figure 13.4 illustrates the role of generative AI in personalized medicine for neurodegenerative disorders.

13.6 Virtual Brain Models for Generative AI in Neurodegenerative Disorders

This section will concentrate on the innovations, perspectives, and challenges that are central to analyzing the topic. Virtual brain models, which are digital simulations of the human brain, utilize advanced computational techniques. These models are emerging as powerful tools in the study and treatment of neurodegenerative diseases, providing a safe, controlled environment to examine how the disease behaves and interacts with other variables. Generative AI plays a pivotal role in enhancing these models by enabling the simulation of realistic brain functions and generating synthetic data for deeper analysis.

13.6.1 New developments applied on virtual brain with generative intelligence

Personalized brain simulations: Generative AI enables the creation of brain models tailored to each individual. These models integrate personal data such as genetic profiles, brain imaging, and medical history, providing a detailed representation of neurodegenerative disease progression in a specific patient. This personalized approach reveals deeper insights into disease behavior and patient-specific responses to treatment.

Simulation of disease progression: Generative AI allows virtual brain models to incorporate various neuropsychiatric conditions, simulating the onset and progression of neurodegenerative disorders. These simulations offer researchers the ability to observe disease development over time, helping to identify early signs or key indicators that might not be readily detectable in clinical settings.

Integration of multi-modal data: By combining data from sources like MRI, PET scans, and genetic information, generative AI can construct a virtual brain that offers a comprehensive view of both structural and functional changes characteristic of neurodegenerative diseases. This approach enables a holistic understanding of brain health.

Drug discovery and testing: Virtual brain models can be utilized to simulate the effects of potential drugs on brain function. Generative AI enhances these models by predicting how different treatments may influence the brain's structure and physiology. This approach accelerates drug development, reduces the need for animal testing, and refines therapeutic strategies.

Realistic brain activity simulations: Certain generative AI models can replicate real-life brain activities, including electrical brain oscillations, synaptic communication, and the overall function of neural networks. These simulations are invaluable for studying the impact of neurodegenerative diseases on brain activity and for developing theories about underlying disease mechanisms.

13.6.2 Obstacles and challenges

Model complexity and accuracy: Creating an accurate and functional representation of the human brain is an incredibly complex task that requires a deep understanding of its anatomical, physiological, and pathological features. While Generative AI can replicate certain brain functions, fully capturing the intricacies of the human brain remains a significant challenge.

Data quality and availability: High-quality data is essential for building virtual brain models. However, data specific to neurodegenerative diseases is often limited due to the rarity of these conditions. Additionally, issues like inaccurate data collection, inconsistent measurements, and problems during processing can affect the reliability of the models.

Computational resources: Simulating a virtual brain, particularly when factoring in multiple data sources and potential disease processes, demands substantial computational resources. Accessing these resources can be difficult, especially for smaller research institutions with limited funding and infrastructure.

Validation and standardization: For virtual brain models to be used in clinical settings, they must undergo extensive validation and standardization processes. This involves collaboration across multiple disciplines, including neuroscience, computer science, and medicine, making it a time-consuming and resource-intensive effort.

Integration with clinical practice: Bringing virtual brain models into routine clinical practice poses significant challenges. Clinicians must be trained to understand and use these models effectively, and there must be seamless compatibility between the models and existing medical systems and workflows.

Virtual brain models, powered by Generative AI, represent a significant breakthrough in diagnosing and treating neurodegenerative disorders. These models offer the potential to track disease progression, tailor treatments

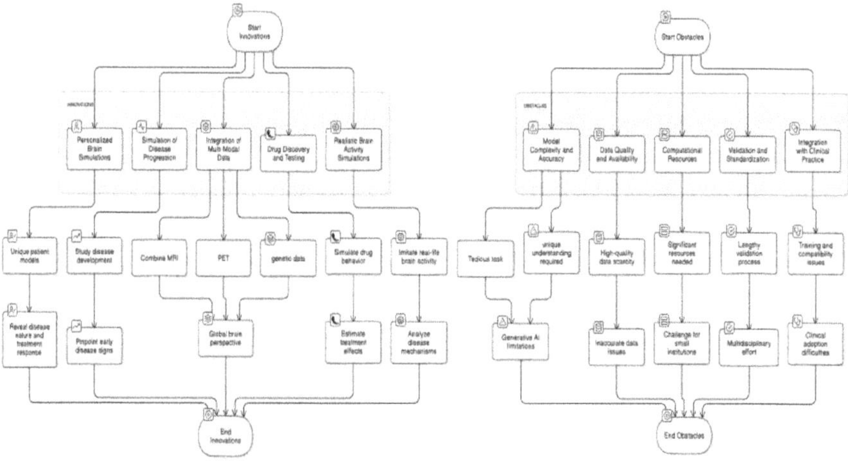

Figure 13.5 Virtual brain models for generative AI in neurodegenerative disorders.

to individual patients, and accelerate drug discovery. However, challenges related to model accuracy, data quality, computational demands, and clinical integration must be addressed to unlock their full potential. As we continue to advance in this field, virtual brain models may become indispensable in the fight against neurodegenerative diseases. Figure 13.5 illustrates the use of virtual brain models in Generative AI for neurodegenerative disorders.

13.7 Automated Diagnosis Systems for Generative AI in Neurodegenerative Disorders

13.7.1 Innovations, perspectives, and challenges in development

Generative AI has the potential to transform diagnostic systems for neurological disorders such as Alzheimer's, Parkinson's, and Huntington's disease. These advanced systems utilize sophisticated machine learning techniques to process medical data, identify patterns, and provide diagnoses faster and more efficiently than traditional methods. This section explores recent innovations in automated diagnostic systems, the perspectives of key stakeholders, and the challenges that must be addressed to fully realize these advancements.

13.7.2 New concept in automated diagnosis systems

Advanced machine learning algorithms: Generative adversarial networks (GANs) are utilized to generate synthetic data, which enhances diagnostic models by supplementing limited datasets. This is particularly beneficial for neurodegenerative disorders, where gathering large datasets can be challenging.

Variational autoencoders (VAEs): VAEs enable the creation and analysis of latent representations of vast medical datasets. This helps in identifying relationships related to neurodegenerative diseases that may not be immediately apparent or easily identifiable.

Integration of multi-modal data: Automated diagnostic systems leverage multiple data sources, such as imaging (MRI, PET scans), genetic information, and clinical records, to reach more accurate diagnoses.

Real-time diagnosis: AI accelerates the diagnostic process by continuously analyzing data from a patient's condition, allowing for faster decision-making. This is particularly valuable in clinical situations where timely diagnosis is critical, especially for neurodegenerative disorders.

Predictive modeling: Generative AI models are used not only for diagnosing current conditions but also for predicting disease progression. These models simulate potential disease trajectories, helping clinicians forecast future developments and reduce diagnostic errors.

Personalized diagnostics: AI systems consider genetic information, clinical history, and lifestyle factors to provide comprehensive, individualized diagnoses. These systems offer tailored recommendations for treatment, ensuring more accurate and personalized patient care.

13.7.3 Obstacles and challenges

Data quality and availability: The effectiveness of automated diagnostic systems relies heavily on the availability of diverse and high-quality datasets. In the case of neurodegenerative disorders, such data is often limited and difficult to obtain, which creates challenges in training robust AI models. The quality of data can vary significantly depending on the source, further complicating the development of accurate diagnostic tools.

Model interpretability: A significant challenge with many AI models, including those used for diagnosis, is that they often function as a "black box," making it difficult to understand how they arrive at their conclusions. For clinicians to trust and effectively use these systems, they need to comprehend the decision-making process behind the AI. Efforts are being made to improve model transparency, but this remains a complex issue.

Regulatory and ethical concerns: The use of AI in medical diagnostics raises several regulatory and ethical challenges. Legal compliance, particularly in terms of safety, efficacy, and fairness, is essential for diagnostic tools. Ethical issues such as obtaining informed consent and ensuring patient data protection are also critical considerations.

Integration into clinical practice: For AI-powered diagnostic systems to be widely adopted, they must seamlessly fit into the current healthcare framework. This requires not only technical innovations but also proper training for clinicians and adjustments to healthcare systems to support these technologies.

Bias and generalization: AI models trained on biased or limited datasets may not perform well in broader, more diverse patient populations. One of the main challenges is ensuring that these systems do not exacerbate existing inequalities in healthcare but instead contribute to fairer and more equitable outcomes.

The incorporation of generative AI in automated diagnostic systems holds great potential for improving the diagnosis and management of neurodegenerative diseases. Advances in data acquisition, multi-modal data integration, and off-site diagnosis are driving significant progress in this area. However, to fully realize the benefits of these systems, challenges such as model interpretability, data quality, regulatory compliance, and ethical considerations must be addressed. As this field continues to evolve, it will be crucial for AI researchers, clinicians, patients, and regulators to collaborate in developing trustworthy and effective AI-driven diagnostic tools.

13.8 Variational Autoencoders (VAEs)

Variational autoencoders (VAEs) are emerging as a powerful tool in both the fields of generative artificial intelligence and neurodegenerative disease research. As a type of generative model, VAEs are designed to learn underlying data patterns and generate new examples that closely resemble those from the training data. Their application in the study of neurodegenerative diseases is growing, driving innovation and prompting new considerations in the field [19].

13.8.1 Innovations

Enhanced data generation: VAEs excel in producing highly realistic synthetic data samples that mimic the patterns of image distributions. This makes them particularly useful in generating lifelike scans related to neurological disorders, cognitive assessments, and other physiological data, which can aid in the study and diagnosis of neurodegenerative diseases.

Improved disease modeling: VAEs create a condensed latent space representation of data, enhancing the ability to model disease progression and variability. This enables researchers to investigate the influence of various factors on the onset and progression of diseases like Alzheimer's and Parkinson's.

Personalized medicine: VAEs, through their capacity to encode variability in the latent space, can be leveraged to develop patient-specific models. This feature allows for the design of treatment plans tailored to individual patients by predicting how they might respond to specific therapies.

Data augmentation: One of the key benefits of VAEs is their capability to generate additional data samples, which proves invaluable when real-world datasets are limited. This helps overcome data scarcity issues in research.

13.8.2 Obstacles

Data quality and bias: VAEs rely heavily on the quality of the training data they are provided. If the data contains biases or is limited in any way, the model may not accurately reflect the complexity of real-world situations. This could lead to generating recommendations that do not align with the patient's actual condition or, in some cases, result in no viable treatment options being suggested.

Complexity of implementation: Implementing VAEs requires substantial expertise, both in selecting appropriate machine learning models and in understanding the specific domain. Fine-tuning these models to achieve optimal accuracy and reliability is a complicated process that can pose significant challenges, even for experienced researchers.

Computational resources: Training VAEs, particularly on high-dimensional medical datasets, demands significant computational power. This presents a barrier for institutions that do not have easy access to high-performance computing infrastructure, limiting their ability to fully leverage this technology.

Interpretability: Although VAEs are capable of identifying intricate patterns within data, interpreting the output and understanding the latent space representations can be quite difficult. Achieving clinically meaningful and interpretable results remains a challenge with current methods.

In conclusion, variational autoencoders (VAEs) have shown great promise as a generative AI tool in the study of neurodegenerative diseases. Their advancements in data generation, disease modeling, and personalized treatment hold significant potential. However, key challenges such as data quality, implementation complexity, and interpretability still need to be addressed. Ongoing research in this field offers the possibility of breakthroughs that could transform the management of neurodegenerative conditions.

13.9 Diffusion Models

Diffusion models represent another breakthrough in generative AI, offering significant advancements in the study of neurodegenerative diseases. These models work by gradually transforming random noise into meaningful features, making them particularly useful in medical imaging and disease prediction, such as for conditions like Alzheimer's and Parkinson's. Their ability to generate clear, high-quality data contributes to their effectiveness in these areas.

13.9.1 Innovations

Diffusion models have revolutionized how we diagnose and evaluate neurodegenerative diseases and their progression. By transforming noise into realistic data, these models can generate high-resolution medical images, simulate disease development, and even create virtual brain models.

This enhanced capability provides a more robust foundation for understanding disease progression and developing diagnostic strategies for conditions like Alzheimer's and amyotrophic lateral sclerosis (ALS). These models are frequently used to identify biomarkers, offering valuable insights by integrating data such as genetics and brain imaging (BIRG). This approach not only aids in diagnosing diseases more accurately but also paves the way for more effective treatment methods through modern technological advancements.

13.9.2 Views

The integration of diffusion models into neurodegenerative disease research is widely considered a significant breakthrough. For researchers and clinicians, these models offer the ability to handle large datasets and generate highly realistic simulations of disease progression. This is especially valuable for tracking changes in the brain over time, which is crucial for conditions like Alzheimer's and Parkinson's that develop gradually. Moreover, these models provide deeper insights into the mechanisms driving neurodegenerative disorders. By enhancing our understanding of disease complexity, they open doors for discovering new therapeutic options and refining existing treatments.

13.9.3 Obstacles

Despite the advancements brought by diffusion models, they are not without challenges. One major issue is the need for large datasets to effectively train these models. In the study of neurodegenerative diseases, obtaining such datasets can be difficult due to the rarity of some conditions and the complexity of gathering relevant data.

Another concern revolves around the interpretability of the models and their outcomes. While diffusion models can create impressive simulations, understanding how these simulations align with actual pathology remains a significant hurdle. This lack of clarity can be problematic in clinical settings, where diagnostic results must be both highly reliable and easy to interpret.

Ethical issues also arise, particularly regarding the generation of synthetic data. The creation of artificial data brings risks related to data privacy and potential misuse. Ensuring that these models are applied ethically, with strict measures in place to protect patient identities, is crucial.

In summary, diffusion models represent a cutting-edge trend in generative AI with great promise for advancing the analysis and treatment of neurodegenerative diseases. While tools like OICR and ADMET offer valuable solutions for modeling disease progression, addressing the challenges of data availability, interpretability, and ethical use will be essential for their adoption in clinical practice.

13.10 Synthetic Data Generation

The use of generative AI to create synthetic data has emerged as an innovative approach in the study of neurodegenerative disorders. Like other AI technologies, it relies on sophisticated algorithms to produce artificial data that simulates real-world conditions. This not only provides valuable insights for research but also enhances clinical applications.

Innovations: Advances in generative AI continue to drive progress in creating synthetic datasets that simulate various aspects of neurodegenerative diseases, such as Alzheimer's, Parkinson's, and amyotrophic lateral sclerosis (ALS). Techniques like generative adversarial networks (GANs) and variational autoencoders (VAEs) have been used to generate realistic brain images and models of disease progression. These models enable researchers to explore disease development, forecast outcomes, and tailor individual treatment plans with greater accuracy.

Additionally, generative models have contributed to the development of virtual brain models that help visualize and analyze neural interactions and disease processes. Of particular importance are simulations of cognitive decline and other disease symptoms, which may enhance diagnostic precision for conditions like sclerosis and lead to more effective therapeutic strategies.

13.10.1 Views

The application of generative AI in neurodegenerative disorder research is widely seen as a significant advancement. Many experts believe that synthetic data can help address the issue of limited patient data, aiding in the generalization of AI models. This technique allows for the creation of more

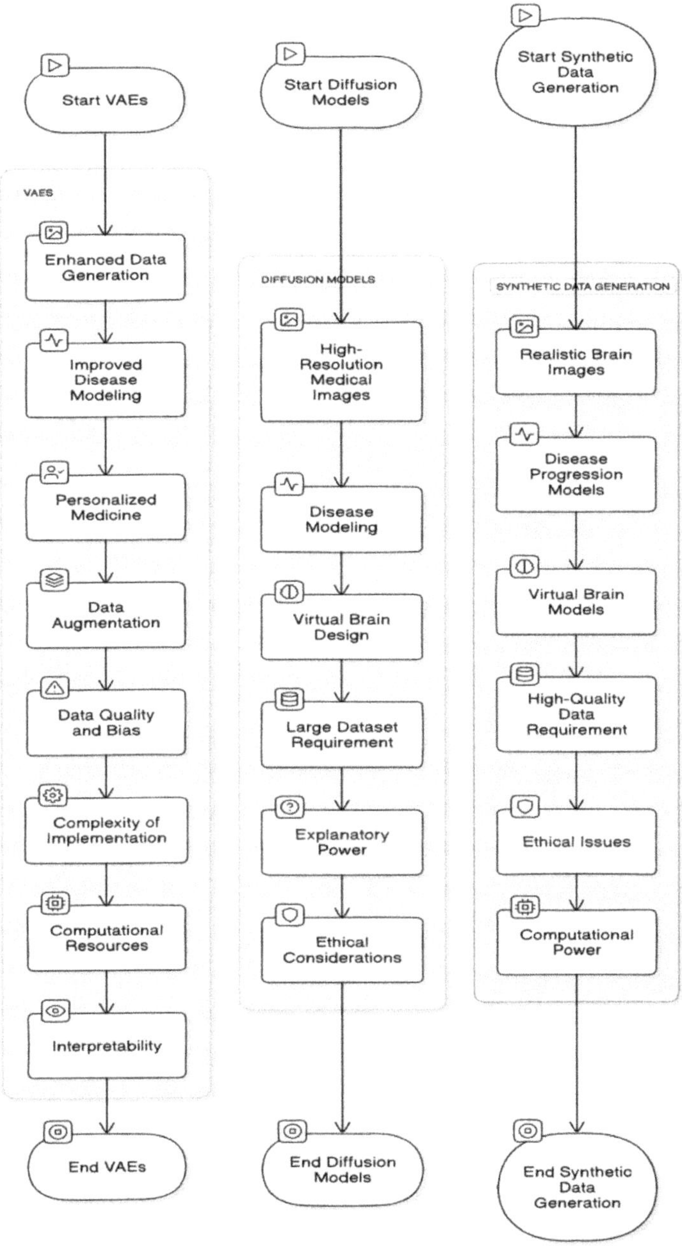

Figure 13.6 Other techniques.

diverse data samples, which enhances the stability of predictive algorithms and contributes to the discovery of new biomarkers.

There is also growing support for the idea that generative AI could enhance the implementation of personalized medicine. By generating patient-specific data, treatments can be tailored to fit the unique characteristics of each case. This personalized approach has the potential to improve patient outcomes and elevate the quality of care.

13.10.2 Obstacles

The use of generative AI in neurodegenerative disorder research does come with challenges, as outlined below. One of the key concerns is the ability to produce high-quality, realistic synthetic data. For this data to be effective it must closely mirror actual patient data; any deviation could result in misdiagnosis or incorrect treatment plans.

There are also ethical concerns related to synthetic data, such as data privacy and the potential misuse of the generated information. Since generative models treat synthetic data as realistic patient information, questions arise regarding how this data might be exploited and whether it accurately represents patients without introducing bias.

Additionally, the computational power required to train and validate these models poses a challenge, particularly for research institutions with limited resources. Ensuring that these technologies can be accessible to institutions or individuals with smaller budgets is essential for their widespread adoption.

In conclusion, generative AI offers great promise in advancing research and treatment for neurodegenerative disorders by generating synthetic data. However, to fully harness its potential, it is crucial to address the accompanying challenges and ethical concerns, ensuring the technology is used responsibly and effectively. Figure 13.6 illustrates the other techniques modern diagnosing methods.

13.11 Conclusion

The integration of generative AI for creating synthetic data enhances the prospects for advancing research and treatment of neurodegenerative diseases. While the potential benefits of these solutions are promising, addressing the associated challenges and ethical concerns is crucial to fully harness the advantages and maximize their positive impact.

References

[1] G. Litjens, T. Kooi, B. E. Bejnordi, et al., "A survey on deep learning in medical image analysis," Medical Image Analysis, vol. 42, pp. 60-88, 2017.

[2] S. Rathore, M. Habes, M. A. Iftikhar, et al., "A review on neuroimaging-based classification studies and associated feature extraction methods for Alzheimer's disease," Frontiers in Neuroscience, vol. 11, p. 10, 2017.

[3] M. van der Schaar, A. M. Alaa, A. Floto, "How artificial intelligence and machine learning can help healthcare systems respond to COVID-19," The Lancet, 2020.

[4] E. E. Bron, M. Smits, W. M. van der Flier, et al., "Standardized evaluation of algorithms for computer-aided diagnosis of dementia based on structural MRI: the CAD Dementia challenge," NeuroImage, vol. 111, pp. 562-579, 2015.

[5] I. Goodfellow, Y. Bengio, A. Courville, "Deep Learning," MIT Press, 2016.

[6] M. Crisanto-Nieto, J. Villanueva, C. Navarro, "Generative Adversarial Networks for Medical Image Augmentation: A Comprehensive Review," Computers in Biology and Medicine, vol. 136, p. 104730, 2021.

[7] A. E. Fetit, J. D. Novakovic, J. T. O'Brien, "AI in the diagnosis of neurodegenerative diseases: Approaches and challenges," Trends in Cognitive Sciences, vol. 25, no. 2, pp. 93-104, 2021.

[8] E. J. Topol, "High-performance medicine: the convergence of human and artificial intelligence," Nature Medicine, vol. 25, pp. 44-56, 2019.

[9] D. Zhang, D. Shen, Alzheimer 's disease Neuroimaging Initiative, "Predicting future clinical changes of MCI patients using longitudinal and multimodal biomarkers," PLoS ONE, vol. 7, no. 3, p. e33182, 2012.

[10] K. J. Geras, S. Wolfson, Y. Shen, "Artificial intelligence in healthcare: The hope, the hype, the promise, the peril," Nature Medicine, vol. 26, pp. 31-38, 2020.

[11] S. Schaefer, E. Fernandez, "Generative AI in Neurodegenerative Disease Research: Innovations and Challenges," Neuroinformatics, vol. 21, no. 1, pp. 27-40, 2023.

[12] M. S. Hossain, N. Mahmood, "Advancements in Generative AI for Alzheimer's Disease: A Review," Journal of Alzheimer's Disease, vol. 86, no. 1, pp. 1-15, 2024.

[13] J. Lee, H. Park, "Generative Models for Predicting Disease Progression in Neurodegenerative Disorders," Frontiers in Neuroscience, vol. 17, p. 743122, 2023.
[14] L. Yang, Z. Wang, "AI-Driven Biomarkers for Neurodegenerative Diseases: Insights from Generative Models," Computational Intelligence and Neuroscience, 2023, p. 9876543.
[15] A. Kumar, R. Sharma, "Generative AI for Early Diagnosis of Parkinson's disease: Opportunities and Challenges," Parkinsonism & Related Disorders, vol. 96, pp. 15-22, 2024.
[16] T. Miller, M. Lee, "Exploring Generative Adversarial Networks for Brain Imaging Data in Neurodegenerative Disorders," IEEE Transactions on Medical Imaging, vol. 42, no. 4, pp. 978-989, 2023.
[17] X. Zhang, J. Zhang, "Generative AI in Predicting Disease Progression: Case Studies in Dementia and ALS," Journal of Biomedical Informatics, vol. 134, p. 104249, 2024.
[18] Y. Chen, Z. Chen, "Generative Models for Simulating Cognitive Decline in Neurodegenerative Diseases," Neuropsychology Review, vol. 33, no. 2, pp. 211-225, 2023.
[19] R. Singh, A. Gupta, "Generative AI and Neuroimaging: Enhancing Diagnosis and Personalization in Alzheimer's Disease," Frontiers in Aging Neuroscience, vol. 16, p. 678945, 2024.
[20] H. Smith, C. Brown, "Challenges in Applying Generative AI to Neurodegenerative Disease Biomarkers," Artificial Intelligence in Medicine, vol. 120, p. 102237, 2023.
[21] N. Patel, H. Desai, "Generative AI Models for Personalized Medicine in Neurodegenerative Disorders: A Systematic Review," Journal of Personalized Medicine, vol. 14, no. 5, p. 374, 2024.
[22] T. Nguyen, H. Nguyen, "Virtual Brain Models and Generative AI: Innovations in Neurodegenerative Disease Research," Brain Research, vol. 1802, pp. 147-158, 2023.
[23] K. Takahashi, T. Suzuki, "Overcoming Obstacles in Generative AI for Neurodegenerative Disease Imaging: Current Perspectives," Medical Image Analysis, vol. 86, p. 102582, 2024.
[24] D. Anderson, C. Lee, "Ethical Considerations and Limitations of Generative AI in Neurodegenerative Disease Research," AI Ethics Journal, vol. 5, no. 3, pp. 65-78, 2023.
[25] P. Williams, M. Garcia, "The Role of Generative AI in Advancing Neurodegenerative Disorder Research: A Comprehensive Review," Journal of Neuro engineering and Rehabilitation, vol. 21, no. 1, pp. 58-71, 2024.

[26] R. Y. Rani, M. L. Prasad, I. S. Reddy, I. A. Tayubi, G. Sultan and P. C. S. Reddy, "Early Prediction and Diagnosis Cardiovascular Disease Using Deep Learning Models," *2024 International Conference on Emerging Technologies in Computer Science for Interdisciplinary Applications*, India, pp. 1-6,.2024,

[27] A. Gadupudi, M. L. Prasad, S. Kedar Nadgaundi, P. C. Shaker Reddy, S. Sharma and N. Sharma, "A Deep Learning Framework For Human Disease Prediction Using Microbiome Data," *2024 International Conference on Integrated Circuits and Communication Systems*, India, pp. 1-6.2024.

[28] S. Sampath, M. L. Prasad, M. M. Hussain, R. Parameswari, D. Anil Kumar and P. C. S. Reddy, "Ensemble Nonlinear Machine Learning Model for Chronic Kidney Diseases Prediction," *2023 IEEE 3rd Mysore Sub Section International Conference* , India, pp. 1-6., 2023.

[29] B. Sudhakar, P. A. Sikrant, M. L. Prasad, S. B. Latha, G. R. Kumar, S. Sarika, and P. C. S. Reddy, "Brain Tumor Image Prediction from MR Images Using CNN Based Deep Learning Networks," *International Journal of [Journal Name]*, vol. vol.16 no.1, pp. 45-60, 2024.

[30] C. K, M. L. Prasad, A. Kiran, P. C. Shaker Reddy, G. C. Babu and N. Partheeban, "Skin Cancer Classification using A Hybrid Convolutional Neural Network with SVM Classifier," *2023 Global Conference on Information Technologies and Communications*, Bangalore, India, pp. 1-6, 2023.

14

AI-driven Innovations: Revolutionizing the Management of Neurodegenerative Disorders

Amrutha T. V.[1], Nabeeha Koya[1], Sarasa Meenakshi[1], Ved Prakash[2], Nitesh Kumar[1], Nikhilesh Anand[3], Santhosh Kumar[4], and Krishna Murti[1]

[1]National Institute of Pharmaceutical Education and Research (NIPER), India
[2]Indira Gandhi institute of medical sciences (IGIMS), India
[3]School of Medicine, University of Texas, USA
[4]Carver College of Medicine, University of Iowa, USA
E-mail: amruthatv1996@gmail.com; nabeehakoya@gmail.com; sarasameenakshi@gmail.com; vedprakashims@gmail.com; niteshkumar43@gmail.com; nikhilesh.anand@utrgv.edu; santosh-kumar@uiowa.edu; krishnamurti@niperhajipur.ac.in

Preface

AI's incorporation into cognitive and physical rehabilitation marks a substantial advancement in medical treatment, especially for those with neurodegenerative diseases. This chapter is crucial because it highlights how AI technology might improve patient outcomes, encourage independence, and enhance the general quality of life for those living with diseases like Parkinson's and Alzheimer's. The chapter highlights the potential of multidisciplinary methods to significantly enhance rehabilitation tactics by examining state-of-the-art applications such as robots for physical therapy and virtual reality (VR) for cognitive rehabilitation. It emphasizes how important it is to create individualized treatment programs that are specific to each patient's needs and how AI can successfully customize therapeutic approaches. The chapter also addresses the ethical issues and difficulties surrounding AI in

DOI: 10.1201/9788743801764-14

healthcare, giving readers a more sophisticated grasp of the difficulties in using these technologies. In addition to providing information, the discussion of AI's possible applications in the treatment of neurodegenerative diseases sparks interest in the field's current advancements and future prospects. This chapter encourages readers to actively participate in the quickly changing field of artificial intelligence in healthcare. By presenting a strong case for AI's critical role in transforming rehabilitation and improving the lives of individuals impacted by neurodegenerative illnesses, it seeks to stimulate more research and cooperation. Through linking AI developments to real-world uses, this story invites readers to consider the significant implications for the future of healthcare and the possibilities that lie ahead.

Abstract

Neurodegenerative disorders (NDDs), such as Alzheimer's, Parkinson's disease (PD), amyotrophic lateral sclerosis (ALS), multiple sclerosis (MS), and polyglutamine (polyQ) diseases, are becoming a global health crisis, particularly with aging populations. These diseases cause progressive neuronal deterioration, leading to severe cognitive and motor impairments. The World Health Organization estimates that around 50 million people are affected by NDDs, with Alzheimer's and Parkinson's being the most common. The rising prevalence of these conditions presents a significant public health challenge, compounded by economic strain on healthcare systems. Current diagnostic methods often fail to detect NDDs early, hindering efforts to slow progression, while treatments focus primarily on symptom management rather than cures. Artificial intelligence (AI) offers transformative potential in managing NDDs, with systems designed to improve early diagnosis, create personalized treatment plans, and enhance clinical decision-making. AI can analyze large datasets, including medical histories, lab results, and imaging studies, providing predictive insights that enable earlier interventions. Additionally, AI can improve clinical efficiency by automating routine tasks and reducing administrative burdens, allowing healthcare professionals to focus on patient care. The integration of AI in telemedicine further expands access to care, particularly for patients in remote areas. To fully harness AI's potential, challenges such as data privacy, patient trust, and seamless integration into clinical workflows must be addressed. Future AI tools will need to be adaptable, transparent, and secure to ensure widespread acceptance and effective use in healthcare.

Keywords: Neurodegenerative Disorders, Early Diagnosis, Predictive Analytics, Artificial Intelligence, Personalized Treatment, Cognitive Rehabilitation.

14.1 Introduction

14.1.1 Neurodegenerative disorders: A comprehensive overview

Neurodegenerative disorders are a range of complicated and advanced ailments that cause the nervous system's structure and function, particularly the brain and spinal cord, to deteriorate over time. These disorders are frequently connected with the buildup of misfolded proteins, resulting in neuronal death and the resultant impairment of cognitive, motor, and sensory functioning [1] & Kalakota, 2019; [3, 4]. One of the defining features of neurodegenerative illnesses is the selective degradation of certain neuronal populations, which results in unique clinical manifestations [5]. These situations have a negative impact on millions of people globally and eventually result in the collapse of brain networks necessary for human function. These disorders are incurable; however, several issues can be managed to alleviate symptoms, enhance the quality of life, or slow the progression of the disease [5, 6]. Aging has been linked to a higher chance of developing neurodegenerative conditions, and the incidence of these disorders has increased in recent decades. In the coming decades, as the population ages, it is anticipated that the burden of Alzheimer's disease and associated dementias would increase significantly, particularly in low- and middle-income nations (Table 14.1) [7, 8]. As the global population ages, it is crucial to treat and manage these disorders effectively [1, 6, 9]. Neurodegenerative disorders include Alzheimer's disease (AD), Parkinson's disease (PD), amyotrophic lateral sclerosis (ALS), multiple sclerosis (MS), and polyglutamine (polyQ) diseases [6, 10, 11]. Common characteristics of these disorders include pathological aggregation of proteins, malfunction of synapses and brain networks, inadequate protein synthesis, cytoskeletal defects, changed metabolism of energy, errors in DNA and RNA, inflammatory conditions, and death of neurons [6, 9]. Alzheimer's disease is marked by the deterioration of neurons in the hippocampus and cerebral cortex, resulting in impaired memory and a decline in cognitive function. As the condition progresses, individuals become more dependent on others for daily activities [12]. AD can cause patients to lose communication skills, recognize loved ones, and control their movements which significantly affects people, families, and society at large [1]; Swaab et al., 2011; [13]. Parkinson's disease is characterized by motor impairments such as tremors and rigidity and is correlated with the death of dopaminergic neurons in the substantia nigra [14, 15]. Dopamine deficiency causes PD-specific symptoms related to the muscles including tremors, bradykinesia (slow movement), muscle rigidity, and instability of posture [16]. PD can induce cognitive impairment, depression, and sleep difficulties, in addition to reduced motor function [16, 17]. ALS, is a motor neuron disease described by degeneration of upper motor neurons in the motor cortex and lower motor neurons in the brain stem and spinal cord, resulting in progressive degeneration of voluntary muscles [18]. Multiple sclerosis is a chronic immune-mediated inflammatory condition of the central nervous system (CNS) that causes demyelination and neuronal death. The immune system, in reality, begins to recognize CNS myelin constituents as foreign bodies and damages myelin sheets, resulting in disease progression [19]. PolyQ diseases are a group of rare neurodegenerative disorders which include Huntington's disease, spinocerebellar ataxias, spinal and bulbar muscular atrophy [20]. Huntington's disease is characterized by a polyQ expansion in the huntingtin protein, a key signal regulator in the neurological system. The key characteristic is the significant degradation of a part of the brain known as the striatum, which narrows to a fraction of its initial dimension [21].

Table 14.1 Comparison of the prevalence and economic burden of major neurodegenerative diseases globally.

Neurodegenerative disorders	Global prevalence	Economic burden
Alzheimer's disease (AD)	In 2020 , there were around 50 million cases, which are expected to rise to 152 million by 2050 .	Estimated at $1.3 trillion in 2019 and expected to reach $2 trillion by 2030.
Parkinson's disease (PD)	Globally, there are approximately 6 million cases and are expected to increase to 12-17 million by 2040 .	Estimated at $51.9 billion in the United States in 2017 and anticipated to approach $79 billion by 2037.
Amyotrophic lateral sclerosis (ALS)	The U.S. has approximately $20,000 - 30,000$ cases; however, the prevalence varies worldwide.	In the United States, the annual expenditure of ALS and related ailments is expected to be $655 billion (2020).
Spinal muscular atrophy (SMA)	Approximately one in every 10,000 live births; the prevalence varies globally.	Part of the greater economic burden of ALS and comparable ailments; particular expenses are unclear.
Huntington's disease (HD)	Impacts are generally $5 - 10$ per 100,000 people; prevalence varies worldwide.	The economic burden is unclear but significant to the overall expenditures related to neurodegenerative disorders.

The progressive traits of neurodegenerative conditions have been linked to a common underlying process that leads to excessive inflammation. Substantial evidence suggests that the interactions between damaged neurons and dysfunctional, overactivated microglia develop a self-propagating cycle of chronic inflammation, which promotes the ongoing degradation of the nervous system [1, 6, 9, 11]. This chronic inflammation is believed to be a key factor in the development of various neurodegenerative diseases, including AD, PD, and ALS [22].

14.1.2 The need for advanced management tools in neurodegenerative disorders

In view of the complexities and progressive nature of neurodegenerative disorders such as AD, PD, and ALS, there is a growing recognition of the need for improved management techniques. As the global population ages, the prevalence of these ailments rises, demanding new approaches to diagnosis, treatment, and patient care [9]. Emerging technologies, particularly AI and ML, are proving that they are critical for the early diagnosis and monitoring of neurodegenerative disorders. These techniques may evaluate large volumes of information from a different source, which includes neuroimaging and biofluid analysis, to discover abnormalities that standard diagnostic methods might not identify. For instance, artificial intelligence can improve Alzheimer's disease diagnosis accuracy by detecting small changes in brain imaging that correspond to early-stage symptoms [23]. Advanced management tools make it easier to develop personalized treatment plans. Biosensors and wearable technology enable healthcare providers to keep up with the wellness of patients in real time. This constant monitoring enables rapid revisions to treatment strategies depending on the patient's present condition and reactions to medicines [9, 24]. Wearable gadgets, for example, can follow motor symptoms in those with Parkinson's disease, providing crucial data to help clinicians make decisions [25]. Besides diagnostics and therapy, enhanced management technologies are critical to improving supportive care. Technologies that help patients with daily tasks, such as communication aids for speech impairments, can dramatically improve their quality of life. Furthermore, advanced care planning (ACP) training programs for healthcare providers can prepare them to initiate essential discussions about patient needs and goals as the condition develops [9, 26]. Ongoing research into innovative treatment possibilities, with tailored medication delivery systems and gene treatment, indicates the promise for new approaches that address the fundamental causes of neurological disorders rather than simply treating symptoms [9]. These improvements demand sophisticated management tools to ensure their successful application in clinical settings as shown in Table 14.1.

14.2 AI in Revolutionizing Neurological Care

AI algorithms can analyze brain scans, MRIs, and CT scans to find abnormalities and help diagnose disorders such as tumors, ischemic attacks, and neurodegenerative diseases more accurately and quickly [27]. Machine learning models can anticipate the progression of diseases and clinical results, allowing physicians to create tailored regimens and interventions. AI speeds up the identification of possible medication candidates for neurological conditions by analyzing large datasets and modelling molecular interactions [28, 29]. AI-powered robots and virtual reality systems aid in the physical and cognitive rehabilitation of people regaining from strokes or brain damage. Wearable gadgets and smartphone apps equipped with AI can monitor patient symptoms, adherence to medications, and overall health state, allowing for prompt treatments and lowering hospital readmissions [30].

Artificial intelligence systems can analyze clinical data and scientific literature to generate evidence-based therapy recommendations, allowing neurologists to make more educated judgments. AI systems can detect small trends in patient data, potentially allowing for earlier identification of disorders like AD or PD when prior indications appear [25]. AI can analyze factors related to genes, the environment, and lifestyle to customize treatment strategies for each patient, boosting outcomes and lowering adverse effects [27, 29]. AI-powered solutions can analyze medical records and patient data to glean key insights and help with neurology research [30]. AI technology assists neurosurgeons in designing challenging therapies and provides real-time advice during surgery, enhancing accuracy and patient safety. These AI technologies alter neurological care through better diagnosis, medication, and supervision of patients, eventually leading to improved results and quality [25, 28].

14.2.1 AI and machine learning in healthcare

Artificial intelligence (AI) is a rapidly expanding topic in the field of information technology. AI involves generating intelligent technology that can learn and demonstrate intelligence comparable to human intellect. AI technology is built on algorithms that allow robots to learn from experience on their own.

As the system accomplishes tasks repeatedly, incremental modifications help to facilitate this learning process [27]. AI in healthcare is the application of natural language processing, machine learning, supervised learning, and other AI technologies to improve the interactions of both healthcare workers and patients [3, 31]. ML is a form of statistical analysis for adapting models to data and learning by training models on data. ML is one of the most common kinds of AI. It is a wide approach that is crucial to many AI approaches, and there are numerous variations of it [2]. This involves acquiring knowledge, making inferences, updating and enhancing the knowledge base, and developing algorithms [31]. AI algorithms can analyze medical data, such as imaging and electronic health records, to help healthcare workers diagnose diseases more precisely and rapidly. Investigations have shown that AI might surpass human radiologists in detecting tumors and other anomalies in medical imaging [2]. The drug development process is generally long and costly. Artificial intelligence can drastically cut the time necessary for drug research by predicting potential drug candidates, optimizing clinical trial concepts, and locating suitable volunteers [4, 31]. AI-powered robotic devices assist surgeons with complicated procedures, improving precision and control. This device has shortened recovery durations for patients and lessened the issues. AI can automate many repetitive tasks, including appointment scheduling, billing, and data entry, allowing healthcare professionals to focus on caring for patients rather than dealing with administrative tasks [32, 33].

AI systems improve healthcare operations' efficiency by rapidly processing large volumes of data. This capacity enables rapid decision-making and utilization of resources in medical facilities [34]. The adoption of AI can result in significant cost savings by eliminating needless tests, minimizing human error, and streamlining procedures [35]. For example, using artificial intelligence in diagnostics has the potential to reduce medical expenses by up to 50% while increasing health outcomes by 40%. AI allows for a more personalized approach to therapy by analyzing individual patient data and recommending individualized medicines. This shift to precision medicine tries to enhance therapeutic efficacy and patient satisfaction [23, 30, 32, 34].

14.2.2 Key technologies driving AI in healthcare

Machine learning is a key component of AI that allows computers to gain knowledge from information and develop periodically without any explicit programming. It is commonly used for predictive analytics and medical imaging. Predictive analytics characterized by machine learning algorithms use historical data to forecast patient outcomes, illness development, and therapy responses. In medical imaging, ML improves the accuracy of image processing, providing faster and more exact diagnoses in radiology and pathology [26, 28, 29, 33]. Deep learning (DL), a form of ML that makes use of multi-layered neural networks, is especially useful for analyzing vast amounts of unstructured data [23, 30]. DL systems excel at recognizing patterns within medical images, allowing for early identification of illnesses such as cancer. Natural language processing (NLP) helps AI systems comprehend and interpret human language, allowing for better administration of clinical documentation and interaction with patients [2, 23, 30, 31]. NLP enables AI to process and analyze massive volumes of written content from electronic health records (EHRs), medical records, and scientific articles. This technology improves clinical decision support and patient engagement. NLP tools can extract meaningful information from unstructured data, allowing healthcare practitioners to make informed judgments [2]. AI-powered chatbots with NLP can provide individuals with personalized information and support, boosting their entire experience. AI-powered robotic devices are widely used in surgical processes to improve precision and shorten recovery durations. Key advantages include minimally invasive surgery and automation of routine tasks [2, 3, 32]. Robots help surgeons achieve greater accuracy, which leads to fewer complications and faster patient recovery. Robots can automate repetitive chores in hospitals, allowing medical personnel to focus on more sophisticated patient care duties [2, 3, 4, 28, 34].

14.3 AI for Early Diagnosis of Neurodegenerative Disorders

Various data sources are analyzed for early indicators of neurodegenerative disorders using machine learning and deep learning techniques. Early detection using ML and DL includes medical imaging, biomarker identification, and electroencephalogram (EEG) analysis [36]. AI algorithms examine MRI, CT, and PET scans for small changes in brain structure that could signal early-stage dementia. Convolutional neural networks (CNNs) have provided great accuracy in identifying sequences linked with illnesses such as AD and PD before clinical symptoms onset (Table 14.2) [23, 36]. ML analyses genomic, proteomic, and metabolomic data to help find possible biomarkers. This enables researchers to detect early signs of disease and intervene before substantial neurodegeneration occurs. AI is being used in EEG assessments to detect aberrant brain wave patterns linked with neurodegenerative disorders.

Table 14.2 List of AI algorithms used in biomarker discovery for neurodegenerative diseases and their applications.

AI algorithm	Description	Applications
Convolutional neural networks (CNNs)	A deep learning algorithm designed primarily for image analysis.	Used to evaluate neuroimaging data (e.g., MRI) to find early biomarkers of AD and PD. Accomplished great accuracy in differentiating disease phases.
Deep neural networks (DNNs)	A multi-layered neural network capable of modeling complex data interactions.	Designed to evaluate gene expression data for AD, resulting in great accuracy in predicting disease occurrence and severity.
Support vector machines (SVM)	A supervised learning algorithm that distinguishes data by identifying the most appropriate hyperplane.	MRI data is evaluated for minor brain structural changes that indicate early AD, which enhances the accuracy of diagnosis.
Recurrent neural networks (RNNs)	A neural network was developed to process data sequentially.	Time-series data from monitoring devices worn by patients were investigated to track cognitive and motor impairments in neurodegenerative conditions.
Logistic regression	A statistical approach used to solve challenges with binary classification.	Clinical studies have employed it to determine the likelihood of acquiring AD based on a variety of clinical and genetic markers.

According to studies, AI can improve the processing of EEG data, making it easier to diagnose illnesses like AD at an early stage [23, 36, 37]. The use of digital biomarkers in data acquired via wearable devices and mobile apps allows the creation of predictive models for neurodegenerative disorders. AI systems analyze data from such gadgets to detect minor changes in behavioral or cognitive function that could indicate disease onset [38]. Cognitive decline detection can be characterized by monitoring reaction times, walking patterns, and facial expressions, which can reveal information about cognitive health, which enables earlier evaluation and therapeutic planning. Eye tracking can be done using artificial intelligence to analyze eye movements, and blinking rates can help in prediction of the progression of neurodegenerative disorders like AD and PD [38, 39].

AI is playing an important role in improving biomarker analysis for neurodegenerative disorders such as AD and PD. In diagnostic biomarkers, AI algorithms analyze complicated datasets such as genetic sequences, medical pictures, and digital biomarkers to detect early signs of neurodegenerative illnesses before clinical symptoms occur. This allows for timely intervention and better patient outcomes [36]. In prognostic biomarkers analysis, AI uses predictive modelling approaches to analyze longitudinal patient data, enabling personalized disease care plans based on patient health profiles [38]. AI techniques use a variety of data types, including neuroimaging, genomics, and digital phenotyping, to identify new meta-biomarkers. This integration improves the predictive value of biomarkers and helps generate more effective medicines [38, 40] as shown in Table 14.2.

14.4 AI in Monitoring Disease Progression

14.4.1 Wearable technology and AI for monitoring

The internet of things (IoT) broadly means to anything that can exchange information and communicate with other devices across network architecture. Any integrated device or sensor with system interaction capabilities to collect information on motions, image recognition, patient heart rates, and location might be considered an object or item in this context [41]. The wearable gadget is among the main elements supporting the IoT. Wearable computing has also brought about new methods, more efficient procedures, and innovative products in entertainment, sports, and many other fields [42]. But no other industry anticipates and uses wearable technology to the same extent as the healthcare sector, whose interests range from chronic patient care and other medical disciplines to well-being and disease prevention. This is because a wearable gadget paired with a mobile app might serve as a useful healthcare service, functioning as an intelligent personal assistant for the patient [43, 44]. With the introduction of wearable technology in the past few years, healthcare professionals are now more motivated and able to work outside of the hospital or workplace to help identify and assess health hazards, track the development of diseases, such as AD, and provide therapy or guidance [43]. The tests used to diagnose neurodegenerative disorders are widely established, although they are often less effective in detecting abnormalities that arise early in the course of cognitive loss. In the quest for gold standards for AD evaluation, the creation of readily accessible digital biomarkers that take advantage of developments in consumer-grade mobile and wearable technologies is becoming more and more crucial [45]. These gadgets are especially equipped to investigate physical and cognitive capacities or symptoms, and because they are being utilized by expanding sectors of

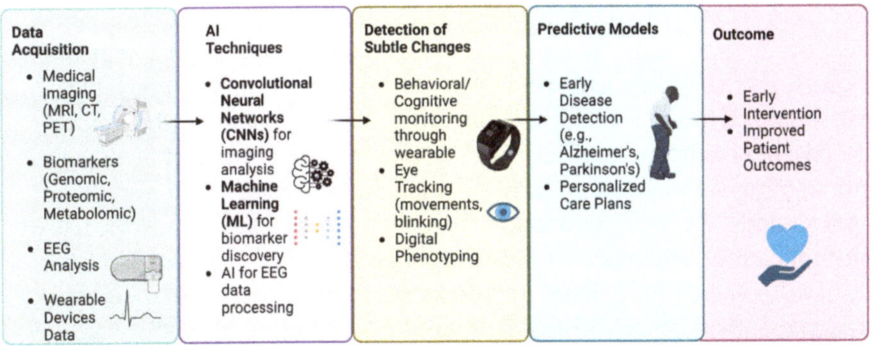

Figure 14.1 AI-Driven Early Detection and Prediction of Neurodegenerative Disorders.

the public, they have a substantial impact on the load on the healthcare system and considerably reduce the stress placed on patient caregivers. These factors make mobile and wearable technologies an exceptional chance to promptly identify neurodegenerative illnesses in a timely and cost-effective manner. Advancement and the range of onboard sensors at the core of these systems allow for significant approach flexibility by providing metrics via active or passive measurements [46]. With time, there has been a major evolution in the technologies utilized for Parkinsonism disease (PD) diagnosis and monitoring. Most significantly, such tools have advanced from lab settings to the home or daily environment, allowing additional information collection on Parkinson's disease symptoms [47]. Wearable devices with accelerometers and gyroscopes were also used to measure other PD symptoms [48]. As tremor analyses included more and more wearable accelerometers, they began to be used outside of the lab and assisted in differentiating between patients with vital tremor, Parkinson's disease, and other control groups [49] as shown in Figure 14.1.

14.4.2 Personalized monitoring systems

Physicians, medical specialists, and medical assistants will need to engage with computer systems and use specialized apps as computerized patient observation systems grow to assist with remote monitoring and medical tasks. This will ensure that patients receive high-quality healthcare services [50]. Healthcare apps save expenses, broaden the breadth and reach of medical facilities, improve service quality, and allow information sharing between physicians and patients or between institutions. The new medical devices have sensors, RFID chips, microcontrollers, actuators wireless communication devices, nano pumps, and other features that enable patients, physicians, and other medical specialists to deliver more timely, convenient, and personalized health monitoring, diagnosis, and treatment all while reducing the cost of healthcare services [51]. The fastest-growing area of healthcare is remote patient monitoring (RPM), which helps doctors in a variety of hospital settings. By using wearable technology, contact-based sensors, telehealth applications, and other novel IoT approaches in the healthcare industry, this is accomplished [52]. RPM is frequently used to assess vital signs or other physiological characteristics like motion recognition in order to aid in clinical decisions and treatment options for issues like movement disorders or psychological ailments [53]. They can improve treatment and provide a rapid, simple, and cost-effective solution. Patients with Parkinson's disease are better able to be distinguished from comparable conditions when they are observed for a predefined period of time while the severity of their symptoms is evaluated (Table 14.3) [51]. Information and communication technologies and the IoT enable the creation of personalized home management and healthcare solutions. The ability to gather patient evaluation and measurement data wirelessly using innovative approaches permits individuals to perform self-testing [54].

Table 14.3 AI algorithms used in personalized treatment strategies for neurodegenerative disorders.

Component	Data source	Description
Wearable devices	Smartwatches, accelerometers, gyroscopes	Devices equipped with sensors to track signals like tremor, gait, and balance
Predictive models	Symptoms tracking	AI algorithms that predict problems or the development of symptoms based on trends in past data
Mobile app	Self-reported systems	Patient tracking of symptoms, medication adherence, and health insights can be facilitated through mobile app interfaces
Telehealth support	Data from wearables, clinical assessment	Virtual communication for monitoring and treatment modifications with medical professionals
Data analytics	Patient reported outcomes, patient history	Tools for data analytics to produce useful insights from clinical and wearable data

14.5 AI-Enhanced Treatment Strategies

14.5.1 AI-guided drug discovery and development

AI is turning the biopharmaceutical industry's approach to creating new treatments on a completely new level. AI is now an important component in the drug discovery process [55]. Modern drug design and discovery are now operating under drastically different paradigms as a result of the rapid proliferation of advanced AI approaches [56]. This change offers a faster confirmation of the drug target and optimization of the drug structure design, and it has permeated nearly all critical phases of drug discovery, from early hit identification to lead determination [57]. The emergence of a plethora of AI-driven CADD tools has also been made possible by these advancements. The ligand-based quantitative structure-activity relationship (QSAR) modeling and structure-based molecular docking are two examples of these techniques. Furthermore, the rise of deep generative techniques has led to the revival of de novo drug design methodologies [56]. Finding novel treatments for the central nervous system (CNS) is a very costly process with several special difficulties that result in low effectiveness and significant attrition. Virtually every part of life has been impacted by data-driven technologies like AI and ML in the information age due to the proliferation of data. In the case of drug discovery, the advent of a large amount of information through genetic, proteomic and biochemical technologies has resulted in the collaboration of pharmaceutical giants with AI-focused startups to revolutionize the process and increase its efficiency. These advances have given new impetus and direction to research on treatments for conditions like Parkinsonism, Alzheimer's disease, and schizophrenia. AI and ML have been used in the design of CNS treatments and in both structure- and ligand-based drug development [58].

14.5.2 AI in optimizing treatment plans

The rapid advancement of AI technology presents opportunities for its application in medical institutions and has the capacity to completely alter how healthcare is provided. As a result of current developments in AI, computational methods for diagnosis and monitoring that are created with the use of machine learning algorithms can be of great assistance. AI systems have the ability to forecast the diagnosis and prognosis of AD by analyzing genetic information from patients. The investigation of genetic interactions, gene activity patterns, and genetic variants in AD have benefited greatly by the application of AI technology (machine learning algorithms) over the past ten years [59]. Using patient genetic data, AI algorithms were utilized to forecast the diagnosis and outcome of AD. The development of AD stratification tools is also being aided by the use of ML to group patients according to shared genetic traits. Additionally, the analysis of protein signatures in patient samples can help identify biomarkers, which will likely enhance the diagnosis of the illness i.e., the Alzheimer's disease biomarker APOE-e4 gene variation. Large genetic datasets have been used to train models to find patterns linked to the beginning and development of Alzheimer's disease. AI can forecast the course of a disease by comparing a patient's genetic makeup to that of other people who have the same ailment. This makes it easier to determine which therapy may work better based on genetic predispositions and when to begin interventions [59, 60, 61]. AI can evaluate clinical data, such as MRI, PET, and results from cognitive tests, to find early signs of Alzheimer's disease even before symptoms appear. Machine learning algorithms trained to detect patterns in amyloid plaques and brain shrinkage can produce early warning systems that guide treatment decisions [62, 63]. Based on clinical data from electronic health records (EHRs), AI can forecast how patients with similar medical histories have responded to various medicines, such as cholinesterase inhibitors or NMDA receptor antagonists. Therefore, based on real efficacy data, AI can recommend treatments to patients with similar clinical characteristics [61]. AI uses information from wearables and patient reports on diet, exercise, and sleep habits to make decisions about how a patient's disease progresses. It offers customized lifestyle adjustments, including frequent exercise or mental activities that may slow the loss of cognitive function. AI combines clinical, genetic, and lifestyle data from each patient to create personalized treatment plans based on their unique profile. AI simulations can help determine the optimal course of action with the fewest adverse consequences of simulating treatment outcomes [61, 64] as shown in Table 14.3.

14.6 AI in Cognitive and Physical Rehabilitation

AI's revolutionary potential in cognitive and physical rehabilitation for neurodegenerative disorders like Alzheimer's is becoming more widely acknowledged. AI improves diagnosis, treatment planning, and patient monitoring by utilizing sophisticated algorithms and data analysis, which eventually results in a higher quality of life. AI systems are capable of analyzing a wide range of data sources, such as clinical notes and photos of patients, to help with the early identification and precise diagnosis of Alzheimer's disease [65]. The utilization of ML methodologies facilitates the identification of biomarkers and forecasting the course of disease progression, hence enabling prompt therapies [60].

14.6.1 Virtual reality (VR) and AI for cognitive rehabilitation

AI-powered rehabilitation initiatives apply tailored strategies to improve mental and physical capacities, combining interdisciplinary techniques from psychology and neurology. By meeting both cognitive and emotional demands, artificial intelligence-powered digital communication solutions increase patient engagement and adherence to rehabilitation methods [63, 66] . The fields of neuroscience, neuropsychology, and cognitive rehabilitation have been paying more and more attention to virtual reality (VR), a game-changing technology that immerses users in surroundings that are multimodal and interactive [67]. Virtual reality has the potential to fundamentally alter the way that we approach cognitive rehab by offering fresh possibilities for enhancing cognitive abilities, promoting brain plasticity, and, eventually, enhancing the quality of life for persons with cognitive disabilities [68]. VR is revolutionizing cognitive rehabilitation by offering immersive, customized environments designed for patients with neurological conditions including AD and stroke. With particular applications like multiplayer VR for social skill development in autism and motor function recovery in Alzheimer disease, it improves engagement and rehabilitation outcomes [69]. Moreover, VR provides real-time data recording, which enables prompt feedback and modifications to rehabilitation tactics, enhancing overall efficacy. Studies show that VR interventions lead to significant cognitive improvements, with a focus on enhancing the transfer of skills to daily activities [70]. Through real-time personalization and plan adaptation depending on patient performance in virtual reality exercises, AI improves cognitive rehabilitation [71]. AI systems employ predictive analytics to identify targeted cognitive impairments, modify the difficulty of tasks, and recommend successful remedies [72]. VR and AI integration enables adaptive VR scenarios that are customized to the individual needs of each patient as well as immersive data collection [66, 71, 72, 73]. Personalized training regimens can be created using AI-driven technologies like NeuroAIreh@b and AI-Rehab, which leverage machine learning [71, 73]. Another example would be apps like Livongo, which use wearable data to generate customized recommendations [74]. VR technology provides a flexible variety of tools for cognitive rehabilitation, spanning from non-immersive to highly immersive situations. Non-immersive setups, which usually consist of normal PCs, tablets, cellphones, and television screens, are at one extreme of this spectrum [75]. These configurations are accessible to a broad spectrum of users and, although not as immersive, nonetheless offer beneficial cognitive workouts. In this instance, the third person perspective allows the user to perceive both the real world and the virtual environment without fully submerging in it [68]. The combination of VR and AI presents exciting new opportunities for cognitive rehabilitation.

14.6.2 Robotics and AI in physical therapy

Daily activities are hampered by the cognitive, physical, and functional impairments caused by neurodegenerative diseases. As a means of improving the self-sufficiency and standard of living for people with certain illnesses, intelligent assistive technologies such as robots that can perform repetitive activities or help with socialization show promise. Using a range of robots and sensors in conjunction with machine intelligence techniques, it provides assistance to the elderly and people with impairments. Socially supportive robots can lessen isolation, improve communication, and lessen the effects of sensory loss [76]. Robots have been widely used in a variety of clinical settings for physical rehabilitation applications, such as helping stroke victims regain their movement and enhance or replace lost function [77, 78]. One such device that encourages patients to move and advance is an exoskeleton, which is used for hands, legs, and arms in videogames. AI might assist therapists in obtaining the resources and support they need to give their patients the appropriate attention and care [79]. Limited AI is being developed to evaluate mobility, gait, upper extremity recovery, motor function, and functional status in conjunction with robotic-assisted therapy. AI created a knee exoskeleton AI that combines force, motion, and pressure signals obtained from the exoskeleton's detectors to give intelligent support when needed for walking. Another created a robotic knee system with AI human-robot interactive control that uses electromyography impulses to assist in mobility, such as walking, as necessary [79, 80]. Giving patients tactile, aural, and visual input is another important function of robotic systems. By using actuators to provide tactile sensations through motions, forces, and vibrations that mimic real-world interactions, haptic feedback incorporates the sense of touch into digital encounters. This technology supports robotic systems, improves user interface interactions during therapeutic exercises, and accelerates the process of neuroplasticity by using sophisticated materials and precise control algorithms to produce accurate and responsive tactile inputs [81]. For neurological patients undergoing physiotherapeutic rehabilitation, such as those with Parkinson's disease, AI may be a useful therapeutic choice.

14.7 Ethical Considerations and Challenges

14.7.1 Ethical issues in AI for healthcare

With the advent of AI come ethical concerns that must be recognized and appropriately resolved in the most efficient and evidence-based way feasible. The moral dilemmas raised by AI in healthcare are numerous and intricate [82]. Recent evaluations of the impact of AI in public health have urged caution when it comes to the implementation of AI in healthcare, while additional study is needed to ensure ethical AI design and deployment. AI may have the potential to improve people's health and additionally contribute to the health systems' sustainability and resilience [83]. Even though the use of AI in healthcare is growing, there is not yet a widely recognized, broad framework for directing the development and use based upon artificial intelligence decision support within the industry. Importantly, there are still a lot of unanswered ethical questions that could apply to a variety of technological advancements and algorithmic applications. Concerns including biases (i.e., using subpar or inadequate datasets for training and testing can lead to subpar or unfavorable results when creating AI systems), safeguarding patient privacy, and earning the faith of physicians and patients are inherent to AI [83]. Professionals in related fields and policymakers have been searching for ways to manage the ethical hazards that come with the development of AI [84]. For example, sensing algorithms are used for autopilot cars in automated transportation systems; algorithms based on genes are used to foresee the outcomes for terminally ill patients; and natural language processing (NLP) is integrated alongside ML to support virtual education. Explainability can increase engagement and trust in AI, which is crucial for ethical AI. The judiciary, the government, and the media are among the societal bodies that have called for algorithmic openness and explainability [85, 86]. Understandably, there are concerns that artificial intelligence (AI) could damage the relationship between patients and providers, lead to the deskilling of healthcare professionals, compromise transparency, misdiagnose, or treat patients inappropriately due to hard-to-detect errors in AI decision-making, exacerbate preexisting cultural or social biases, or create algorithmic bias that will be difficult to find. Conventional research techniques, namely the comparative legal approach with a focus on general and particular techniques, were selected. The AI must be trained in order to function, and it is currently gaining knowledge from a variety of sources. Health data, or sensitive personal data, makes up the majority of the data used to train AI. Given the importance of the information included and the significant risks of a leak, personal data is classified as sensitive personal data, which highlights the need for tighter regulation and control [87].

14.7.2 Challenges in implementing AI in neurodegenerative disorder management

The science of ML, implementation logistics, and planning that takes into account adoption barriers and required sociocultural or clinical pathway modifications are among the main obstacles to the integration of AI systems in healthcare. These factors all undermine clinical relevance and usefulness. A significant obstacle is the dependence on extensive neurological exams, which often entail manual evaluations of sensory and motor abilities, additionally gait, cerebellar, and cognitive impairments [88]. Accurate diagnosis and disease monitoring may be hampered by the inadequacies of virtual platforms in capturing these subtleties. Further impediments to the senior population's effective participation in telehealth programs may come from difficulties relating to technological literacy and access for those suffering from AD or different types of dementia, including dementia caused by PD [89]. Maintaining continuous and dependable teleneurology services is made more difficult by the absence of established procedures for remote neurological exams and the possibility of inconsistent internet access. ML and DL algorithms still have a lot of drawbacks despite their great potential for use in the diagnosis of degenerative nerve diseases. While some of these restrictions apply to ML and DL systems, some are more particular than others. Nearly all models encounter the major issue of having a little or incomplete dataset [90] and the requirement for reliable and understandable models [91]. For rare medical conditions like ALS or Huntington's disease, which frequently struggle with a lack of substantial and appropriate datasets, this issue is severe. Datasets with degenerative nerve disorders frequently have biases. Because of the small sample size and potential overfitting, models' capacity for generalization is frequently overstated [92]. Patient privacy is an important social concern that must be respected by any computer assistant system [90]. The possible legal liability that medical centers incur while using AI to treat patients makes collaboration and openness with vendors essential to

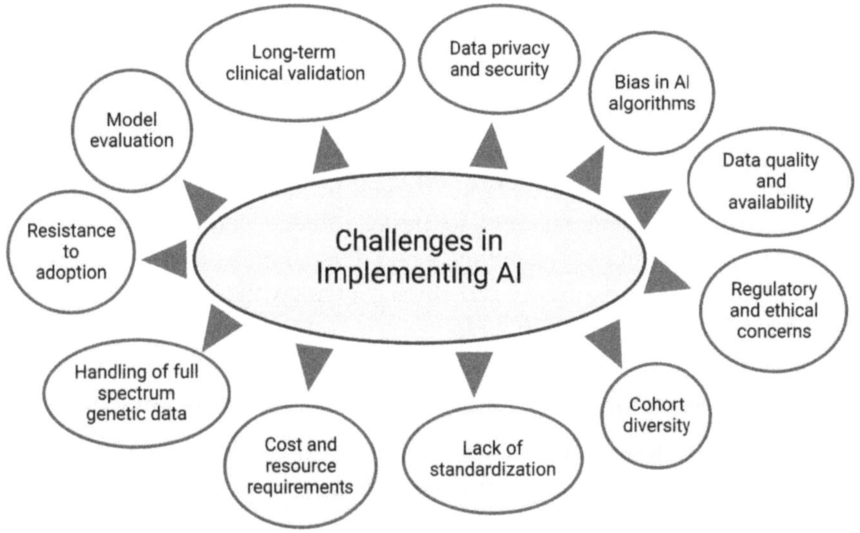

Figure 14.2 Challenges in Implementing AI.

the successful implementation of industry-developed AI. Determining how to evaluate various AI platform vendors is one of the challenges facing individual enterprises. Specifically, the absence of well-established AI vendors can leave the healthcare industry open to firms overstating their capabilities and having no idea of how to integrate AI into healthcare requirements. Features like interconnection and interaction with current digital networks and electronic medical record systems may be missing from early AI offerings [93]. Additionally, early AI solutions will inevitably have limited therapeutic utility due to regulatory issues, whereas a wider use case and product could be most advantageous to the organization and society. Thus, there are numerous prospects for codesigning systems that are most clinically beneficial for providers by industry and health systems [94] as shown in Figure 14.2.

14.8 Future Directions

Advanced health informatics using DL will be beneficial to most biomedical research domains. Even though biomedical data analysis has advanced significantly due to applications for ML and DL for the identification of new targets for therapy and biomarkers, there is still much work to be done in order to use integrated data to create more individualized and effective treatments. The biomedical area is showing signs of promise in big data analytics, as evidenced by the increasing number of initiatives aimed at standardizing the integration of many sources of information and exchanging data, particularly in neurodegenerative disease research. Modern healthcare is built on precision medicine, and AI is essential to customizing therapy for each patient [95]. When applied within the context of precision medicine, DL can be extremely useful in identifying new targets for therapeutic intervention as well as early biological markers for more effective clinical treatment and diagnosis of individuals with complex and diversified neurodegenerative diseases. Enhancing AI's resilience and efficacy in many therapeutic contexts is the main goal of future research.

14.8.1 Next-generation AI tools for neurodegenerative disorders

Neuroimaging is exploding over a wide range of fields, from autonomous diagnosis of medical images to improving the quality of upstream image data. For neurodegenerative disease, there are numerous applications ranging from synthesizing missing data through cross-modality transformation to improving the classification of disease states and current and future biomarkers; in many cases, these applications will improve access to neuroimaging technology at lower cost and risk [96]. In the case of neuroimaging, functional MRI (fMRI) research has advanced significantly. More accurate and quick scans are now possible due to recent developments, which are crucial for capturing the dynamic activity of the brain. These advancements are especially noteworthy when it comes to learning more about how certain brain regions are involved in various cognitive tasks and how neurodegenerative diseases impact these regions. Modern fMRI technologies have made it possible to identify and monitor functional changes in the brain that indicate the early stages of diseases like Parkinson's and Alzheimer's [97]. Neurodegenerative disorders differ from person to person. It can be very difficult to deal with and process medical data. Differently formatted data requires special normalization before processing. To comprehend and handle the research challenge, complex medical data demands specialized understanding. With the development of numerous learning neural networks, including convolutional, recurrent, and visual geometry group (VGG) networks, AI has evolved into multidimensional processing. The network must be trained on the data in order to determine which network is most appropriate for processing the input and producing the desired outcomes [98]. AI is now involved in the discovery of novel biomarkers for neurodegenerative diseases. By analyzing large datasets that include genetic, proteomic, and metabolomic information, AI tools can identify biomarkers that may be useful for early detection, tracking the development of diseases, or forecasting the outcome of treatment.

14.8.2 Integrating AI into clinical practice

Among the most significant benefits of AI in clinical practice is its ability to accurately evaluate large volumes of datasets. As a result, numerous apps that have enhanced patient outcomes and lessened the strain for medical personnel have been developed. AI can help medical professionals diagnose patients more accurately and create individualized treatment regimens [99]. AI is evolving quickly, creating opportunities for its application in clinical settings and potentially revolutionizing the way healthcare is provided. Knowledge on the technology's use in clinical settings must be documented and disseminated in order to give healthcare workers the tools and resources they need to successfully incorporate AI into patient care [74]. Early identification of AD is essential since it enables proper therapy approaches and preventive actions to limit the progression of the illness. AI is starting to show promise as a tool for raising the precision and promptness of AD diagnosis. Currently, AI's most widely used use in AD is the analysis of massive volumes of medical dataset, especially brain imaging tests, to find preliminary disease symptoms. Deep learning methods for brain image analysis can be used to detect anatomical anomalies in certain regions of the brain, which is utilized to distinguish AD patients from healthier individuals and patients with additional neurodegenerative disorders [100]. Applications known as clinical decision support (CDS) tools are designed to give clinicians filtered information at the point of care in an effort to improve patient outcomes. A CDS tool is essentially an application that helps doctors make clinical decisions by filtering and translating empirical facts into a format that is immediately useful. Through the integration of patient-specific parameters (such as genetics and biomarker profiles), precision management therapies can be guided by CDS applications [101].

14.9 Conclusion

AI has the potential to revolutionize both clinical treatment and neuroscience research. The integration of AI into medical sciences has ushered in a new era in healthcare, with neurodegenerative disease research benefiting significantly. AI enables the analysis of vast amounts of medical data from multiple sources, facilitating tailored treatment strategies, enhanced diagnostic accuracy, and predictive modelling. These advancements offer unprecedented opportunities for early diagnosis, personalized therapies, and monitoring disease progression. The convergence of explainable AI, digital biomarkers, precision medicine, and advanced neuroimaging analysis is enabling better patient outcomes and more effective treatments. ML techniques have been instrumental in the significant progress made in neurodegenerative disease research, particularly in neuroimaging and motor function analysis. This marks a paradigm shift in how the medical field approaches and treats complex neurological disorders, rather than just incremental improvements. AI holds enormous potential to deliver more personalized, effective, and efficient treatment plans for neurodegenerative diseases.

Acknowledgments

The authors are thankful to the Department of Pharmaceuticals, Ministry of Chemicals and Fertilizers, Government of India. All the figures are from https://www.biorender.com.

Credit Authorship Contribution Statement

Sarasa Meenakshi, Krishna Murti, Ved Prakash: Conceptualization, Amrutha TV, Nabeeha Koya, Sarasa Meenakshi, Nitesh Kumar: Writing – original draft preparation, Visualization, Sarasa Meenakshi, Ved Prakash, Nitesh Kumar, Nikhilesh Anand, Santhosh Kumar, Krishna Murti: Supervision, Writing – review & editing.

Declaration of Competing Interest

The authors declare no competing or financial interests relevant to this article.

References

[1] Gao, H.-M., & Hong, J.-S. (2008. Why neurodegenerative diseases are progressive: uncontrolled inflammation drives disease progression. Trends in immunology, 29(8), 357-365.

[2] Davenport, T., & Kalakota, R. (2019). The potential for artificial intelligence in healthcare. Future healthcare journal, 6(2), 94-98.

[3] Keeratihuttayakorn, K., Chavanotai, N., et al. (2021). Medical System and Artificial Intelligence: How AI assists hospital-dependent patients. Int. J. Med. Phar. Drug Re, 5.

[4] Lee, D., & Yoon, S. N. (2021). Application of artificial intelligence-based technologies in the healthcare industry: Opportunities and challenges. International Journal of Environmental Research and Public Health, 18(1), 271.

[5] Wilson, D. M., Cookson, M. R., et al. (2023). Hallmarks of neurodegenerative diseases. Cell, 186(4), 693-714.

[6] Gupta, A. (2021). Human Caspases and Neuronal Apoptosis in Neurodegenerative Diseases.Academic Press.

[7] Nandi, A., Counts, N., et al. (2022). Global and regional projections of the economic burden of Alzheimer's disease and related dementias from 2019 to 2050: A value of statistical life approach. 51.

[8] Chudzik, A., Śledzianowski, A., et al. (2024a). Machine learning and digital biomarkers can detect early stages of neurodegenerative diseases. 24(5), 1572.

[9] Palanisamy, C. P., Pei, J., et al. (2023). New strategies of neurodegenerative disease treatment with extracellular vesicles (EVs) derived from mesenchymal stem cells (MSCs). Theranostics, 13(12), 4138.

[10] Kirschbaum, C., Hellhammer, D., et al. (2000). Encyclopedia of stress. In Salivary Cortisol. (pp. 379-384). Academic Press San Diego: CA.

[11] Verkhratsky, A., & Butt, A. (2023). Chapter 11-Neurodegenerative diseases. Neuroglia. 1st ed. Academic Press: New York, 563-598.

[12] Swaab, D. F., Fliers, E., et al. (2011). Aging of the Brain and Alzheimer's Disease.Elsevier.

[13] Brill, M. T. (2005). Alzheimer's Disease.Marshall Cavendish.

[14] Duarte, J. M., Schuck, P. F., et al. (2014). Metabolic disturbances in diseases with neurological involvement. Aging and disease, 5(4), 238.

[15] Dugger, B. N., & Dickson, D. W. (2017). Pathology of neurodegenerative diseases. Cold Spring Harbor perspectives in biology, 9(7), a028035.

[16] Poewe, W. (2008). Non-motor symptoms in Parkinson's disease. European journal of neurology, 15, 14-20.

[17] Váradi, C. (2020). Clinical features of Parkinson's disease: the evolution of critical symptoms. Biology, 9(5), 103.

[18] Mead, R. J., Shan, N., et al. (2023). Amyotrophic lateral sclerosis: a neurodegenerative disorder poised for successful therapeutic translation. Nature Reviews Drug Discovery, 22(3), 185-212.

[19] Gironi, M., Arnò, C., et al. (2016). Multiple sclerosis and neurodegenerative diseases. In Immune rebalancing (pp. 63-84). Elsevier.

[20] Fan, H.-C., Ho, L.-I., et al. (2014). Polyglutamine (PolyQ) diseases: genetics to treatments. Cell transplantation, 23(4-5), 441-458.

[21] Vonsattel, J.-P., Myers, R. H., et al. (1985). Neuropathological classification of Huntington's disease. Journal of Neuropathology & Experimental Neurology, 44(6), 559-577.

[22] Zhang, W., Xiao, D., et al. (2023). Role of neuroinflammation in neurodegeneration development. Signal transduction and targeted therapy, 8(1), 267.

[23] Bakkar, N., Kovalik, T., et al. (2018). Artificial intelligence in neurodegenerative disease research: use of IBM Watson to identify additional RNA-binding proteins altered in amyotrophic lateral sclerosis. Acta neuropathologica, 135, 227-247.

[24] Plus, E. S. (2022). Towards Modern-Age Advanced Sensors for the Management of Neurodegenerative Disorders: Current Status, Challenges and Prospects.

[25] Asakawa, T., Sugiyama, K., et al. (2019). Can the latest computerized technologies revolutionize conventional assessment tools and therapies for a neurological disease? the example of Parkinson's disease. Neurologia medico-chirurgica, 59(3), 69-78.

[26] Giordano, A., De Panfilis, L., et al. (2022). Advance care planning in neurodegenerative disorders: a scoping review. International Journal of Environmental Research and Public Health, 19(2), 803.

[27] Kuo, C.-L. (2023). Revolutionizing Healthcare Paradigms: The Integral Role of Artificial Intelligence in Advancing Diagnostic and Treatment Modalities. International Microsurgery Journal (IMJ).

[28] Patel, U. K., Anwar, A., et al. (2021). Artificial intelligence as an emerging technology in the current care of neurological disorders. Journal of neurology, 268, 1623-1642.

[29] Hussain, I., & Nazir, M. B. (2024). Mind Matters: Exploring AI, Machine Learning, and Deep Learning in Neurological Health. International Journal of Advanced Engineering Technologies and Innovations, 1(4), 209-230.

[30] Hebold Haraldsen, I. R., Hatlestad-Hall, C., et al. (2024). AI-Mind: Revolutionizing Personalized Neurology Through Automated Diagnostics and Advanced Data Management. Drug Repurposing, 1(1), 20240005.

[31] Panesar, A. (2019). Machine learning and AI for healthcare.Springer.

[32] Bajwa, J., Munir, U., et al. (2021). Artificial intelligence in healthcare: transforming the practice of medicine. Future healthcare journal, 8(2), e188-e194.
[33] Jiang, F., Jiang, Y., et al. (2017). Artificial intelligence in healthcare: past, present and future. Stroke and vascular neurology, 2(4).
[34] Sharma, A. (2024). Artificial intelligence in healthcare. In Revolutionizing the Healthcare Sector with AI (pp. 1-25). IGI Global.
[35] Wilson, T. (2017). No longer science fiction, AI and robotics are transforming healthcare. PWC Accessed October, 31, 2021.
[36] Feng, T. (2023). Applications of Artificial Intelligence to Diagnosis of Neurodegenerative Diseases. Studies in Health Technology and Informatics, 308, 648-655.
[37] Stefano, G. B. (2023). Artificial intelligence as a tool for the diagnosis and treatment of neurodegenerative diseases. In (Vol. 13, pp. 938): MDPI.
[38] Chudzik, A., Śledzianowski, A., et al. (2024b). Machine learning and digital biomarkers can detect early stages of neurodegenerative diseases. Sensors, 24(5), 1572.
[39] Beheshti, I., Sone, D., et al. (2023). State-of-the-art artificial intelligence methods in neurodegeneration. In (Vol. 13, pp. 1112639): Frontiers Media SA.
[40] Khaliq, F., Oberhauser, J., et al. (2023). Decoding degeneration: the implementation of machine learning for clinical detection of neurodegenerative disorders. Neural regeneration research, 18(6), 1235-1242.
[41] Alghamdi, A. A. J. J. o. E., & Sciences, A. (2022). A Comparative Analysis to Advancing the National Cybersecurity Strategy in Saudi Arabia. 9(1).
[42] Gupta, M., Gupta, K. K., et al. (2021). An intelligent session key-based hybrid lightweight image encryption algorithm using logistic-tent map and crossover operator for internet of multimedia things. 121(3), 1857-1878.
[43] Amft, O. J. I. P. C. (2018). How wearable computing is shaping digital health. 17(1), 92-98.
[44] Salehi, W., Gupta, G., et al. (2022). IoT-Based Wearable Devices for Patients Suffering from Alzheimer Disease. 2022(1), 3224939.
[45] Kourtis, L. C., Regele, O. B., et al. (2019). Digital biomarkers for Alzheimer's disease: the mobile/wearable devices opportunity. 2(1), 9.

[46] Doraiswamy, P. M., Narayan, V. A., et al. (2018). Mobile and pervasive computing technologies and the future of Alzheimer's clinical trials. 1(1), 1.
[47] Chandrabhatla, A. S., Pomeraniec, I. J., et al. (2022). Co-evolution of machine learning and digital technologies to improve monitoring of Parkinson's disease motor symptoms. 5(1), 32.
[48] Phan, D., Horne, M., et al. (2018). Measurement of axial rigidity and postural instability using wearable sensors. 18(2), 495.
[49] Cole, B. T., Roy, S. H., et al. (2010). Dynamic neural network detection of tremor and dyskinesia from wearable sensor data. 2010 Annual International Conference of the IEEE Engineering in Medicine and Biology,
[50] Tan, J., Mas, F. G. S., et al. (2005). E-PUBLIC HEALTH INFORMATION SYSTEMS. 127.
[51] Chiuchisan, I., & Geman, O. J. W. T. o. S. (2014). An approach of a decision support and home monitoring system for patients with neurological disorders using internet of things concepts. 13(1), 460-469.
[52] Farias, F. A. C. d., Dagostini, C. M., et al. (2020). Remote patient monitoring: a systematic review. 26(5), 576-583.
[53] Vegesna, A., Tran, M., et al. (2017). Remote patient monitoring via non-invasive digital technologies: a systematic review. 23(1), 3-17.
[54] Vermesan, O., & Friess, P. (2013). Internet of things: converging technologies for smart environments and integrated ecosystems.River publishers.
[55] Huang, D., Yang, M., et al. (2024). AI-DRIVEN DRUG DISCOVERY:: ACCELERATING THE DEVELOPMENT OF NOVEL THERAPEUTICS IN BIOPHARMACEUTICALS. 3(3), 206-224.
[56] Shen, C., Song, J., et al. (2024). DrugFlow: An AI-Driven One-Stop Platform for Innovative Drug Discovery. 64(14), 5381-5391.
[57] Mak, K.-K., Wong, Y.-H., et al. (2023). Artificial intelligence in drug discovery and development. 1-38.
[58] Gautam, V., Gaurav, A., et al. (2023). Artificial intelligence and machine-learning approaches in structure and ligand-based discovery of drugs affecting central nervous system. 27(2), 959-985.
[59] Mishra, R., Li, B. J. A., et al. (2020). The application of artificial intelligence in the genetic study of Alzheimer's disease. 11(6), 1567.

[60] Myszczynska, M. A., Ojamies, P. N., et al. (2020). Applications of machine learning to diagnosis and treatment of neurodegenerative diseases. 16(8), 440-456.

[61] Johnson, K. B., Wei, W. Q., et al. (2021). Precision medicine, AI, and the future of personalized health care. 14(1), 86-93.

[62] Alvarado, M., Gómez, D., et al. (2023). Implementation of an Early Detection System for Neurodegenerative Diseases Through the use of Artificial Intelligence. 2023 IEEE XXX International Conference on Electronics, Electrical Engineering and Computing (INTERCON),

[63] Krishna, K. S., Sarma, K. J., et al. (2023). Alzheimer Disease Detection using AI with Deep Learning based Features with Development and Validation based on Data Science.

[64] Malcangi, M. J. A. N. N. (2021). AI-based methods and technologies to develop wearable devices for prosthetics and predictions of degenerative diseases. 337-354.

[65] Dabbaghi, K. G., Khosravirad, Z., et al. (2023). The Use of Artificial Intelligence in the Management of Neurodegenerative Disorders; Focus on Alzheimer's Disease. 12, 1.

[66] Khalid, U. b., Naeem, M., et al. (2024). Impact of AI-powered solutions in rehabilitation process: Recent improvements and future trends. 943-969.

[67] Wen, D., Lan, X., et al. (2018). The study of evaluation and rehabilitation of patients with different cognitive impairment phases based on virtual reality and EEG. 10, 88.

[68] Catania, V., Rundo, F., et al. (2023). Virtual Reality for the Rehabilitation of Acquired Cognitive Disorders: A Narrative Review. 11(1), 35.

[69] Quan, W., Liu, S., et al. (2024). A Comprehensive Review of Virtual Reality Technology for Cognitive Rehabilitation in Patients with Neurological Conditions. 14(14), 6285.

[70] Buele, J., Varela-Aldás, J. L., et al. (2023). Virtual reality applications based on instrumental activities of daily living (iADLs) for cognitive intervention in older adults: a systematic review. 20(1), 168.

[71] Sirsat, Y. A. M. S., i Badia, S. B., et al. AI-Rehab: A Framework for AI Driven Neurorehabilitation Training The Profiling Challenge.

[72] Bazarbekov, I., Razaque, A., et al. (2024). A review of artificial intelligence methods for Alzheimer's disease diagnosis: Insights from neuroimaging to sensor data analysis. 92, 106023.

[73] Faria, A. L., Almeida, Y., et al. (2024). NeuroAIreh@ b: an artificial intelligence-based methodology for personalized and adaptive neurorehabilitation. 14, 1258323.

[74] Alowais, S. A., Alghamdi, S. S., et al. (2023). Revolutionizing healthcare: the role of artificial intelligence in clinical practice. 23(1), 689.

[75] Georgiev, D., Georgieva, I., et al. (2021). Virtual Reality for Neurorehabilitation and Cognitive Enhancement. Brain Sci. 2021, 11, 221. In: s Note: MDPI stays neu-tral with regard to jurisdictional clai-ms in . . . .

[76] Sylvester, A., Temesgen, E., et al. (2023). Ethical robot design considerations for individuals suffering from a neurodegenerative disease. Workshop Geriatronics: AI and Robotics for Health & Well-Being in Older Age at IROS,

[77] Pattanshetty, R. B., Khan, S. J. I. J. o. P. T., et al. (2022). A Shifting Paradigm from Human Intelligence to Artificial Intelligence in Rehabilitation: A Descriptive Review. 4(1), 8-13.

[78] Perju-Dumbrava, L., Barsan, M., et al. (2022). Artificial intelligence applications and robotic systems in Parkinson's disease (Review). Exp Ther Med, 23(2), 153. https://doi.org/10.3892/etm.2021.11076

[79] Lyu, M., Chen, W.-H., et al. (2019). Knee exoskeleton enhanced with artificial intelligence to provide assistance-as-needed. 90(9).

[80] Fulk, G. (2023). Artificial Intelligence and Neurologic Physical Therapy. 47(1), 1-2. https://doi.org/10.1097/npt.0000000000000426

[81] Banyai, A. D., & BriŞan, C. (2024). Robotics in physical rehabilitation: Systematic Review. Healthcare,

[82] Murphy, K., Di Ruggiero, E., et al. (2021). Artificial intelligence for good health: a scoping review of the ethics literature. 22, 1-17.

[83] Karimian, G., Petelos, E., et al. (2022). The ethical issues of the application of artificial intelligence in healthcare: a systematic scoping review. 2(4), 539-551.

[84] AI, H. J. E. g. f. t. A. (2019). High-level expert group on artificial intelligence. 6.

[85] Shin, D. J. I. j. o. h.-c. s. (2021). The effects of explainability and causability on perception, trust, and acceptance: Implications for explainable AI. 146, 102551.

[86] Li, F., Ruijs, N., et al. (2022). Ethics & AI: A systematic review on ethical concerns and related strategies for designing with AI in healthcare. 4(1), 28-53.

[87] Boris, E., Alexey, B., et al. (2024). The Use of AI in Medicine: Health Data, Privacy Risks and More. (2), 57-79.

[88] Fereshtehnejad, S.-M., & Lökk, J. (2023). Challenges of Teleneurology in the Care of Complex Neurodegenerative Disorders: The Case of Parkinson's Disease with Possible Solutions. Healthcare,

[89] Gosse, P. J., Kassardjian, C. D., et al. (2021). Virtual care for patients with Alzheimer disease and related dementias during the COVID-19 era and beyond. 193(11), E371-E377.

[90] Bhachawat, S., Shriram, E., et al. (2023). Leveraging computational intelligence techniques for diagnosing degenerative nerve diseases: a comprehensive review, open challenges, and future research directions. 13(2), 288.

[91] Kumar, A. V., Kumar, S., et al. (2023). Future perspectives for automated neurodegenerative disorders diagnosis: Challenges and possible research directions. In Data Analysis for Neurodegenerative Disorders (pp. 255-267). Springer.

[92] Shusharina, N., Yukhnenko, D., et al. (2023). Modern methods of diagnostics and treatment of neurodegenerative diseases and depression. 13(3), 573.

[93] Lehne, M., Sass, J., et al. (2019). Why digital medicine depends on interoperability. 2(1), 79.

[94] Singh, R. P., Hom, G. L., et al. (2020). Current challenges and barriers to real-world artificial intelligence adoption for the healthcare system, provider, and the patient. 9(2), 45-45.

[95] Li, X., Zeng, L., et al. (2023). A review of artificial intelligence in the rupture risk assessment of intracranial aneurysms: applications and challenges. 13(7), 1056.

[96] Zaharchuk, G. (2023). Artificial Intelligence Approaches to the Imaging of Neurodegenerative Diseases. In Molecular Imaging of Neurodegenerative Disorders (pp. 207-219). Springer.

[97] Akram, A. S., Grezenko, H., et al. (2024). Advancing the Frontier: Neuroimaging Techniques in the Early Detection and Management of Neurodegenerative Diseases. 16(5).

[98] Priya R, K., Al Shahri, A., et al. (2024). Integration of Artificial Intelligence in the Diagnosis and Prevention of Neurodegenerative Disease: An Update. In Handbook of Neurodegenerative Disorders (pp. 1-12). Springer.

[99] Karalis, V. D. J. A. B. (2024). The integration of artificial intelligence into clinical practice. 3(1), 14-44.

[100] Angelucci, F., Ai, A. R., et al. (2024). Integrating AI in fighting advancing Alzheimer: diagnosis, prevention, treatment, monitoring, mechanisms, and clinical trials. 87, 102857.
[101] Miller, J. B., Shan, G., et al. (2018). Biomedical informatics applications for precision management of neurodegenerative diseases. 4, 357-365.

15

Generative AI for Enhancing Cognitive Rehabilitation in Patients with Neurodegenerative Disorders

Manisha Sharma[1], Amit Dholakia[2], Shenson Joseph[3], and Ram Chandra Sachan[4]

[1,2]Department of Political Science, Maharaja Sayajirao University of Baroda, India
[3]University of North Dakota, USA
[4]Independent researcher, USA
E-mail: manishasharma78889@gmail.com; acrosstoamit@gmail.com; shenson.joseph@gmail.com; ramchandra.sachan@gmail.com

Abstract

Generative AI is emerging as a transformative tool in cognitive rehabilitation, offering innovative solutions for enhancing cognitive functioning in patients with neurodegenerative disorders such as Alzheimer's disease, Parkinson's disease, and amyotrophic lateral sclerosis (ALS). By utilizing advanced machine learning models, particularly generative models like GPT and GANs, AI systems can simulate personalized cognitive training programs, adapt to patient progress, and provide real-time feedback. These AI-driven interventions are designed to promote neuroplasticity, slow cognitive decline, and improve the quality of life for patients by delivering targeted exercises tailored to individual needs. Moreover, AI systems can analyse vast datasets to identify patterns in cognitive decline, offering insights for developing more effective rehabilitation strategies. Despite the potential benefits, ethical considerations such as patient privacy, data security, and the accuracy of AI-generated recommendations must be addressed. This chapter reviews the current advancements in generative AI applications in

DOI: 10.1201/9788743801764-15

cognitive rehabilitation, explores their potential impact on patient outcomes, and highlights the challenges that remain in clinical implementation.

Keywords: Generative AI, Cognitive Rehabilitation, Neurodegenerative Disorders, Machine Learning, Personalized Therapy, Neuroplasticity, Alzheimer's Disease.

15.1 Introduction

Generative AI basically deals with various technological aspects including contents, synthetic data, audio-visual aids images and much more creating a high-quality interface for its users in just a matter of seconds. There is a huge gap between generative AI and applied AI. Generative AI emphasizes new sources by learning methods, which is mainly concerned with certain creative output and content generation. Whereas, the goal of applied AI is to address actual issues in the real world by tailoring AI solutions to the distinctive issues faced by various sectors. Moreover, cognitive rehabilitation is a therapeutic approach maintaining the cognitive functions such as memory, attention, problem-solving, and executive functioning in individuals with cognitive impairments. In the context of neurodegenerative diseases, it seeks to enhance patients' ability to manage everyday tasks, thereby promoting independence and improving overall quality of life. Again, neurorehabilitation is an important as well as a difficult medical treatment that emphasizes to cure the injury of nervous system and to compensate for any functional alterations resulting from it.

It is important to note that the rise of generative artificial intelligence (AI) has revolutionized the landscape of cognitive rehabilitation. Generative AI is a subset of machine learning that enables systems to create new content, such as text, images, or data, based on the patterns it has learned from existing datasets. In the context of neurodegenerative diseases, generative AI has opened up new possibilities for creating personalized, adaptive, and scalable cognitive rehabilitation programs tailored to the specific needs of individual patients. Unlike traditional rehabilitation, which is often one-size-fits-all, generative AI can create personalized rehabilitation plans by analysing patient-specific data, including cognitive assessments, medical histories, and real-time performance feedback. This allows the AI to generate interventions that are specifically designed to target the individual patient's deficits. For instance, a patient with early-stage Alzheimer's disease may require memory exercises tailored to their current cognitive state, while a patient with Parkinson's disease might benefit from motor tasks that improve coordination and reduce tremors. Generative AI can dynamically adjust these tasks as the patient's abilities change over time.

The impact of AI in neurorehabilitation is something that is interrelated to the general backdrop of AI. Here, a major role shall be played by the international organizations and the creators of various AI systems to regulate as well as to usher the problems and prospects of the process of AI implementation. It also recommended around 30 suggestions in terms of generative AI and beyond it enhancing a fast response in the field of neurorehabilitation.

Generative AI offers the ability to create tailored interventions that adapt to the unique needs of each patient, enhancing real-time feedback and continuous adjustments to the rehabilitation process. Moreover, AI-driven cognitive rehabilitation has the potential to be delivered remotely, significantly expanding access to care and alleviating the burden on healthcare systems. As this technology continues to evolve, it represents a promising frontier in the fight against neurodegenerative diseases, offering new hope for improving patient outcomes and maintaining independence.

15.2 Neurodegenerative Disorders: An Overview

Neurodegenerative disorders refer to a group of diseases that involve the progressive degeneration of nerve cells (neurons) in the brain. These disorders can affect movement, cognition, behavior, and various other bodily functions depending on the specific areas of the nervous system that are damaged [20]. Therefore, Table 15.1 elaborates certain neurodegenerative diseases along with their features.

Table 15.1 Neurodegenerative disorders and their features.

Sl.no.	Diseases	Features
1	Alzheimer's disease	Primarily affects memory, thinking, and behavior, often leading to dementia [12]
2	Parkinson's disease	Affects movement, causing tremors, stiffness, and issues with balancing and coordination [19]
3	Amyotrophic lateral sclerosis (ALS)	It is also known as Lou Gehrig's disease, which impacts the motor neurons, leading to muscle weakness and eventual paralysis [22]
4	Huntington's disease	A genetic disorder that leads to cognitive decline, uncontrolled movements, and emotional disturbances [21]
5	Multiple sclerosis (MS)	Involves damage to the myelin sheath, the protective covering of nerves, leading to various physical and cognitive impairments [5]

Source: Author's understanding from different sources mentioned in the brackets

Figure 15.1 illustrates that Alzheimer's disease (AD) is classified into three stages according to the severity of the ailment. Stage one deals with mild stage including memory loss, mood dysfunctions, and problems with language. Stage two is the moderate stage that includes dementia (at the

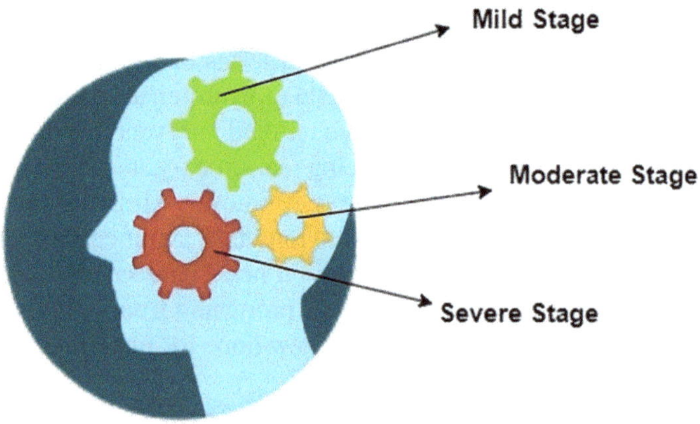

Figure 15.1 Classifications of Alzheimer's disease (AD) into stages.

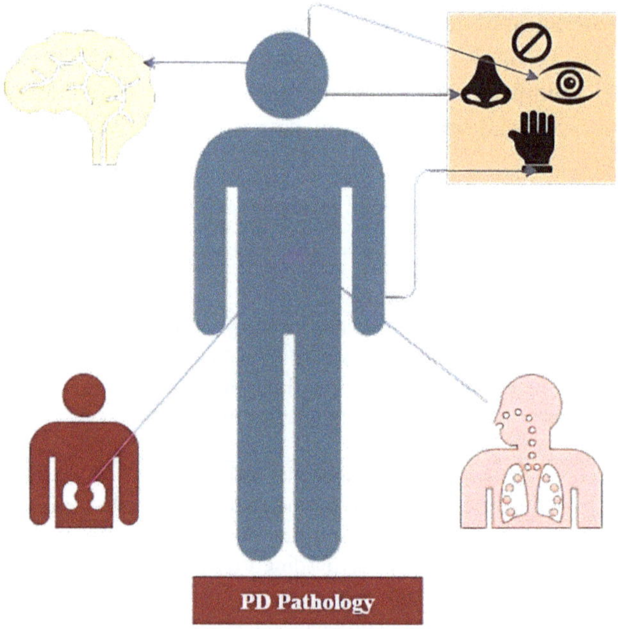

Figure 15.2 Clinical symptoms of Parkinson's disease (PD).

starting), anger and difficulty in doing daily chores. The final stage is the severe stage that involves with severe dementia, lack of communication as well as sleeping. It is due to inadequate choline supply in synapses, amyloid beta plaques, and tau hyperphosphorylation which are the primary genotypic manifestations in individuals with Alzheimer's disease.

Figure 15.2 illustrates the prevalent clinical symptoms of Parkinson's disease (PD) and the underlying molecular pathology contributing to its aetiology. The primary motor symptoms of Parkinson's disease encompass tremor, stiffness, bradykinesia, and postural instability. The identified pathophysiological characteristics include reactive oxygen species (ROS) and genomic modifications. A decrease in dopamine leads to misfolded proteins that contribute to the aetiology of Parkinson's disease, ultimately resulting in neurodegeneration.

Figure 15.3 portrays a summary of Huntington's disease (HD): This figure indicates that mostly over 35 repeats of the CAG mutation predominantly contribute to the aetiology of Huntington's disease by inducing neuronal

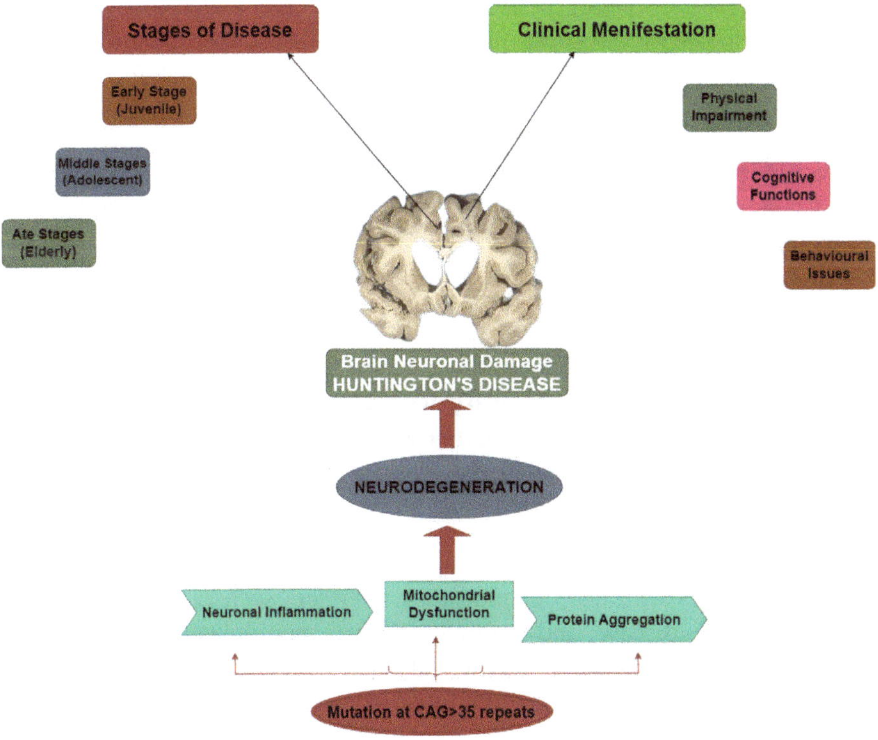

Figure 15.3 Potential significant clinical signs in Huntington's disease (HD) patients.

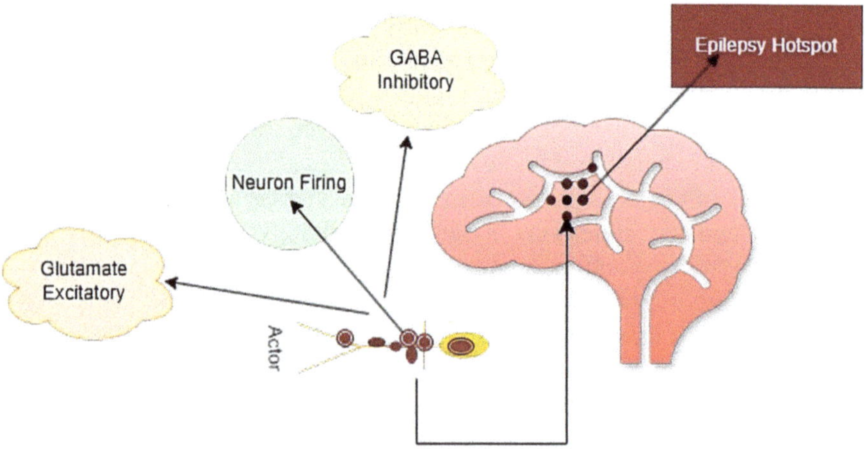

Figure 15.4 Symptoms and stages of epilepsy.

inflammation, mitochondrial failure, or protein aggregation. Typically, HD is categorised into three stages. 1. Initial phases (Juvenile cohorts); 2. Intermediate phases (Adolescent groups); 3. Advanced phases (Elderly cohorts). This image also highlights the potential significant clinical signs reported in HD patients.

Figure 15.4 shows the symptoms and stages of epilepsy which are influenced by both genetic and environmental variables, including neuroinfection, genetic predisposition, metabolic issues, and brain injury as potential etiological contributors. Additionally, it has been demonstrated that the suppression of GABA neuronal activity results in the phenotypic symptoms observed in epileptic patients.

15.3 Enhancing Neuroplasticity in Context of Neurodegenerative disorders and the Role of AI in promoting Neuroplasticity

Neuroplasticity is a remarkable ability of the brain to adapt itself by forming new neural connections, which is central to the process of cognitive rehabilitation. In patients with neurodegenerative disorders such as Alzheimer's disease, Parkinson's disease, and multiple sclerosis, neuroplasticity offers a glimmer of hope, allowing for some recovery of cognitive functions even as neurons deteriorate. Generative artificial intelligence (AI) has emerged as a promising tool to harness and enhance neuroplasticity in these patients by delivering personalized and adaptive cognitive training programs.

Now if we look at the understanding of neuroplasticity in the context of neurodegenerative disorders, it can be observed that neuroplasticity is the brain's inherent ability to modify its structure and function in response to external stimuli, learning, and injury. It is significant in cognitive rehabilitation, mainly in the context of neurodegenerative diseases, where the progressive loss of neurons leads to declines in memory, attention, and executive functions [9]. Neuroplasticity allows the brain to compensate for these losses by forming new connections between neurons and even recruiting different regions of the brain to take over impaired functions [18]. For example, in Alzheimer's disease, areas of the brain responsible for short-term memory may deteriorate, but with the right intervention, other regions can be trained to support memory recall. Cognitive rehabilitation aims to enhance this natural plasticity by stimulating specific neural pathways through repetitive and targeted cognitive exercises.

Moreover, certain models of generative AI, such as generative adversarial networks (GANs) and generative pre-trained transformers (GPT), are playing an increasingly important role in developing cognitive rehabilitation strategies that promote neuroplasticity. These AI systems can analyse vast amounts of data on patient performance, identify areas of cognitive decline, and generate tailored interventions that stimulate specific neural pathways.

For instance, a patient with Parkinson's disease may experience difficulties with motor skills and cognitive tasks related to attention and memory. Generative AI can develop exercises that challenge these cognitive domains, progressively increasing the difficulty as the patient improves. These adaptive programs are crucial for stimulating the brain and promoting neuroplasticity because they ensure that the patient is always working at the edge of their capabilities – enough to foster new neural connections, but not so much as to cause frustration or disengagement [26]. One of the major features of generative AI is its ability to provide real-time feedback and adjustments to cognitive exercises based on the patient's progress. This dynamic adaptability helps to maintain the optimal level of challenge needed to promote neuroplasticity. As the patient engages in these personalized tasks, the brain is continuously forced to adapt and reorganize, thereby reinforcing neural pathways and fostering the development of new ones [25]. By keeping the brain in a constant state of learning, generative AI accelerates the process of neuroplasticity, which can slow the progression of cognitive decline and even restore some cognitive functions.

15.4 Generative AI and Cognitive Rehabilitation

Generative artificial intelligence or Generative AI has become a significant tool in cognitive rehabilitation, particularly for individuals with neurological illnesses like Alzheimer's, Parkinson's, and multiple sclerosis. Cognitive rehabilitation aims to improve or restore cognitive functions, such as memory, attention, and problem-solving, which are often compromised in these conditions. Generative AI can deliver personalized, adaptive, and scalable cognitive training programs, offering distinct benefits compared to conventional approaches.

One of the primary benefits of generative AI in cognitive rehabilitation is its ability to provide tailored cognitive training regimens suited to individual needs. Generative AI models, such as generative pre-trained transformers (GPT) and generative adversarial networks (GANs), can analyse extensive datasets, including patient-specific data, to create tailored exercises that target specific cognitive impairments. This approach addresses cognitive deficiencies while engaging patients in significant activities, enhancing motivation and compliance with rehabilitation methods.

Generative AI systems can change in real time, so the AI can keep learning from how the patient is doing and adjust the therapy program to match. This makes sure that patients are not too stressed out by jobs that are too hard or too bored by activities that are too easy. AI-powered apps give patients immediate feedback, pointing out areas where they can improve and offering new ways to practice. This fast feedback method keeps patients more interested and speeds up their cognitive improvement.

Generative AI greatly improves neuroplasticity, which is an important idea in cognitive rehabilitation, by making activities that correctly test the brain and help new neural networks form. AI-driven cognitive rehabilitation can enhance neuroplasticity by tailoring tasks that focus on regions of the brain impacted by neurodegeneration, thereby preventing cognitive deterioration.

Another benefit of generative AI is its ability to augment patient involvement and motivation. By creating engaging and interactive rehabilitation programs tailored to patients' preferences and skills, AI can alleviate irritation and diminished desire, enabling them to participate in activities they find enjoyable. Real-time feedback from AI systems can also help clinicians monitor illness progression, providing a more comprehensive understanding of the impact of neurodegenerative disorders on cognitive performance.

15.5 Ethical and Clinical Challenges of Generative AI in Cognitive Rehabilitation

The integration of generative AI into cognitive rehabilitation holds immense promise for enhancing neuroplasticity and improving cognitive functions in patients with neurodegenerative disorders. However, along with its potential benefits, the use of AI in healthcare, particularly in sensitive areas like cognitive rehabilitation, presents several ethical and clinical challenges. These challenges need to be carefully considered to ensure that AI-driven interventions are safe, effective, and ethically sound. The major concerns include issues related to patient data privacy, algorithmic bias, clinical validation, and patient consent depending upon AI systems.

15.5.1 Data privacy and security concerns

One of the most pressing ethical challenges in implementing generative AI in cognitive rehabilitation is the issue of patient data privacy and security. Generative AI models focus on the large amounts of data to generate personalized cognitive training programs, often drawing from sensitive health information, such as patient history, cognitive assessments, and real-time performance data. This reliance on personal health data raises significant concerns about how this information is collected, stored, and used [9].

The storage of large datasets in centralized or cloud-based systems makes patient information vulnerable to data breaches or unauthorized access, potentially exposing sensitive details about the medical history of a patient and its cognitive impairments. In healthcare, privacy is a critical issue governed by stringent laws, such as the Health Insurance Portability and Accountability Act (HIPAA) in the United States and the General Data Protection Regulation (GDPR) in Europe. Breaches of these laws can result in severe legal and financial results for healthcare providers and developers of AI technologies [18].

Moreover, the anonymization of data is another key concern. Although many AI systems aim to anonymize patient data to protect privacy, the complexity of the data used – such as detailed health profiles, behavioural data, and unique cognitive patterns – can make re-identification possible. This can lead to privacy violations if AI-generated insights are inadvertently linked back to individual patients. Ensuring robust anonymization and encryption protocols, as well as maintaining transparency about how data is used, is essential to safeguarding patient privacy [26].

15.5.2 Algorithmic bias and fairness

Another critical ethical issue in the use of generative AI for cognitive rehabilitation is the risk of algorithmic bias. AI models are trained on historical data, and if that data is unrepresentative or biased, the AI system could produce biased outcomes. For example, if an AI model is primarily trained on cognitive data from a specific demographic group – such as individuals of a particular age, ethnicity, or socio-economic status – it may generate rehabilitation programs that are less effective for individuals outside that group [9].

Algorithmic bias can lead to discrepancies in the quality of care provided to different patient populations. For instance, an AI system that is biased toward a younger, more affluent population might generate exercises that are not well-suited for older patients or those with lower cognitive baselines. This bias can reduce the effectiveness of cognitive rehabilitation for underrepresented groups and perpetuate health inequities. To mitigate this risk, it is significant for developers to ensure that the training datasets used for AI systems are diverse and representative of the population as a whole [18].

In addition, ongoing auditing as well as monitoring of AI algorithms are essential to detect and correct any biases that emerge during real-world use. This requires collaboration between data scientists, clinicians, and ethicists to ensure that AI-driven cognitive rehabilitation programs are equitable and effective for all patients [25].

15.5.3 Clinical validation and efficacy

While generative AI holds great potential for cognitive rehabilitation, one of the most significant clinical challenges is the lack of rigorous validation. Cognitive rehabilitation is a complex and highly individualized process, and although AI can generate personalized interventions, these interventions must be clinically tested to determine their effectiveness. Without proper validation through randomized controlled trials (RCTs) and other clinical studies, there is a risk that AI-driven programs may not deliver the desired therapeutic outcomes, or worse, they may harm patients by providing inappropriate or ineffective interventions [23].

AI-generated cognitive exercises are often based on patterns identified in large datasets, but these patterns may not always translate to meaningful clinical improvements for individual patients. Additionally, the complexity of neurodegenerative diseases means that different patients may respond to interventions in highly variable ways. It is critical that AI-driven cognitive rehabilitation programs undergo extensive clinical testing to ensure their safety and efficacy across diverse patient populations [26].

Moreover, generative AI systems need to be continuously updated and validated as new data becomes available. Cognitive rehabilitation is an evolving field, and new insights into neuroplasticity and brain function may necessitate changes to AI-generated interventions. Without ongoing validation, there is a risk that AI systems may become outdated or provide interventions that are no longer supported by the latest clinical evidence [25].

15.5.4 Patient consent and autonomy

Another ethical issue in the use of generative AI in cognitive rehabilitation is ensuring informed consent and patient autonomy. AI-driven interventions can be complex and difficult for patients to understand, especially in cases where patients are experiencing cognitive decline. It is essential that patients are fully informed about how AI systems will be used in their treatment, including how their data will be collected, analysed, and used to generate personalized rehabilitation programs [18].

Patients must have the opportunity to make informed decisions about whether they wish to participate in AI-driven rehabilitation programs. This includes understanding the potential risks and benefits, as well as any limitations of the AI system. In some cases, patients may prefer more traditional rehabilitation methods, and their preferences must be respected. Ensuring that patients retain control over their treatment choices is a foremost ethical principle in healthcare, and it is particularly important when using AI systems that may not yet be fully understood by the general public [9].

Additionally, in cases where patients have cognitive impairments that limit their ability to provide informed consent, it is important to involve family members or legal guardians in the decision-making process. Clear communication about the role of AI in rehabilitation, its limitations, and the potential for unforeseen outcomes is essential to maintaining patient autonomy and trust in AI-driven healthcare [23].

15.5.5 Over-reliance on AI and the role of human clinicians

While generative AI can enhance cognitive rehabilitation by providing personalized and adaptive interventions, there is a risk of over-reliance on AI systems. Healthcare providers may be tempted to rely too heavily on AI-generated insights and recommendations, potentially sidelining the role of human judgment and clinical expertise. AI systems, while powerful, are not infallible, and they may fail to capture the nuances of individual patient needs or the complexities of neurodegenerative diseases [26]. It is critical that AI is used as a tool to support, instead of human clinicians. Cognitive rehabilitation is a deeply personal and context-dependent process, and human clinicians play a vital role in interpreting patient responses, providing emotional support, and making adjustments to treatment plans based on clinical expertise. Ensuring that AI systems are used in conjunction with, rather than in place of, human clinicians is essential to providing high-quality, patient-centred care [18].

Despite of facing the above challenges, it can be understood that generative AI is playing an increasingly important role in cognitive rehabilitation for patients with neurodegenerative disorders. By offering personalized, adaptive, and data-driven solutions, AI-driven cognitive training programs can promote neuroplasticity, enhance engagement, and improve treatment outcomes. The ability of generative AI to tailor exercises to individual needs, provide real-time feedback, and continuously adapt rehabilitation programs based on patient progress marks a significant advancement over traditional cognitive rehabilitation methods. While challenges related to privacy, data security, and clinical validation remain, the integration of AI into cognitive rehabilitation holds tremendous promise for boosting the quality of life for patients with neurodegenerative diseases.

15.6 Role of Generative AI in Enhancing Cognitive Function

Generative AI can target several cognitive functions that are often affected by neurodegenerative disorders, such as, memory, attention, executive function, and language processing. Each of these cognitive domains relies on specific neural circuits, and by delivering targeted exercises, AI systems can help strengthen these circuits, encouraging the brain to adapt.

Memory: Memory impairment is one of the hallmark symptoms of many neurodegenerative disorders, particularly Alzheimer's disease. AI-driven cognitive rehabilitation programs often include memory exercises designed to reinforce both short-term and long-term memory recall. For example, generative AI can create exercises that challenge patients to recall specific details of recent events or sequences of information, which helps to strengthen the hippocampus and other areas of the brain associated with memory processing [23].

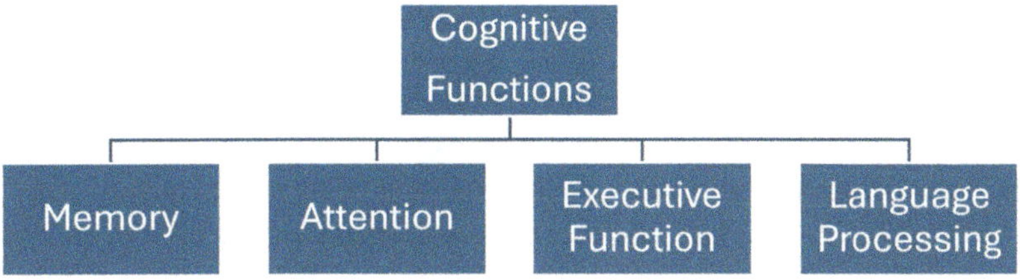

Figure 15.5 Some cognitive functions which can be affected by neurodegenerative disorders.

Attention: Many patients with neurodegenerative diseases experience difficulties with sustained attention and focus. Generative AI can develop exercises that require patients to deal with specific stimuli while filtering out distractions, a process that strengthens neural circuits involved in attentional control. These exercises are particularly useful in conditions like Parkinson's disease, where cognitive decline often begins with attentional deficits [9].

Executive function: These are related to problem-solving, planning, and decision-making processes which are often impaired in neurodegenerative disorders. Generative AI can generate exercises that involve multi-step problem-solving tasks or simulations that require patients to make decisions in real time. These exercises engage the prefrontal cortex, a region critical for executive function, and encourage the brain to reorganize and improve its efficiency in processing complex tasks [26].

Language processing: Speech and language impairments are common in diseases like ALS and frontotemporal dementia. AI-generated rehabilitation exercises can focus on language processing tasks, such as word recall, sentence construction, and verbal fluency. These tasks stimulate neural circuits associated with language production and comprehension, potentially slowing the decline in verbal communication skills [18].

15.7 Conclusion

Apart from all the challenges and issues, it is important to note that one of the most significant benefits of using generative AI in cognitive rehabilitation is its ability to continuously adapt to the patient's progress, ensuring that the exercises remain challenging yet achievable. This dynamic approach is essential for fostering neuroplasticity, as it ensures that the brain is always in a state of learning and adaptation. When patients reach a plateau in their rehabilitation, generative AI can increase the complexity of tasks or introduce new types of cognitive challenges, preventing stagnation and promoting continuous neural growth [25]. For example, a patient undergoing rehabilitation for memory loss might start with basic recall exercises, such as remembering a short list of words. As their memory improves, AI can progressively introduce more complex tasks, such as recalling sequences of events or solving problems that require both memory and reasoning. This gradual increase in difficulty encourages the brain to form new neural connections, thereby enhancing cognitive resilience [9].

The use of generative AI in cognitive rehabilitation presents numerous ethical and clinical challenges that must be inscribed to ensure that AI-driven interventions are both effective and ethical. Data privacy, algorithmic bias, clinical validation, patient consent, and the risk of over-reliance on AI are all significant concerns that require careful consideration. By addressing these challenges through robust clinical testing, transparency, and ongoing monitoring, healthcare providers can harness the power of AI to improve cognitive rehabilitation while maintaining patient trust and ensuring equitable access to care.

Generative AI offers unprecedented opportunities to enhance cognitive rehabilitation for patients with neurodegenerative disorders. By leveraging advanced machine learning algorithms, AI systems can deliver personalized, adaptive cognitive exercises that promote neuroplasticity and slow cognitive decline. While there are ethical and clinical challenges to address, the integration of generative AI into rehabilitation programs holds a progressive nature to improve the quality of life for individuals suffering from neurodegenerative diseases. As AI technology continues to advance, it will likely become an integral part of therapeutic strategies for cognitive rehabilitation.

References

[1] Archi Dubey, Kishor Kumar Reddy C, Srinath Doss and Marlia Mohd Hanafiah, "Exploring the Advancements and Future Directions of Digital Twins in Healthcare 6.0, IGI Global, 2024

[2] Balarajan Y, Selvaraj S, Subramanian SV. Health care and equity in India. Lancet. 2011;377:505-515

[3] Kishor Kumar Reddy C., Patlolla Sathvika Reddy, P. R. Anisha, Srinath Doss, "Towards smarter Chatbots Unravelling the capabilities of ChatGPT", Cognitive Machine Intelligence CRC Press, August 2024, https://doi.org/10.1201/9781003500865

[4] Chirra M, Marsili L, Wattley L, et al. Telemedicine in neurological disorders: opportunities and challenges. Telemed J E Health. 2019; 25:541-550

[5] Dobson R, Giovannoni G. Multiple sclerosis – A review. Eur J Neurol. 2019;26(1):27-40. doi:10.1111/ene.13819

[6] Erkkinen MG, Kim MO, Geschwind MD. Clinical neurology and epidemiology of the major neurodegenerative diseases. Cold Spring Harb Perspect Biol. 2018;10(4): a033118. doi:10.1101/cshperspect.a033118

[7] Fiorente N, Mojdehdehbaher S, Salvatore Calabrò R. Artificial intelligence and neurorehabilitation: fact vs. fiction. Innov Clin Neurosci. 2021;21: PMC10941864. doi:10.1093/pmc/articles/PMC10941864

[8] Garg D. Specific considerations for epilepsy in India. Curr Med Issues. 2020; 18:105-110

[9] Graham JE, Karmarkar AM. Artificial intelligence and cognitive rehabilitation: current trends and future directions. Front Neurol. 2021; 12:635705. doi:10.3389/fneur.2021.635705

[10] Kishor Kumar Reddy C, Aarti Rangarajan, Deepti Rangarajan, Mohammed Shuaib, Fathe Jeribi and Shadab Alam, "A Transfer Learning Approach: Early Prediction of Alzheimer's Disease on US Healthy Aging Dataset", MDPI Mathematics, July 2024, 2204. https://doi.org/10.3390/math12142204

[11] Krucoff MO, Rahimpour S, Slutzky MW, et al. Enhancing nervous system recovery through neurobiologics, neural interface training, and neurorehabilitation. Front Neurosci. 2016; 10:584

[12] Lane CA, Hardy J, Schott JM. Alzheimer's disease. Eur J Neurol. 2018;25(1):59-70. doi:10.1111/ene.13439

[13] Lawton G. What is generative AI? Everything you need to know. https://www.techtarget.com/searchenterpriseai/definition/generative-AI.Published2023

[14] Li C, Larsen B, Halopé H, Velasco L. The Presidio Recommendations on Responsible Generative AI. World Economic Forum. https://www3.weforum.org/docs/WEF_Presidio_Recommendations_on_Responsible_Generative_AI_2023.pdf. Published June 2023. Accessed January 9, 2023

[15] Nadig R, Namapally USK, Sarma GRK, et al. Outpatient burden of neurological disorders: a prospective evaluation of 1500 patients. Neurol India. 2019; 67:708-713

[16] P R Anisha, Kishor Kumar Reddy C, Marlia Mohd Hanafiah, B V Ramana Murthy, R Madana Mohana Y V S S Pragathi, "An Intelligent

Deep Feature Based Feature Based Metabolism Syndrome Prediction System for Sleep Disorder Diseases", Multimedia Tools and Applications, Springer, November 2023, DOI: https://doi.org/10.1007/s11042-023-17296-4

[17] Padma MV. "Telestroke": an Indian approach to telemedicine. Pract Cardiovasc Sci. 2017; 3:2-4

[18] Pan Y, Zhang Z. Artificial intelligence in the management of neurodegenerative diseases: progress and challenges. Nat Rev Neurol. 2020;16(12):703-715. doi:10.1038/s41582-020-00400-1

[19] Poewe W, Seppi K, Tanner CM, et al. Parkinson disease. Nat Rev Dis Primers. 2017; 3:17013. doi:10.1038/nrdp.2017.13

[20] Ramanan VK, Saykin AJ. Pathways to neurodegeneration: mechanistic insights from GWAS in Alzheimer's disease, Parkinson's disease, and related disorders. Am J Neurodegener Dis. 2013;2(3):145-175

[21] Ross CA, Tabrizi SJ. Huntington's disease: from molecular pathogenesis to clinical treatment. Lancet Neurol. 2011;10(1):83-98. doi:10.1016/S1474-4422(10)70245-3

[22] Taylor JP, Brown RH, Cleveland DW. Decoding ALS: from genes to mechanism. Nature. 2016;539(7628):197-206. doi:10.1038/nature20413

[23] Topol EJ. High-performance medicine: the convergence of human and artificial intelligence. Nat Med. 2019; 25:44-56. doi:10.1038/s41591-018-0300-7

[24] Vellingiri B. An overview about neurological diseases in India – A theranostics approach. Aging Health Res. 2024;4(1):100177. doi:10.1016/j.ahr.2023.100177

[25] Wang Y, Zhang J. Machine learning approaches in Alzheimer's disease diagnosis and rehabilitation. IEEE J Biomed Health Inform*. 2021;25(10):3692-3702. doi:10.1109/JBHI.2021.3059885

[26] Zhou Q, Li X. AI in neurocognitive rehabilitation: opportunities and challenges in digital therapeutics. J Neuroeng Rehabil. 2022;19(1):85. doi:10.1186/s12984-022-01050-3

Index

About the Editors

Anindya Nag obtained an M.Sc. in Computer Science and Engineering from Khulna University in Khulna, Bangladesh, and a B.Tech. in Computer Science and Engineering from Adamas University in Kolkata, India. He is currently a lecturer in the Department of Computer Science and Engineering at the Northern University of Business and Technology in Khulna, Khulna 9100, Bangladesh. His research focuses on health informatics, medical Internet of Things, neuroscience, and machine learning. He serves as a reviewer for numerous prestigious journals and international conferences. He has authored and co-authored about 47 publications, including journal articles, conference papers, and book chapters, and has co-edited nine books.

Md. Mehedi Hassan is currently a Ph.D. researcher in STEM (Computer and Information Science) at the University of South Australia, working on a fully funded research project. He started his Ph.D. in 2025, building on a strong academic background in computer science and engineering. He holds an M.Sc. in Computer Science and Engineering from Khulna University, Bangladesh, completed in 2024, and a B.Sc. in Computer Science and Engineering from North Western University, completed in 2022. His research spans computer science engineering and data science, with a strong focus on predictive analysis and expert system development. Md. Mehedi Hassan has authored 73 research papers and edited 5 books, actively contributing to the academic community. He serves as a peer reviewer for over 80 prestigious journals and collaborates extensively in interdisciplinary research. As a trainer for the VCourse platform, he has educated over 250 students over the past two years, sharing knowledge in emerging technologies and research methodologies. Beyond publications, he has actively engaged in intellectual property development, with several patents filed and three already granted in his name. His current research interests include computational neuroscience, machine learning for healthcare, and predictive modeling for biometrics.

Asif Karim, Ph.D., is a research active lecturer at Charles Darwin University, Australia. His research interests include applying machine intelligence to fields such as smart contracts and health informatics. Besides being an active researcher, he has considerable industry experience in IT, primarily in software engineering. In addition, Dr. Karim is also involved in active teaching to undergraduate and postgraduate students in a range of different computer science related courses.

Kishor Kumar Reddy C. is currently working as an associate professor with the Department of Computer Science and Engineering, Stanley College of Engineering and Technology for Women, Hyderabad, India. He has research and teaching experience of more than 10 years. He has published more than 50 research papers in national and international conferences, book chapters, and journals indexed by Scopus and others. He is an author for two text books and seven co-edited books. He acted as the special session chair for Springer FICTA 2020, 2022, SCI 2021, INDIA 2022, and IEEE ICCSEA 2020 conferences. He is the corresponding editor of AMSE 2021 conferences, published by IoP Science JPCS. He is the member of ISTE, CSI, IAENG, UACEE, and IACSIT.

For Product Safety Concerns and Information please contact our EU
representative GPSR@taylorandfrancis.com
Taylor & Francis Verlag GmbH, Kaufingerstraße 24, 80331 München, Germany

www.ingramcontent.com/pod-product-compliance
Ingram Content Group UK Ltd.
Pitfield, Milton Keynes, MK11 3LW, UK
UKHW021932250925
463327UK00001B/4

9788743801757